A Good Idea

A Good Idea

The History of The Nutrition Foundation

Charles Glen King, Ph.D.

THE NUTRITION FOUNDATION
New York and Washington

Library of Congress Number 76-44654

Copyright © 1976 by The Nutrition Foundation, Inc.
489 Fifth Avenue
New York, New York 10017

Printed in the United States of America

Contents

Foreword   ix

I The First Decade: Development of a Good Idea   3

A Good Idea—Its Development   3
Organization for Action   3
Appointment of the Scientific Director   13

Program Development   14
Examples of Basic Research Supported   15
Grant Support and Personnel Development   18
NUTRITION REVIEWS—New Journal to Identify
 and Extend Nutrition Knowledge   19
Liaison with Governmental and Scientific Organizations   22
Expanded Foundation Membership and Program   24
Studies of Food Composition   27
Quality of Military Rations and Processing Techniques   29
Studies of Metabolism Under Stress   31

A New National and International Resource: The Food and Nutrition Board   31

A Five-Year Resume   36

Education—Channels and Challenges   37
Scientific Publications   37
General Publications   39
Awards   40
International Union of Nutritional Sciences   44

Nutrition Fact Finding   45
Nutrition is Essentially a Quantitative Science. Why?   45
Toxic Excesses of Vitamins A and D   46
Food Selection in Relation to Need   47
Early Medical School Examples of Nutrition Teaching   48
A New Vitamin   49
Requirements of Other Vitamins   50
Studies of B-Complex Vitamins at Duke University   50
Fat Soluble Vitamins E and A   51
Vitamin B_6 52
Vitamin C   53
Proteins and Amino Acids   53
Carbohydrates, Fats and Total Calories   56
Mineral Metabolism   57
Studies in Relation to Cancer   58
Food Practices During Gestation and Lactation and Their Effect on Child Health   58

Comments of Evaluation   59

Summary of Appropriations for Grants-in-Aid, 1942-1952   60

II The Second Decade: Research, Education, Service 63

Personnel Changes 63

The Spread of the Good Idea 65
    Other National Foundations 65
    International Union of Nutritional Sciences 67

Support of Basic Scientific Advances 69
    Carbohydrates, Fats and Energy 69
    Starches and Sugar 70
    Fats Become Exciting 72
    New Biochemical Aspects of Fats in Nutrition 73
    Vitamins in the Second Decade 74
    Research on Proteins and Amino Acids 79
    Mineral Metabolism 84
    Maternal and Child Development 85
    Vegetarians 87

Education 88

Scheduled Retirement 91

Summary of Appropriations for Grants-in-Aid, 1942-1963 92

III The Third Decade: The Program of the 1960s 93

Program Review, Adjustment and Growth 93

A Poetic Turn 95

Research in the Third Decade 97
    Protein Foods 97
    Minerals 98
    Nutrition and Maternal and Child Health 100
    Taste Perception and "Eating" Areas of the Brain 103

Education 105

IV Reorganization for the 1970s 109

Surveys and Plans 109

Orientation and New Horizons 115
    Review of Activities 116
    Purposes of the Foundation 116
    Nutrition Information 116
    Professional Nutrition Education 118
    Teacher Training, Workshops, Symposia 119
    Research 120

V The Fourth Decade: The Program of the 1970s — 123

Promotion, Exchange and Assessment of Scientific Information — 124
The National Nutrition Consortium 124
Cooperation between National Nutrition Foundations 125
Saccharin 126
Hyperkinesis 126

Improvement of Public Awareness of Nutrition in Relation to Health — 127
Nutrition Labeling 127
Misinformation and Faddism 127
Special Reports to Media 128
Source Material and Educational Publications 128

Encourage Broad Acceptance of Sound Nutrition Principles — 129
Annual Symposia of the Food and Nutrition Liaison Committee 129
Benefit-Risk Decision Making: The Citizens' Commission on Science, Law and the Food Supply 130
Nutrition Foundation Senior Scholar 131
Participation in and Support of Scientific Meetings and Symposia 133

Improvement of Nutrition Education at All levels — 136
Nutrition Education in Medical Centers 136
Nutrition Education in Colleges and Universities 142
Nutrition Education for Teachers 144
Educational Materials and Guides 146
Current Publications 149

Grants for Research and Education — 151
Challenging Opportunities 151
Major Interests 152

World Food and Nutrition Problems 154

VI Appendix — 159

A. Excerpts from the Organizational Meeting of the Board of Trustees, March 12, 1942 — 161
B. Bylaws of the Nutrition Foundation Revised and Adopted, November, 1971 — 170
C. Nutrition in the 1970s: Address to the Board of Trustees of The Nutrition Foundation, November 5, 1971 — 173
D. Selected References Illustrative of Research Supported by The Nutrition Foundation, 1942-75 — 177
E. Future Leader Awardees, The Nutrition Foundation, 1964-75 — 203
F. Recipients of Awards Supported by The Nutrition Foundation — 206
G. The Food and Nutrition Board: 1940-1965—Twenty-Five Years in Retrospect — 210

Foreword

In 1941, the year that saw the birth of The Nutrition Foundation, Dr. Alan Gregg, the distinguished Director for the Medical Sciences at The Rockefeller Foundation, wrote:

... If we take research in medicine to be the function we wish to preserve, we must be prepared to see new institutions appear for this purpose. Indeed, within the past forty years or less a new form of institution has appeared and the relations between it and the older form provide the substance of this ... chapter. The older institution is the university, the new institution is the foundation; the ground they have in common is the furtherance of medical research ...

... A foundation obviously may be more flexible and adaptable in its choice of research to be supported than is a university which is responsible for maintaining established teaching personnel and for preserving knowledge as well as discovering it ...

*Alan Gregg, M.D. "The Furtherance of Medical Research." Yale University Press, New Haven (1941). See Chapter II, "Universities and Foundations," pp. 43-84.

Compared with a government's subsidizing of research, foundations can much more easily work outside national boundaries and support demonstrations of theories not widely enough accepted or fully enough proven to qualify for government support ... they are rarely able to expand on the scale now characteristic of government ...

Compared with learned societies foundations have a much wider choice of fields to aid and are less dominated by specialist or partisan interests ...

In contrast to the individual private donor the foundation is more deliberate, sustained, and dependable, better advised and less personal ...

... Foundations vary with their age, their size, the current economic conditions, their form of organization, their general purposes and their specific fields of interest ... with the personal qualifications and characters of their officers and trustees ...

The first ten years of a foundation's existence determine in large manner its general policies over a much longer period of time. Though resolutely struggling against the formation of tradition the first officers develop precedents

Foreword

and usages in spite of themselves . . . and the first ten years are delightful in the opportunity they afford . . .

Another thoughtful, but unsung man, Mr. Ed Bryan, who devoted his life to the physical construction and maintenance of one of America's important universities, Vanderbilt University, frequently has said to me, "The University is man's most magnificent creation."

Often have I reflected upon the insight and wisdom of both of these men, and reminded myself of the interdependence of universities and foundations. The reader of this history will readily recognize the institutional characteristics of these two great societal institutions described so succinctly by both of these observers.

The concept of the university evolved from medieval schools, *studia generalia*, i.e. places of study open to students without restriction. The modern university organization as it exists in America began to take form in Europe during the twelfth century and emerged first from the church-related function of educating priests and monks beyond the level of the monastic or cathedral schools. The concept of *university* was, in fact, a continuum of the formal institutionalized educational complex that may be traced to the earliest civilizations of Egypt, Mesopotamia, and other cultures. The institutions which flowered during the Renaissance drew heavily upon the precedents for preservation and advancement of knowledge established by the Muslim universities.

The foundation is a much newer instrument developed by society for the advancement of knowledge, education and public good. It is possible to trace historically the foundation concept. Single purpose support in perpetuity for charitable purposes, for relief, for a museum, for ecclesiastical interest, for an academy or library, began as early as the time of ancient Egypt, Greece and Rome. The modern version of the foundation is, however, predominantly a twentieth century United States phenomenon.

Today's American philanthropic foundation, with its profound impact upon society, dates from the gift of the English scientist, James Smithson, which resulted in the creation of the Smithsonian Institution in 1846. The influence of the foundation in the early twentieth century was characterized by the beneficial impact upon research and education supported by large foundations with enormous resources. These foundations possessed broad purposes and flexibility of action assured by an automony of organization. These organized philanthropies, devoted to public good, were endowed with the fortunes of many who had attained great wealth in industry—notably, Andrew Carnegie, John D. Rockefeller, Jr., George Peabody, later Henry Ford, and numerous others. Their contributions to the public good represent one of the great benefits that result from our system of free enterprise. No other system has contributed so widely and wisely to the benefit of mankind.

Apparent on every hand, nationally and internationally, are beneficial influences of the American type of philanthropic foundation on scientific development; medical knowledge and health care; the humanities, arts and human relations; agriculture and food production; education; and upgrading of the general quality of life.

Industry's growth and maturity within the capitalistic system has been manifested by an increasing social awareness, and the development by its leaders of a high sense of corporate citizenship. The Nutrition Foundation is a superb example of the recognition of social responsibility by the food industry and of the willingness of the

Foreword

most highly responsible corporations and executives to accept this responsibility by promoting and supporting research, education and public service in science, medicine, public health and social welfare, and doing so with freedom from any self-serving motivation.

The organizational concepts, the program adjustments, and the enormous contributions of The Nutrition Foundation are told in this history by the distinguished scientist, Charles Glen King, who led the Foundation's development during its initial twenty years. Dr. King has provided an enthralling chronicle of a new philanthropic concept, a new type of Foundation, devoted to one of the basic needs of mankind—food and nutrition.

The pattern, evolved from "the good idea" of those who initially conceived this organization, has now been adopted in other nations—for example, in Sweden, the Swedish Nutrition Foundation; in England, the British Nutrition Foundation. There is a growing consortium of activities among these and other similarly oriented organizations on an international scale —foundations in Switzerland, Holland, Japan, Chile, the Philippines—along with potential interest in developing like organizations in several other countries.

Tomorrow's food needs and nutritional problems are so immense as to make the importance and responsibility of resources such as these of even broader and greater moment than in the past.

Dr. King and The Nutrition Foundation had a part in so many of the significant developments in nutrition that this history of the Foundation becomes a veritable record of the progress of the science and application of nutrition during the past three-and-a-half decades. These decades are an era during which rapid and widespread changes have occurred, changes that permanently will affect human nutrition and health throughout the world.

The reader of this "biography of an institution" will, therefore, glean a perspective concerning the growth of the scientific and technologic knowledge, as well as the organization of the scientific community that supports this field of science in the service of mankind. He will undoubtedly emerge with a profound sense of indebtedness to all of those leaders whose high sense of corporate citizenship was responsible for conceiving and developing, for supporting and expanding The Nutrition Foundation—the original "good idea" conceived as an act in the public welfare.

As current President of The Nutrition Foundation, I express my gratitude to Dr. King for his outstanding leadership in structuring this important organization and for providing in this history a useful perspective of accomplishment and nutrition development. Such perspective will assist the scientific, educational, governmental and industrial communities and international groups better to plan for the most beneficial use of our knowledge and resources to meet the food and nutrition needs of mankind.

William J. Darby, M.D., Ph.D
President
The Nutrition Foundation, Inc.

A Good Idea

The First Decade: Development of a Good Idea

FOOD is so intimately associated with human happiness, health and family budgets in all parts of the world that a good new idea in that realm of thinking is very significant. Such was the story of an idea springing from two, then five, then fifteen thoughtful men talking together—and moving the idea into action. After four years of careful study and growing enthusiasm, The Nutrition Foundation was legally established in December 1941.

A new kind of organization entirely in the public interest had evolved from a farsighted suggestion. The goal was a program of active service in nutrition research and education under the leadership of the foremost independent scientists in universities and government agencies of the United States and Canada. Public-spirited executives in the food industry, with encouragement from their own respective research directors, agreed to support the program without regard to their corporations' specific products or processes. This was industry and democracy at their best.

The basis for this action was the realization that the food industry had an obligation to the public to cooperate with responsible leaders in agriculture, medicine, public health and education to develop and to apply the young and growing science of nutrition for the betterment of mankind.

A determined leader in the initial discussions was Mr. Clarence Francis, President of General Foods Corporation, a community leader of renown. He was long a member of the Economic Development Council of New York City and later chaired the committee of prominent citizens who established the Lincoln Center for the Performing Arts, a multimillion dollar project which immensely benefits the people of New York and the cultural life of America. Let Mr. Francis tell what the first two thoughtful men were discussing in 1938 . . . and how it happened:

> I well recall lunching with Charles Wesley Dunn, General Counsel of the Associated Grocery Manufacturers of America (GMA) many years ago when we were discussing an on-coming annual meeting of that organization. We were searching for an activity on which the industry should and would act in the public welfare. Many ideas were discussed, among which

A Good Idea

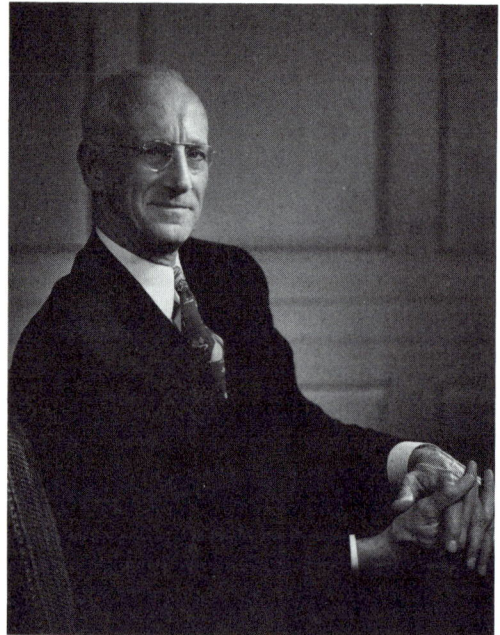
Clarence Francis

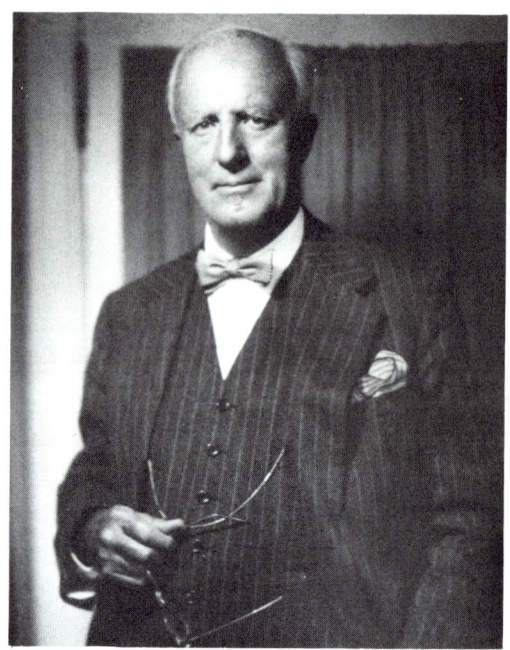
Charles Wesley Dunn

Two men with "A Good Idea"

was nutrition. The more we talked on this subject the more important it became and the idea of a large, intensive program in nutrition was finally agreed upon. We convinced ourselves that the idea was sound and could be sold to the membership.

We discussed the idea with leaders and were surprised with the ready acceptance. Mr. Dunn then proposed the plan at the next annual meeting of GMA and I received the association's blessings as chairman of a committee to move ahead.

At that time there was a big question as to whether or not the public would ever believe that profit-minded industries would be unselfish enough to spend time and money on anything that detracted from profits.

To offset this it was thought advisable to procure as chairman someone outside of industry whose character and reputation were beyond reproach and to develop an organization with bylaws and controls which would insure that the monies contributed by industries be used for the benefit of the public.

The original plan was to centralize the operation in a university. Yale was selected and approached and we received considerable encouragement as to their willingness to cooperate. Then came the task of financing. We felt we must get a five-year commitment if we were to persuade qualified people to join in this endeavor. We got two commitments and then trouble arose, and the idea seemed doomed. Time lagged, no money was forthcoming, but questions were continually asked about the movement.

Finally the real cause for lack of support came to light. Industry executives were not impressed with centralizing in any one university. They felt, and time has proven rightly so, that this subject of nutrition was so vital and broad that instead of trying to bring experts to one location that the most capable men should be found anywhere in the world and that they should be supported to work on their respective problems independently on their home grounds. The money should be spent for talent, not brick and mortar.

The First Decade

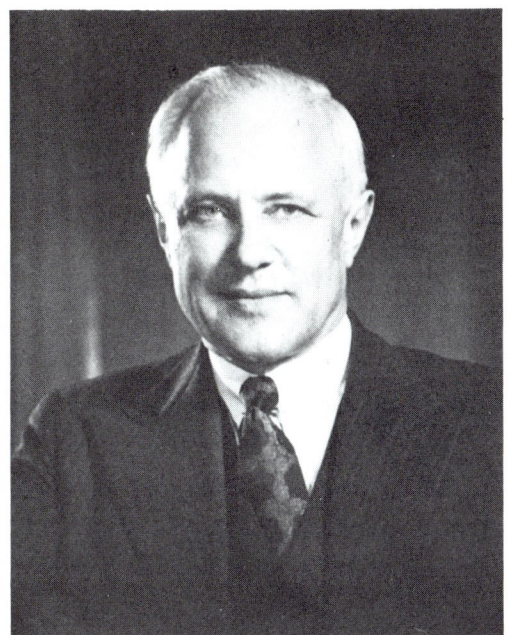
Karl Compton

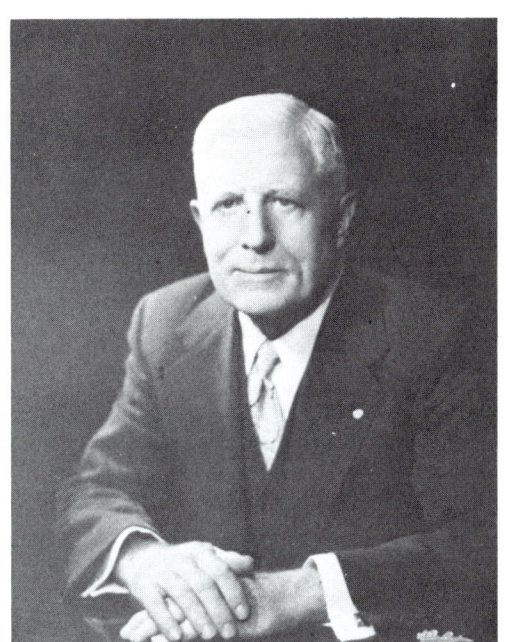
John Holmes

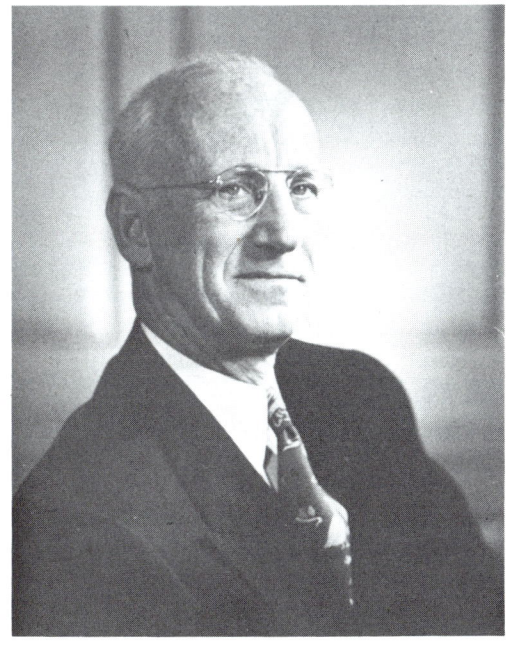
Clarence Francis

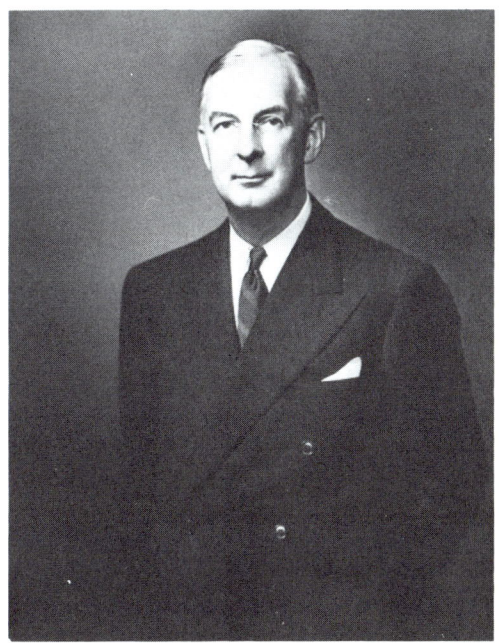
Morris Sayre

The Organizing Committee of The Nutrition Foundation

A Good Idea

That finding gave new impetus to the movement and under the forceful and intelligent leadership of Morris Sayre, then President of Corn Products Refining Company, and John Holmes, then President of Swift & Company, finances were procured. To those men must go great credit for bringing the Foundation into being.

With this idea of a Nutrition Foundation and a suggested set of bylaws in hand and financing assured, we approached Dr. Karl Compton, President of Massachusetts Institute of Technology, and were encouraged by his statement that we were setting a new and broad policy for industry and by his acceptance of the chairmanship. His leadership was outstanding.

One of the first great services rendered by Dr. Compton was persuading Dr. Glen King to leave his important and secure post at the University of Pittsburgh to accept the position of Scientific Director of the Foundation.

I shall stop here with appreciation for the privilege of having participated in this movement which, for the good of all humanity, should spread its influence beyond our national borders.

The spirit and the work envisioned were exciting to scientists and laymen alike. Administrative personnel in industry, agriculture, education, public health and government agencies would have more extensive and more reliable guideposts by which better to serve the public. Both nationally and internationally there would be an accelerated development of new information and of greater numbers of well-trained leaders in nutrition research, education, medical practice and food technology.

On Christmas Eve, 1941, the official certificate of incorporation was filed with the New York Department of State. The initial fifteen members of the Board of Trustees who served until the first annual meeting were:

James S. Adams, Standard Brands, Inc.;
Frederick Beers, National Biscuit Company;
Carlysle H. Black, American Can Company;
Carle C. Conway, Continental Can Company;
Daniel W. Creeden, Libby, McNeill & Libby;
Alfred W. Eames, California Packing Corporation;
Clarence Francis, General Foods Corporation;
Henry J. Heinz, II, H. J. Heinz Company;
John Holmes, Swift & Company;
J. Preston Levis, Owens-Illinois Glass Company;
James McGowan, Jr., Campbell Soup Company;
J. Stafford Ellithorp, Jr., Beechnut Packing Company;
Russell G. Partridge, United Fruit Company;
Morris Sayre, Corn Products Refining Company;
R. Douglas Stuart, Quaker Oats Company.

These men were top-level executives in their respective companies, they had studied the project with great care, and they proved to be sincere in their motivation of public service.

There was enthusiastic agreement that Dr. Karl T. Compton, President of the Massachusetts Institute of Technology and a former professor of physics at Princeton University, should serve as Chairman of the Board of Trustees and also on a steering committee with John Holmes (Chairman), Clarence Francis and Morris Sayre, to select officers and move ahead in developing the organization, structure and policies. Morris Sayre served without compensation as Treasurer. George A. Sloan, then Commissioner of Commerce in New York City, was invited to be President on a part-time basis with a special responsibility for membership promotion.

The First Decade

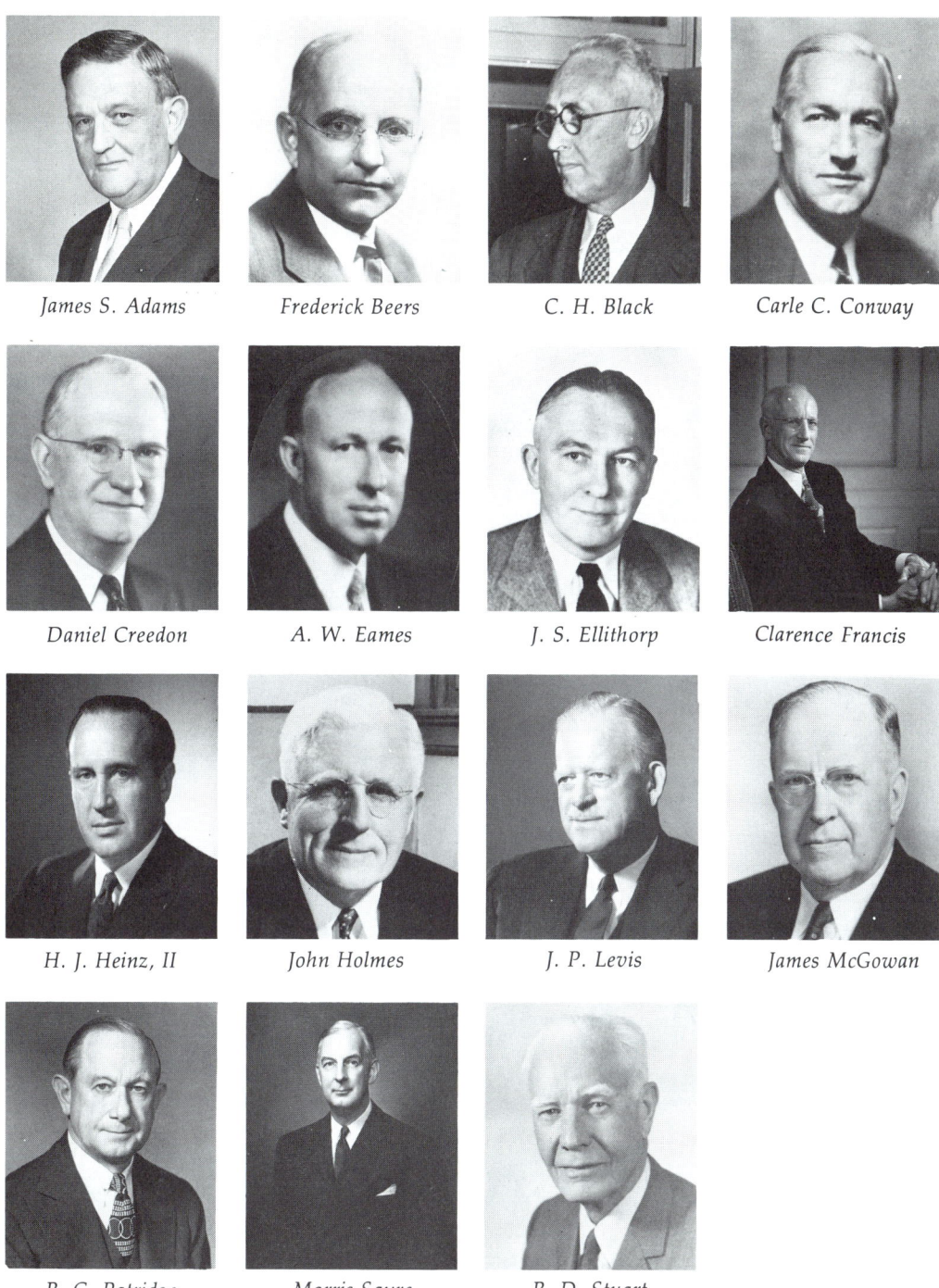

Members of the Initial Board of Trustees of The Nutrition Foundation

A Good Idea

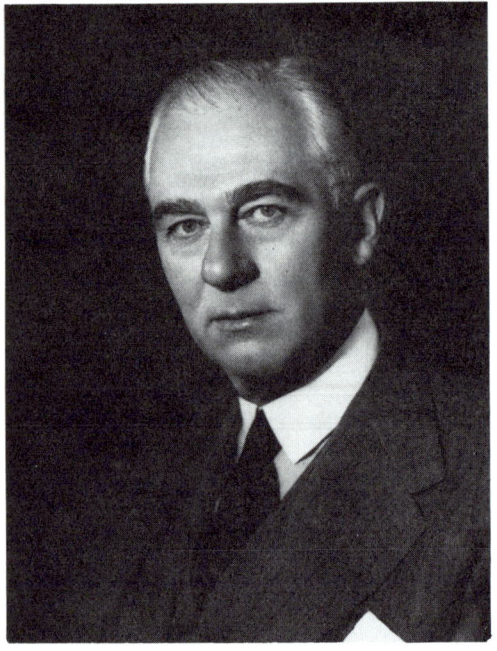

George A. Sloan —First President of The Nutrition Foundation

As Professor of Chemistry and Director of the Buhl Foundation Program in Chemistry, Physics and Biology at the University of Pittsburgh, I was invited to be the full-time Scientific Director in charge of the program. Ole Salthe, who had been associated with Senator Copeland in revision of the Federal Pure Food and Drug Law and as a senior staff member in the New York City Department of Health, was asked to become Executive Secretary, and Miss Irene Magnus became Senior Secretary. The administrative offices were established in the Chrysler Building in New York City.

Through January and February 1942, Dr. Compton worked closely with the officers and steering committee to provide for a strong and independent program in research and education. The Scientific Director was designated as Chairman of a Scientific Advisory Committee and authorized

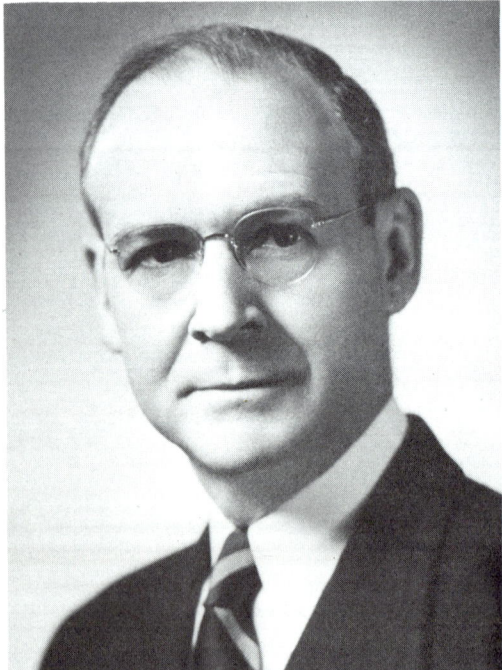

Charles Glen King—The First Scientific Director and Full-Time President of The Nutrition Foundation

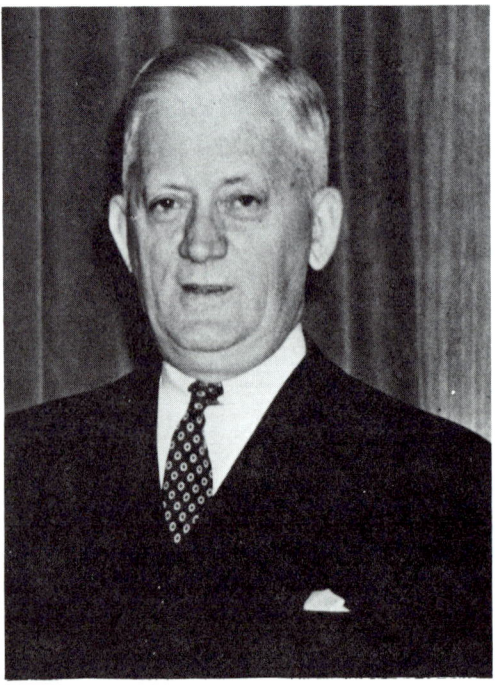

Ole Salthe—First Executive Secretary of The Nutrition Foundation

The First Decade

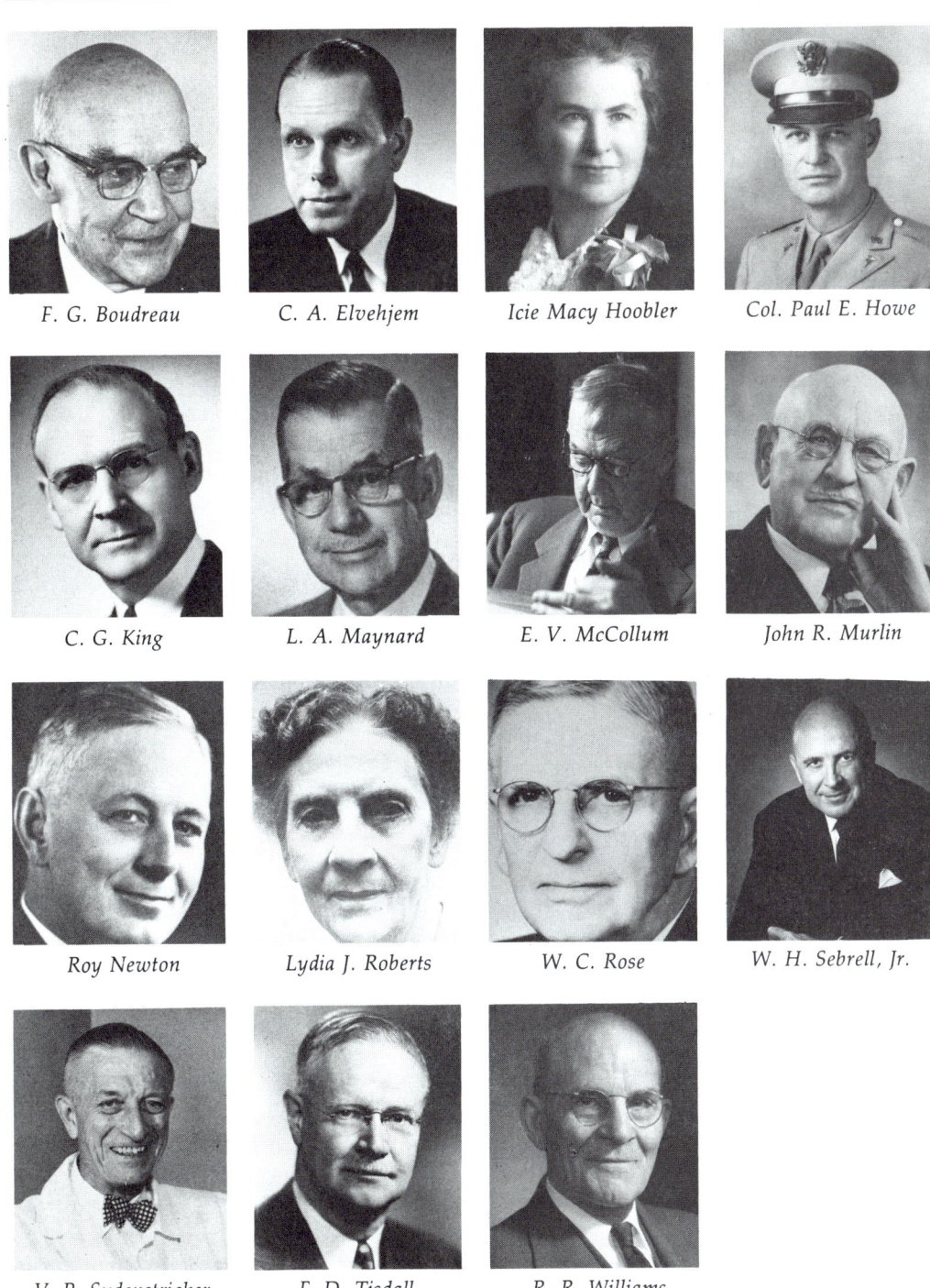

F. G. Boudreau   C. A. Elvehjem   Icie Macy Hoobler   Col. Paul E. Howe

C. G. King   L. A. Maynard   E. V. McCollum   John R. Murlin

Roy Newton   Lydia J. Roberts   W. C. Rose   W. H. Sebrell, Jr.

V. P. Sydenstricker   F. D. Tisdall   R. R. Williams

Original Scientific Advisory Committee of The Nutrition Foundation

A Good Idea

jointly with the Board Chairman to recommend nominations for membership on this committee for approval by the Trustees. Similarly, recommendations for grants in support of research and education were transmitted to the trustees only on authorization of the Director and the Scientific Advisory Committee.

Applications for grants were reviewed and evaluated independently by all members of the Scientific Advisory Committee in advance of their meeting as a group twice each year to reach final decisions on recommendations. Group discussions at committee meetings were particularly useful for evaluating progress on grants underway, for reviewing new proposals on the agenda, and—a highly important role—in looking forward to identify individuals capable of doing important work and of making good selections of young scientists for training. The work of this committee and its rapport with the Trustees were of such a quality that no grant recommendation to the Board of Trustees was denied or restricted in any way during my 21 years of experience as Director or President. Requests for information and frank discussion of the significance of recommendations, however, were always welcomed and encouraged. The sincerity of mutual interest in human service and the complete confidence in Dr. Compton's leadership made meetings of the committees and of the Board of Trustees a pleasure, and reflected a true sense of responsible participation by everyone involved.

To provide both administrative guidance and active liaison with universities, government agencies and other representatives of the public, the following public members were elected to the Board of Trustees at their first formal meeting:

Karl T. Compton, President, Massachusetts Institute of Technology (chairman)
Cason J. Callaway, Agricultural Publisher (vice chairman)
Hugh O'Donnell, President of Notre Dame University (vice chairman)
Frank G. Boudreau, Executive Director of the Milbank Fund and chairman of the Food and Nutrition Board, National Academy of Sciences-National Research Council
Oliver C. Carmichael, Chancellor, Vanderbilt University
W. C. Coffee, President, University of Minnesota
Charles Wesley Dunn, Counsel, Grocery Manufacturers' of America
Charles Glen King (scientific director)
Thomas Parran, Surgeon General, U.S. Public Health Service
George A. Sloan (president)
Ray Lyman Wilbur, President, Stanford University
M. L. Wilson, Chief of Nutrition Service, U.S. Department of Agriculture, and
Stephen S. Wise, Rabbi, Free Synagogue, New York City

Each member company in the Foundation designated a representative on the Food Industries Advisory Committee—usually a vice president in charge of research or with comparable responsibility. This group had an important liaison role for interpretation of the program to personnel within their respective companies and for designation of persons to whom reprints, other technical reports and educational materials could be sent for direct use or distribution. At annual meetings of this committee scientists from universities and government agencies were invited to present informal discussions of their published work or the work of others and its apparent significance. The point of emphasis in these meetings was in relation to health or to significant progress in basic research. It is a great satisfaction to report the fact

The First Decade

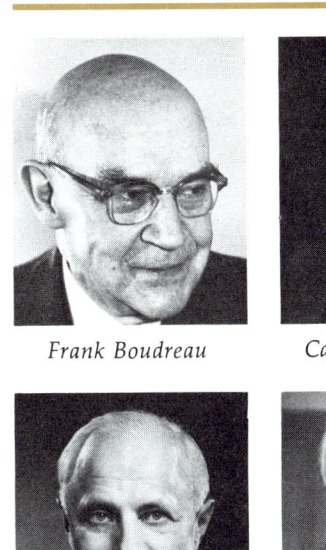
Frank Boudreau

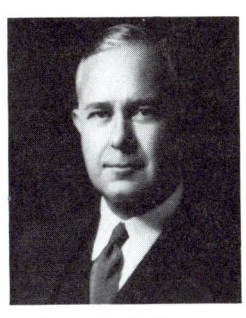
Cason J. Callaway

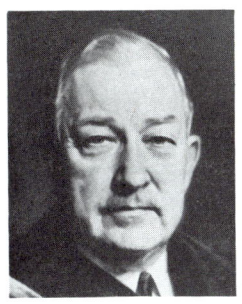
O. C. Carmichael

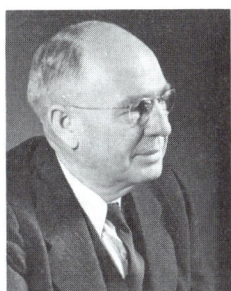
Walter C. Coffery

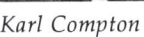
Karl Compton

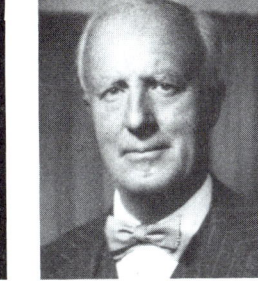
Charles Wesley Dunn

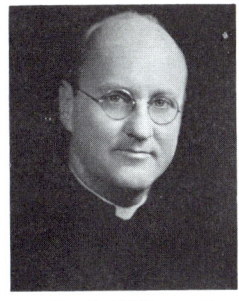
Hugh O'Donnell

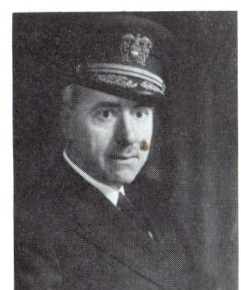
Thomas Parran

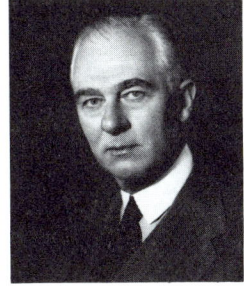
George A. Sloan

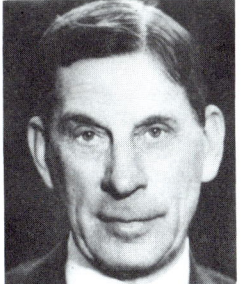
Ray Lyman Wilbur

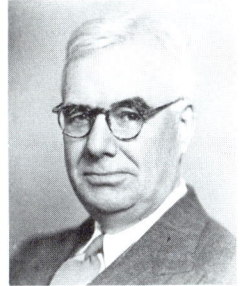
M. L. Wilson

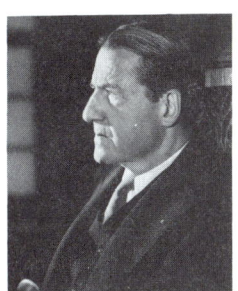
Rabbi Stephan S. Wise

Initial Public Members of the Board of Trustees of The Nutrition Foundation
The Scientific Director, Charles Glen King (Photograph, p. 8), also was an initial Public Trustee

that in no instance during 21 years of service did a member of this committee or the Board of Trustees suggest undertaking any grant or other activity that would work selfishly in the particular interest of his own organization or against any other worthy organization. That experience is a measure of the citizenship of which members of the Foundation can be proud. There has been maintained complete loyalty to the concept that the public and the industry are best served as a result of increased knowledge and education in the science of nutrition.

At the May 1942 meeting of the Board of Trustees Dr. Boudreau, from his rich national and international experience in medicine and public health, gave a stimulating challenge to us, saying with great earnestness: "Much more has been done for animals than for human beings.

A Good Idea

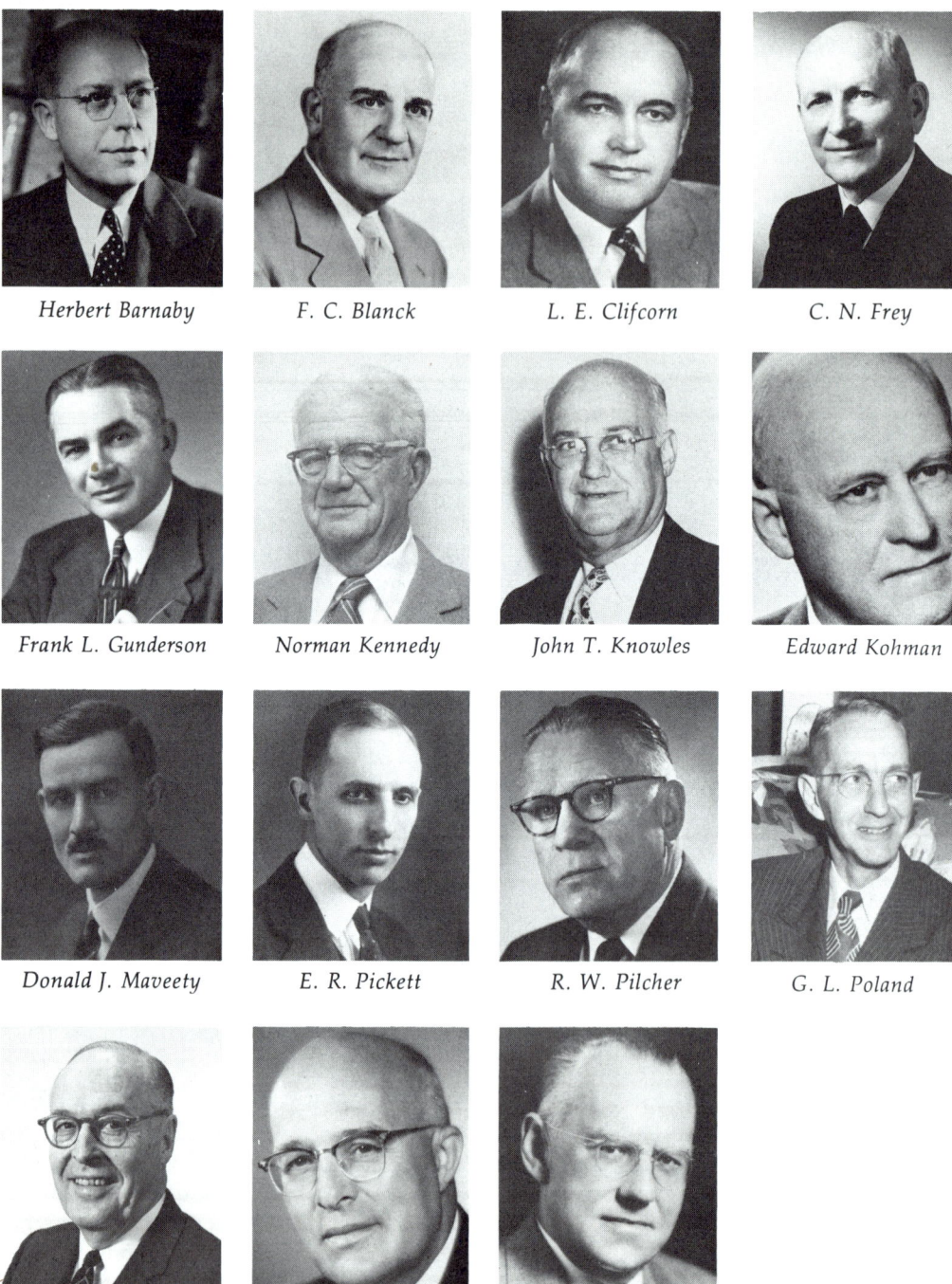

Herbert Barnaby — F. C. Blanck — L. E. Clifcorn — C. N. Frey

Frank L. Gunderson — Norman Kennedy — John T. Knowles — Edward Kohman

Donald J. Maveety — E. R. Pickett — R. W. Pilcher — G. L. Poland

A. C. Richardson — H. E. Robinson — Lewis W. Waters

Members of The First Food Industries Advisory Committee of The Nutrition Foundation

The First Decade

Scientific feeding of livestock has paid high dividends. Scientific feeding of human beings would pay big dividends of a different kind. If all that we know about nutrition were applied to modern society the result would be enormous improvement in public health."

Each member company initially pledged $50,000 in support of the Foundation, payable in one sum or $10,000 annually for five years. Each year members were invited to extend their pledge one year to permit continued stability in the program. This policy permitted research scientists to be in a strong position to attack difficult problems and to support highly qualified graduate students and post-doctoral research personnel in parallel with expenditures for essential equipment and supplies.

After demonstrating the success of the general plan as developed by founder members, provision was made for membership on a lesser scale of payments, down to a minimum of $500 per year to permit a broader representation of the industry and to encourage their regard for public health and for the long range value of basic research. Membership payments (less than $10,000 annually) were based on capitalization instead of a flexible scale such as sales or dividends that would vary from year to year.

Appointment of the Scientific Director

A short time after reading in the December 28, 1941, NEW YORK TIMES a report of the formation of The Nutrition Foundation, I wrote to Dr. Compton asking when the office would be ready to welcome applications for research grants and I merely mentioned that possibly some of our work at the University of Pittsburgh would be of interest. Receipt of his reply baffled and shocked me. Instead of mentioning grant applications he asked me to come to Cambridge at the earliest convenient time to talk with him about The Nutrition Foundation, adding that I had been selected by unanimous vote of the Board of Trustees to serve as Scientific Director of the Foundation and that he wanted me to assist in developing plans for the organization.

The challenge worried me. I was completely engrossed in teaching and research at the University of Pittsburgh where the program was growing steadily in cooperation with the departments of chemistry, physics and biology, and in reasonable degree with the schools of medicine and dentistry and the Mellon Institute. The university faculty had elected me to serve as Chairman of the newly formed Faculty Council. The Buhl Foundation in Pittsburgh had become very helpful in support of the interdepartmental work by means of a sizable and increasing fund for graduate and post-doctoral fellowships. This program was having a major impact on the University's development in graduate research. My personal research interest had been chiefly in studies of vitamin C which we had isolated and identified in 1931-32, and in studies of the molecular structure and functions of edible fats, in parallel with an interest in amino acid metabolism by bacteria.

Physical facilities at the university were still relatively limited, however, and teaching loads were diverse and heavy. For many years my teaching schedule included undergraduate lecture courses in general chemistry, industrial chemistry, food and sanitation, and laboratory or recitation classes in organic chemistry, in addition to my major responsibility for graduate lectures, research and a seminar in biochemistry. I was deeply indebted to the university administration and the faculty for their personal friendship and support, and to the Buhl Foundation for friendly encouragement and substantial assistance. Friendships with alumni and students created an additional strong emotional tie.

Fortunately, my service participation in

A Good Idea

professional societies had developed a fairly wide acquaintance with leading scientists in biochemistry, nutrition, food technology and public health. I had been a charter member of the American Institute of Nutrition when it was organized in 1928 and of the Institute of Food Technologists organized in 1939, active in the American Chemical Society and the American Public Health Association, a member of the British Nutrition Society, and for two years Secretary of the American Society of Biological Chemists. The latter responsibility, particularly, afforded me an opportunity to become well acquainted with most of the leading university, government and industrial research scientists working in biochemistry or in medical and animal nutrition. As a member of the initial U.S. National Committee on Foods and Nutrition in 1940-41, which soon became the Food and Nutrition Board of the National Academy of Sciences-National Research Council, I had been closely associated with several national and international food and nutrition matters related to the war situation.

Dr. Compton indicated a strong preference for me to move to a central office in New York, although that was not a condition essential to my appointment. He said that if I wished to continue in a part-time academic position he would inquire in regard to that possibility. Shortly afterward I was invited to a part-time visiting professorship at Columbia University, in close association with Professors H. C. Sherman, Arthur W. Thomas and others in the Department of Chemistry. I was well acquainted also with Professor Hans Clarke in the Medical Center. The University of Pittsburgh extended a year's leave of absence through 1942-43 so that I could accept the challenge on that basis.

Program Development

General information about the Foundation was released to the press early in 1942 and more details were provided directly from the office to nutrition scientists in the United States and Canada. The first public meeting of the Board of Trustees was held in New York, March 12, 1942, and on May 20, the Board approved 36 grants providing a total of $123,890. Sixteen additional grants were approved on November 12, 1942.

It is noteworthy that these awards preceded by several years the establishment of grant programs for basic research in metabolism, nutrition and broad areas of human biology as now financed by the National Institutes of Health and the National Science Foundation.

The National Institutes of Health was brought into existence under the Act of May 26, 1930 as a reorganization and expansion of the old U.S.P.H.S. Hygienic Laboratory. The Social Security Act of 1935 authorized general health grants to states. In 1937 the National Cancer Institute, the first of the categorical research institutes, was established and provided for the first time grants-in-aid to universities or individuals for research in cancer. Not until 1948 was the National Institute of Dental Research established. The National Institute of Mental Health came into being in 1949 and in 1950 the National Institute of Arthritis, Rheumatism and Metabolic Diseases and the National Institute of Neurological Diseases and Blindness. In the latter year authority was provided by the Congress to the Surgeon General to establish one or more additional institutes for particular diseases or groups of diseases. It was in that same year, 1950, that the National Science Foundation was created.

The national and international situation

The First Decade

resulting from the war made it urgent to give special consideration to research relevant to the war effort and to investigations not adequately supported by other sources. Compared with contract sums from government agencies in support of the war effort or with the sums provided in later years from federal agencies, grants from the Foundation seemed very small, yet in many instances they have been highly significant. Grants were planned in close cooperation with the respective scientific staff members of the Army, Navy, Air Force, Public Health Service, Department of Agriculture, the National Academy of Sciences-National Research Council, and some of the other foundations, including especially the Milbank Fund, the Rockefeller Foundation, the Macy Foundation, the Kellogg Foundation and the Williams-Waterman Fund of the Research Corporation. Advisory Committee members who served two or more organizations provided a desirable liaison. In many instances the prompt action that could be taken by the Foundation enabled scientists to initiate research that later expanded with support from slower acting government agencies.

Examples of Basic Research Supported

Illustrations of outstanding research aided by those seemingly small grants are the following examples:

(1) William C. Rose at the University of Illinois was just completing a long-term study in which he had identified the ten protein fragments (amino acids) essential for the growth and normal health of albino rats. These animals have nutrient requirements similar to those of man, but they were also known to have some very marked differences. Dr. Rose recognized the urgency of extending the studies to establish the human requirements, but he had no funds to buy or prepare the quantities of pure amino acids required for the tests. Highly qualified graduate students were willing to serve as experimental subjects, and Mrs. Rose would help him with the preparation of experimental diets.

This information was obviously of extreme importance in relation to feeding humanity in all parts of the world—it would make it possible to estimate the nutritive quality of a food protein by direct chemical analysis instead of long, tedious, expensive tests with human subjects at various ages and under varying circumstances. An initial grant of $3,600 in the spring of 1942, followed by $12,000 in 1943 and 1944, permitted Dr. Rose to advance his program rapidly. It was dramatic to observe healthy young adults begin to lose body stores of protein within 24 hours when a single amino acid was omitted from an otherwise adequate diet, and within 3 to 4 days to show emotional disturbance. When the missing amino acid was restored in the diet, the onset of recovery was clearly evident within the first or second day. This study is recognized as one of the great milestones in the history of nutrition and continues to guide the high priority, worldwide effort to meet the need for good quality protein foods. Dr. Rose later received many honors as one of our greatest nutritional scientists and teachers. He was the recipient of the first Osborne and Mendel Award for basic research in nutrition by the American Institute of Nutrition, the Willard Gibbs Medal of the American Chemical Society, the National Medal from the President of the United States and the Spencer Award of the Midwest Section of the American Chemical Society.

In the developing countries, particularly in tropical and subtropical areas where the population density is destructively high

A Good Idea

and economic resources are extremely low, the lack of good quality protein foods is frequently the most damaging handicap to health and social or economic progress. Agricultural and medical research to solve this problem is greatly accelerated by our ability to utilize rapid chemical analysis for the essential amino acids in each experimental product. Research in genetics and technologies in agriculture or food science would be severely handicapped without this advantage. Eight of the 21 amino acids present in common food proteins are clearly essential to maintaining health in human adults, and other amino acids may exert a sparing action but not a complete substitution for those that are essential. The ratios between the 21 amino acids are also nutritionally important and they vary over wide ranges in the functions of living organisms from single-cell bacteria to man. The contribution by Dr. Rose was a major achievement and the world benefited quickly from his many years of basic research through application of the new knowledge to meet crucial human needs.

(2) Vincent du Vigneaud at Cornell University was particularly interested in one of the essential amino acids (methionine) because of its sulfur content and its unique role in the metabolism of a widely distributed vitamin-like nutrient (choline) that functions in all living cells to sustain life. Deficiencies of methionine and choline result in striking injury to liver, kidney, adrenal, pituitary and other glandular tissues. An initial grant of $3,800, increased to $5,600 per year, enabled him to extend his early studies with rats using isotope labeled compounds and to include related observations on human liver and kidney functions. Later, using much larger funds from other sources, he was successful in establishing the structure and synthesis of insulin, the sulfur-containing protein which is the dominant hormone involved in diabetes. This led him into a study of other protein or protein-like hormones—vasopressin, the blood pressure-raising principle, and oxytocin, the uterine-contracting principle of the posterior pituitary gland. He elaborated the polypeptide structures of these. In 1955 du Vigneaud received the Nobel Prize in Chemistry for his first synthesis of a polypeptide hormone. The fascinating sequence of his interests are instructively revealed in his account: "A Trail of Research in Sulfur Chemistry and Metabolism and Related Fields" (Cornell University Press, Ithaca, 1952).

(3) Another of the initial grants was $6,000 annually to George W. Beadle at Stanford University and, later, at the California Institute of Technology in support of four graduate student fellowships. His research interest was fundamental in the science of genetics and biochemistry. The techniques he developed in studies with molds furnished many new methods of measuring amino acids, vitamins and related nutrients. His contributions were useful not only in analytical work in food and nutrition but they also provided new insights concerning the origin and functions of materials characteristic of every cell in all plants and animals. In 1958 Dr. Beadle shared the Nobel Prize in Physiology and Medicine with his colleagues, Edwin L. Tatum and Joshua Lederberg, for work in biochemical genetics. Subsequently he was elected President of the University of Chicago. In retirement he continues to study the "pre-Columbian" genetic origin of modern types of corn and has served for many years as a public trustee of The Nutrition Foundation.

In addition to his brilliance in research and teaching, Dr. Beadle had another attribute that was illustrated during my first two visits to Stanford University. During the first trip a faculty member in another

The First Decade

department commented, "I don't know Dr. Beadle very well, although I believe he lives on my street." The same man commented when I returned to the campus, "I've discovered why I was so long getting acquainted with George—he passes my house before I finish breakfast and returns home after dark." The delightful sense of humor within his family is recorded in the refreshing book, "These Ruins are Inhabited," by his wife, Muriel. This biography provides an insight into their experiences in 1958, the year in which George Beadle, then a visiting professor at Oxford, received a Nobel Prize.

(4) The Scientific Advisory Committee was unanimous in their conclusion at the first meeting that there was a serious need for research on the detailed composition of milks, both human and cows', obtained under carefully defined conditions. New methods had become available for accurate and extensive analysis, including quantitation of several newly identified nutrients. This research required collaboration between highly qualified personnel from both a medical center and an agricultural center, and special facilities utilizing the best methods of chemical analysis. Agreement was reached for collaboration among three groups. The dairy work was conducted at Cornell University under the supervision of L. A. Maynard and B. L. Harrington, assisted by J. M. Lawrence. The human studies in association with the Children's Fund of Michigan in Detroit, were led by Icie Macy Hoobler in cooperation with H. H. Williams, C. E. Roderick, M. N. Coryell and the medical staff. The detailed analysis of milk fat from both groups was done at the University of Pittsburgh by H. E. Longenecker and A. R. Baldwin. The analytical work covering the vitamins and mineral elements was divided between the two main laboratories on the basis of facilities and experience.

The results provided new guidance for nutrient planning of infant feeding, maternal nutrition practices and modification of cows' milk as a substitute for breast milk. The results demonstrated substantial differences between human and cows' milk in the content of total and specific proteins, essential and non-essential fatty acids, vitamins and minerals that could not be well adjusted by mere dilution of cows' milk with water or the addition of sugar, as then practiced. Although the significance of the differences could only be surmised by reasoning from animal studies, new quantitative information served as a basic guide for improved practices and a stimulus to continuing research on infant feeding.

(5) The University of Pittsburgh was given support for studies of fat utilization by human adults, using the types of fat "hardened" (hydrogenated) for stabilization against rancidity in army rations and in products for civilian use. This work was conducted by B. F. Daubert and A. R. Baldwin in association with Dr. Herbert Longenecker.

Questions of digestibility and the efficiency of utilization of fats with different types of fatty acids were of urgent nutritional interest for three major reasons. One was the problem of stability of foods against rancidity during storage. Another was the uncertainty about the body's capacity to utilize efficiently fatty acids formed during heating and hydrogenation as occurs in food preparation and processing. And third was the question of whether these fatty acids constituted any risk to health.

At least one "polyunsaturated" fatty acid (linoleic) was well documented to be essential for health. It is present in generous quantities in corn oil, cottonseed oil, soybean oil, sesame seed oil and fish oils, but it occurs in much lesser quantities in butterfat, pork, cocoa fat and beef fat. Hence,

A Good Idea

for military rations, even more than for civilian use, questions of nutritive value, stability, digestibility and physical properties were of crucial importance. The Pittsburgh group demonstrated that the fatty acids present in oils subjected to moderate hydrogenation were utilized efficiently and without evidence of metabolic disturbances, but this recognition did not imply any lowering of the requirement for at least a moderate intake of linoleic acid, perhaps in the range of 2 to 3 percent or more of total calories.

It is a pleasure to note the subsequent leadership in the food industry of these two associates; Dr. Daubert with General Foods Company and Dr. Baldwin with Cargill, Inc. Dr. Longenecker became successively Vice President of the University of Illinois, President of Tulane University, and Chairman of the Board of Trustees of The Nutrition Foundation (1965-1972). In this latter role he made important contributions to the reorganization of the Foundation in 1971.

Grant Support and Personnel Development

During 1926-27, I had been assisted by fellowships to permit post-doctoral studies with Professor H. C. Sherman and others at Columbia University and Professor F. Gowland Hopkins at Cambridge University, and had an opportunity to visit other research centers in Europe for half a year in 1929. I knew from this personal experience how much even a small supporting grant could mean. Early post-doctoral years are generally the period when comprehension of knowledge in a given area by an individual can be most effectively combined with creative imagination and a vigorous physical and intellectual drive for accomplishment. The challenge is then strong to push further the exploration of the universe in which man lives and which he would like more fully to understand.

In an informal discussion of this relationship with Karl Compton and Warren Weaver, two of the most competent men in science education during the past half-century, I was thrilled to hear them agree that probably the most significant grant in proportion to size that The Rockefeller Foundation had ever made was the one to establish within the U.S. National Academy of Sciences-National Research Council post-doctoral fellowships for carefully selected young scientists within the universities of the United States.

The Foundation's policy recognized that research expenditures generally would have greatest benefit when given in a manner to support graduate or post-doctoral personnel development. Personal need for assistance by young scientists is usually most acute during those periods of graduate education and early career development; the potential of an individual for professional development can be estimated reasonably well at the same time. Well managed support of scientists during this phase of their career produces a great return in value to university faculties and to society at large. Such grants permitted a reasonable allowance for supplies, but from a relatively limited budget it was not advisable to recommend appreciable sums for equipment or laboratory construction. Institutional "overhead" has never been allowed by the Foundation.

It should be noted that Dr. Weaver was for many years Director of the Division of Natural Sciences of The Rockefeller Foundation. Previously a lack of this kind of support had robbed many young scientists of their best opportunity for personal development and had handicapped the development of faculties in our universities—and hence constituted a serious handicap to our national development. A

The First Decade

significant number of the American students who could afford to spend a year or more in Europe made major contributions to research centers in Europe. Since the professors's name usually came first on research publications, the students' work thus enhanced both his name and the prestige of the European university. National exchanges in both directions are highly desirable, of course, when based on consideration of ability, inspiration, expense and benefit to society.

Among those who received the benefit of an appointment as a National Research Council Fellow in the medical or biological sciences during the period 1919-1944 (list published by the National Research Council, June 30, 1944), one finds the names of leaders well-known among nutrition scientists in later years: Eric G. Ball, George Beadle, William J. Darby, Vincent du Vigneaud, Conrad A. Elvehjem, Karl E. Mason, Harold S. Olcott and George Wald —and in later years, Herbert E. Longenecker.

As recently as 1972-73, somewhere in the notorious "money and politics" jam of negotiations for continued Federal support of research via the National Institutes of Health, the basic need for selective support of pre-doctoral and post-doctoral training was tragically ignored. This critical error has been only partly corrected to date. It is to be hoped that our leaders will act more wisely in the future.

Having received the decisions reached by the Scientific Advisory Committee in regard to research and educational grants, I always found it a challenge to interpret the recommendations to the Board of Trustees, the Food Industries Advisory Committee and, in an Annual Report, to the general public. The vocabulary had to be adapted to the occasion, but I could be confident that service to the public would be the key point of interest and response. A forecast of vocabulary hazards occurred in an earlier experience in Pittsburgh when I had mentioned in a report that "chemically vitamin C is a very active reducing agent". The Director, a former professor of English, commented: "In our office that would mean that it would make fat women thin!"

NUTRITION REVIEWS—New Journal to Identify and Extend Nutritional Knowledge

During the decade 1932-42, there had been phenomenal progress in identifying the number and chemical nature of vitamins, but there was great uncertainty concerning their functions and the amount of each required by humans. Substantial progress had also been made in regard to the "trace" elements such as copper, iodine, fluorine, manganese and cobalt. These elements were known to be required in very small amounts by farm and laboratory animals, but evidence pertaining to human requirements for health was almost completely limited to comparative approximations with test animals calculated on the basis of body weight. These elements were known to be injurious when consumed in excessive quantities.

During these years practical measures for prevention of scurvy, rickets, pellagra, beri-beri, goiter and some forms of blindness had been advanced very rapidly by research on the vitamins and trace elements. At the same time, however, exciting claims and counterclaims, many of which were unfounded, frequently appeared in the literature. These reports created confusion among physicians, educators, food technologists, agriculturists and others who were responsible for public service and safety. Toxic quantities of vitamin D were proclaimed as treatment for arthritis, vitamin A was widely referred to as both "the anti-infection vitamin" and "the anti-cold vitamin," thiamin was "the morale vitamin," and vitamin E was "the fertility vitamin" and "prevented heart attacks." The research literature of nutrition was being published in widely diverse journals, often without competent critical, nutritionally knowledgeable editorial review. Indeed, the JOURNAL OF NUTRITION, established in 1928, was the only U.S. publication in this field; the BRITISH JOURNAL OF NUTRITION was not established until 1947. Accordingly, there was a great need for some coordinating reference source.

At that time the historical background pertinent to foods and nutrition in the United States and Canada somewhat familiar to most technically trained people included:

1. the trememdous decline in death rates that followed the introduction of filtered and chlorinated water supplies in many cities;
2. the rapid decline in goiter among people and livestock in large sections of the northeast, mid-west and northwest areas of the U.S. following the introduction of iodized table salt and stock feed;
3. the steady decline in rickets among children that resulted from the widespread use of cod liver oil and vitamin D milk;
4. the dramatic drop in infant and child death rates due to the introduction of pasteurized milk;
5. the decrease in the incidence of scurvy, roughly in proportion to the increased consumption of citrus fruits, tomatoes and potatoes, with an assist from apples; and
6. the decreased incidence of pellagra in the southern states from an estimated peak incidence of about 200,000 cases per year, as economic progress and education had improved diets among low income groups.

There was much concern within the medical profession and among nutrition scientists, however, in regard to how much health impairment still persisted in the zone between obvious deficiency and intakes that would be in the approximate range of optimum health. Carefully controlled tests with experimental animals indicated that the margin between prevention of deficiency disease and optimal intake level might be wide in some cases as with vitamin C in guinea pigs, vitamin A in rats, and calcium in livestock, but not wide in others, such as fluoride, copper, and vitamin D. Such simple World War I slogans as "don't waste food" and "spare wheat and meat" were no longer adequate for wartime feeding guidance. Likewise, there was much concern for providing the Allied Military Command with the most healthy, wholesome, nutritious rations—a concern reflected in the fact that the first article in the first number of the new NUTRITION REVIEWS was entitled "Feeding the Army and Navy."

There existed a critical need for a publication that would continuously review the current literature and furnish brief reports with references on newly published original research reports that appeared to have substantial significance in relation to nutrition; these reviews should also indicate whether or not claims made appeared to be supported by adequate evidence.

With the approval of the Scientific Advisory Committee a search was made to find whether any established journal would undertake this responsibility if highly qualified nutrition scientists were willing to write frank, critically analytical, interpretive reviews. Upon finding that no existing publication would accept this responsibility, the Foundation began the publication of a new 32 page monthly journal, NUTRITION REVIEWS. The first issue came off the press in November, 1942.

Dr. Frederick J. Stare, (Ph.D., University of Wisconsin; M.D., Washington Univer-

The First Decade

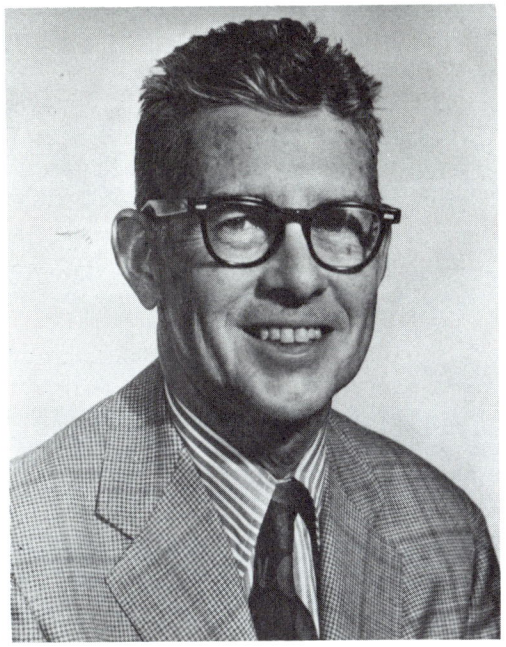
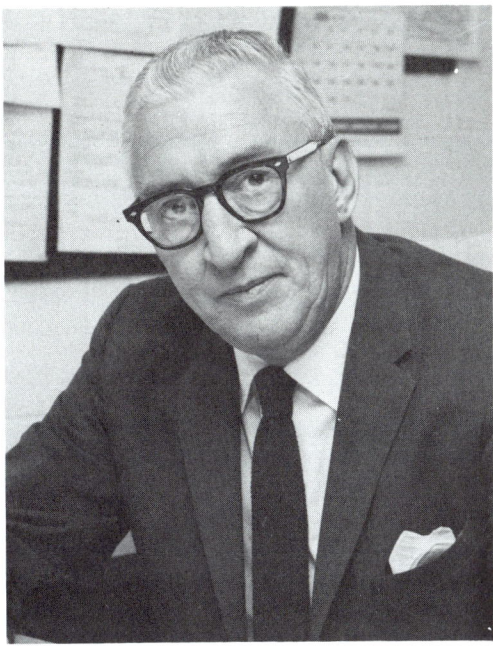

F. J. Stare   *Elmer H. Stotz*

Founding Editor and Associate Editor of NUTRITION REVIEWS

sity, St. Louis), who had recently been appointed to the first professorship in nutrition at Harvard University's Schools of Medicine and Public Health, accepted the position of Editor. Dr. Stare had been the first graduate student to have Professor Conrad A. Elvehjem, co-discoverer of the anti-black tongue, anti-pellagra action of nicotinic acid, as his major adviser in working toward the Ph.D. degree. He also had the strong support of Professor A. Baird Hastings, Chairman of the Department of Biological Chemistry, Harvard University Medical School, in developing the nutrition program at Harvard University.

Ten outstanding nutrition scientists agreed to serve as Assistant Editors and Mrs. Everett Kinsey, a very efficient former secretary in my office at the University of Pittsburgh, served as staff assistant. The Editorial Committee consisted of eleven senior nutritional scientists of international stature. These were:

Assistant Editors - 1942

Esther Batchelder, Ph.D., Bureau of Home Economics, U.S.D.A.

Franklin C. Bing, Ph.D., School of Medicine, Northwestern University

Philip P. Cohen, Ph.D., M.D., School of Medicine, University of Wisconsin, Wisconsin General Hospital, Madison

R. Adams Dutcher, D.Sc., Dept. of Agricultural and Biological Chemistry, Pennsylvania State College

Robert S. Goodhart, M.D., Nutrition Division, Office of Defense, Health and Welfare

Estelle E. Hawley, Ph.D., School of Medicine, University of Rochester

Carl V. Moore, M.D., School of Medicine, Washington University; Barnes Hospital, St. Louis

Paul H. Phillips, Ph.D., Department of Biochemistry, University of Wisconsin

A Good Idea

Elmer H. Stotz, Ph.D., New York Agricultural Experiment Station, Cornell University, Geneva

M. M. Wintrobe, M.D., Ph.D., School of Medicine, University of Utah, Salt Lake City

Editorial Committee - 1942

Reginald M. Atwater, M.D., American Public Health Assn.

Samuel W. Clausen, M.D., University of Rochester

George R. Cowgill, Ph.D., Yale University

Conrad A. Elvehjem, Ph.D., University of Wisconsin

J. Murray Luck, Ph.D., Stanford University

James S. McLester, M.D., University of Alabama

Henry C. Sherman, Ph.D., Columbia University

Russell M. Wilder, M.D., University of Minnesota

John B. Youmans, M.D., Vanderbilt University

J. C. Drummond, D.Sc., University of London
 Correspondent for England

Frederick F. Tisdall, M.D., University of Toronto
 Correspondent for Canada

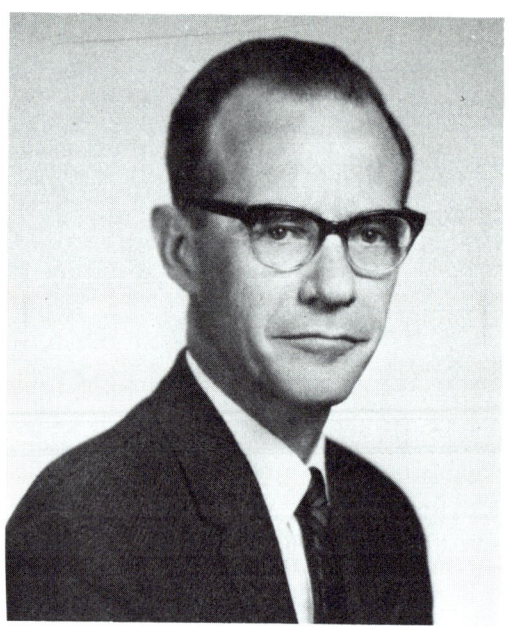

D. Mark Hegsted
Present Editor of NUTRITION REVIEWS

NUTRITION REVIEWS has maintained a worldwide circulation and is today recognized as an outstanding contribution to both professional and lay education. It has the largest paid subscription list of any nutrition journal published, with a significant international circulation. Subscriptions to the journal have always provided about one-half of the cost of publication—the balance is provided by the Foundation as a public service. The journal carries no advertising.

Dr. D. Mark Hegsted, Professor of Nutrition at Harvard University and an associate with Dr. Stare, succeeded him as editor in 1968. Dr. Elmer Stotz, Head of the Department of Biochemistry, University of Rochester, who has served on the editorial staff continuously since 1942, is the associate editor. The unsigned reviews are a composite editorial responsibility. No claims were made for infallibility, but the record has been remarkably good. The lead articles provide an important opportunity for presenting signed summary position papers by distinguished international scientists. The journal occupies a unique position in graduate education in nutrition and recently was cited by the distinguished British biochemist, Sir Frank Young, as a model that usefully could be extended to the many fields of biological endeavors.

Liaison with Governmental and Scientific Organizations

The desirability of promoting informational exchange and coordination of efforts toward nutritional betterment was recognized, and through liaison with various professional, scientific and governmental groups The Nutrition Foundation became a focus of such coordination.

Colonel Paul E. Howe represented the office of the Surgeon General of the Army on the Scientific Advisory Committee, and

The First Decade

close liaison was maintained with the office of the Quartermaster General via Colonel Paul Logan. Both of these men also worked closely with the Food and Nutrition Board of the National Academy of Sciences-National Research Council. The U.S. Public Health Service was represented by the Surgeon General, Dr. Thomas Parran, on the Board of Trustees and by Dr. W. H. Sebrell, Jr. on the Scientific Advisory Committee. I served as a consultant to the above three government offices and as a member of the Executive Committee of the Food and Nutrition Board. On the Board of Trustees also was M. L. Wilson, Chief, Nutrition and Food Conservation Branch, U.S. Food Distribution Administration. There were also informal and helpful meetings with other public, non-government foundations, most of which had administrative offices in New York.

Other means of keeping the Foundation's research and educational program responsive to continuing changes and responsibilities included participation as a member of the best qualified scientific organizations, including the National Academy of Sciences, American Institute of Nutrition, American Society of Biological Chemists, Institute of Food Technologists, American Chemical Society, American Public Health Association, New York Academy of Medicine and the New York Academy of Sciences. Obviously it was necessary to be alert to the time demands in commitments of service among different organizations.

During the war years, competent scientists varied widely in their priorities for emphasis on studies of immediate practical questions such as food composition, cooking and processing losses in nutritive value, nutritional requirements under intense stress, or on research that was more basic to understanding biological functions and therefore more likely to have wider and more enduring applications. It was on one's conscience to follow the course that appeared to have the greatest service value, including consultation with others whose judgments were highly regarded. The Public Health Service was in the best position professionally to advise on needs of the civilian population, but many academic scientists including physicians, biochemists and nutritionists were better prepared in specific aspects of clinical and fundamental principles of nutrition than were most public health personnel —hence a blending of their judgments was advisable and urgent. In regard to food composition and risks of losses in nutritive value during either home or institutional cooking and service, the home economists and dietitians were more knowledgeable than most physicians or biochemists. And the practical aspects of food availability, selection, processing, blending, storage, transportation, costs and market or military acceptance were areas of special competence of food scientists and technologists.

Dr. Russell Wilder, a staff member of the University of Minnesota and of the Mayo Clinic and first Chairman of the National Committee on Foods and Nutrition appointed in 1940, expressed his charge to that committee with his typical sense of urgency: "It is no longer a question of a few experts in our own colleges and research centers talking about vitamins and minerals. What we must do now is make people understand that nutrition is not an academic matter but a thoroughly practical consideration, concerning every person in the country—producers, processors, marketers, consumers, nutritional experts — everyone!"

A great advantage in education and health protection during the war period was the motivation that stimulated an effort to do one's best in conserving health

A Good Idea

along with other resources to meet whatever emergencies the war might create. Doubtlessly, rationing was a strong motivating force. Hence, people in nearly every bracket of life were more willing to learn and to act accordingly in relation to food. Great progress was made in improving military rations as well as in the food practices of the civilian population during the war years. Death rates, especially from cardiovascular disease, and the incidence of tooth decay dropped substantially in the United Kingdom, the United States and the Scandinavian countries during the war period. After the war period the sense of self-discipline sorely slackened, and the deterioration became evident in the resulting health trends and food practices.

There was constant civilian pressure (rumored to stem from Mrs. Eleanor Roosevelt) to meet the demands for emergency and military rations by preparing dry, packaged, water-and-insect-proof "biscuits with all the essential nutrients in one product."

In a military test camp in Colorado, where food acceptance was one of the many features studied, there was a big trench beside the mess hall where "left food" from each meal was recorded and dumped; it was literally "a pile of biscuits." And in another camp used for training ski troops at high altitude the participants were asked to record their opinions on how long they could survive on the ration which was largely biscuits. The essence of reported replies was "longer than I would want to." Such were the challenges of assisting to design improved military rations.

There were many crucial food problems to be met besides supply and distribution for the military services. Nutrient losses had to be estimated for field storage in hot, sun-baked desert areas or in tropical areas of continued rain. Protein quality, vitamin retention, protection from rancidity, and so far as possible, maintaining variety, acceptance and quick service were constantly in the foreground. In addition there was the need to design specialized rations for life-rafts and for aviation personnel. Against a crisis of thirst in a desert or on a life raft, for example, 50 grams of sugar or starch might be more protective than 50 grams of water, because as the carbohydrate "burned" in the body to supply energy it would form water and thereby lessen the drinking water required to meet the kidneys' need for water to dispose of urea formed from "burning" body protein.

And aviation personnel, if exposed to moderate or severe oxygen deficiency, could function better in eyesight, operate instruments with greater skill, and be more alert after eating a lunch or snack high in carbohydrate than if they had no food for a few hours or had eaten food low in carbohydrate. This difference could be crucial when in combat or returning from combat areas.

Colonel Wendell Griffith, a senior nutrition officer attached to our air force in England, reported "There was a distinct improvement in performance of flight personnel when they put into effect a policy of supplying very convenient high carbohydrate food for pre-flight, in-flight and return-flight use, and so far as possible, avoidance of long delays between food intake and combat or take-off and landing periods."

Expanded Foundation Membership and Program

As the nature of the Foundation's program and structure became evident during 1942, membership grew rapidly from 15 to 34 food and related companies. By July 1, 1946, there were 54 members. NUTRITION REVIEWS, as a guide to progress in nutrition research, was in wide circulation, includ-

The First Decade

ing introductory issues in Spanish and Portuguese in Latin America. Research papers with acknowledgements of Nutrition Foundation support were beginning to appear in established scientific journals. The timely publication of these investigations was based in part on accelerated completion of work formerly underway.

Dr. Compton's chairmanship of both the Board of Trustees and the Board's Executive Committee gave strength of leadership and inspired confidence among scientists, business executives and civic leaders alike. His integrity, good judgment and enthusiasm for the program provided an inspiration for everyone in the Foundation. On October 15, 1943, he wrote, "It has been said—'Food will win the war.' Such a generality is an obvious overstatement. We know the war will be won by fighting courage, production, civilian morale and willingness to sacrifice.

"Food, nevertheless, is playing a more important part in this war than in any previous war. Food is essential to the well-being of our armed forces and to the civilian population. Due to scientific advances in nutrition, our armies are better fed and more physically fit, and civilian populations are better able to withstand the rigors of the war's strains and stresses.

"The food industry is a front line industry, confronted with problems which demand the fullest measure of energy and resourcefulness. It is more than this—it is a public service. To that end, leaders in the industry are striving to advance the science of nutrition for the purposes of strengthening the war effort today and building better living for tomorrow."

President George A. Sloan's genuine interest, pride in the work of our staff, and experience with industrial and civic executives through his service to community organizations were always helpful. His view was summarized in saying, "In the recent establishment of this Foundation, the food industry has made an earnest effort to aid in the solution of problems which have arisen in the midst of a war emergency. It has done more than this. It has acknowledged a definite social responsibility and function in making further explorations into the science of nutrition for the betterment of mankind."

Mr. Ole Salthe, Executive Secretary, proved to be one of the most devoted, honest, candid, quiet, and perceptive persons that I have known. His personality showed up quickly when a prominent early visitor from one of the national professional societies called to offer congratulations and advice: "Of course you will have to scratch the back of your member companies occasionally and do little favors according to their interest!"—to which Ole replied with a courteous but icy cool: "Is that the way you would run this organization?"—in a voice so clear and steady that it opened the door outward for the guest's first and last visit.

Miss Irene Magnus had served as secretary in Mr. Salthe's New York City Department of Health office before he was invited to the Foundation staff and agreed to accompany him in the move, with one reservation—that she would not have to be secretary to the Director—but she remained as my very efficient secretary.

By 1943 the Foundation's program was well underway with a constant effort to evaluate work that was to assist directly in the war effort or to accomplish longer range objectives in personnel training and research, the time for application of which could not be predicted. To meet this responsibility the Foundation maintained constant contacts with the most qualified leaders within the military agencies, the National Research Council, university centers in the United States and Canada, and the food and related industries.

A Good Idea

Meetings of the Food Industries Advisory Committee furnished an opportunity for organized but informal discussions with representatives from university and government centers who were highly qualified to discuss research accomplishments and their apparent significance to public health and the practices of consumers and producers. The spirit of these conferences was comparable to faculty seminars, with frankness, courtesy, appreciation and a general sense of challenge in their mutual responsibility to serve the public.

Grants by the Foundation during the period July 1, 1942 to June 30, 1944 could be grouped for general significance in the following categories:

Human requirements for specific nutrients	$ 69,000
Functions of individual nutrients	134,150
Maternal and infant nutrition	26,200
Direct public health problems	106,950
Education and professional training	42,600
Information related directly to the war	151,040
	529,940

Few if any grants carried greater significance than did the support to the National Academy of Sciences-National Research Council made at the request of the president, Professor Ross G. Harrison of Yale University. We were asked to join in providing assistance to the newly organized Food and Nutrition Board. Later discussion will indicate why this $5,000 annual grant proved to be so significant.

A grant of $4,000 per year to Drs. Conrad A. Elvehjem and Paul H. Phillips at the University of Wisconsin permitted initiation of a study of nutrition and food practices in relation to tooth decay. Both military and civilian personnel had been surprised to find that when using the same standards, current rejection from military services on the basis of dental inspection was *greatly in excess* of rejections during World War I. Professionals and laymen alike were shocked into recognizing that something, and perhaps food practices, had grossly deteriorated in that relationship. Yet little significant research had been done and dental schools had not aggressively attacked the situation. The Wisconsin and later Harvard programs included training for leadership in broad areas of dental research, including the use of different kinds of animals for controlled experiments. The work focused attention on the protective role of fluorides and the acceleration of decay by carbohydrates —especially "sweets." Poorly formed teeth were less resistant to decay resulting from acid-forming bacteria. Calcium, phosphates, fluoride and vitamins A, C and D were recognized as notably important for tooth development and defense. The first research fellow trained on the grant, James H. Shaw, became Professor of Nutrition and Director of a training center in the School of Dental Medicine at Harvard University. Also trained on the same grant was B. S. Schweigert, now head of the Department of Food Science and Technology at the University of California in Davis and chairman of the Committee on Nutrition Training in Departments of Food Science and Technology of the International Union of Nutritional Sciences. He also had a leading role in persuading the U.S. Institute of Food Technologists to recommend that their respective departments include a required course in nutrition!

Additional support of research guided by Dr. Elvehjem included extensive studies of vitamin retention in processed foods of special importance to the military forces and studies of the potentially toxic effect of bleached ("agenized") flour. This work was stimulated by the report from Sir Edward Mellanby of the Medical Research Council in England that flour treated with

The First Decade

nitrogen trichloride, "agene," in order to improve its baking quality produced running fits in dogs when fed as a major ingredient of the food intake. Dr. Elvehjem identified the derived product affecting the dogs (a derivative of the amino acid, methionine), and demonstrated that in man it was *non-toxic* and readily metabolizable. Despite this finding, the producers voluntarily interdicted the use of agene in flour and substituted other treatments.

Dr. Elvehjem was one of the most active investigators on the importance of amino acid ratios, including both the broad concept of amino acid imbalance and the specific relationship of imbalance to nicotinic acid requirement to prevent pellagra. Through active participation he gave strong leadership to the Food and Nutrition Board of the National Academy of Sciences-National Research Council and to the Council on Foods and Nutrition of the American Medical Association. The University of Wisconsin increasingly was recognized the world over for its training of outstanding scientists in nutrition and in biochemistry. Dr. Elvehjem became Dean of the Graduate School, then President of the University of Wisconsin, and was welcomed heartily as a Public Trustee of The Nutrition Foundation. An art museum on the Madison campus is named in his honor. In recognition of his "outstanding service to the public," the American Institute of Nutrition annually presents an award that carries his name. It was a deeply moving experience for me in later years (1966) to receive the first in this series of awards supported by the Wisconsin Alumni Research Foundation, and in 1972 to see the new President of the Foundation, Dr. William J. Darby, receive this same award.

Studies of Food Composition

In 1942 the military agencies, the U.S. Department of Agriculture and the Food and Nutrition Board all urged support of intensive research on food composition, including consideration of genetic variations and losses during cooking, processing and storage. Supporting grants for such studies were made available by the Foundation beginning in 1942, to George R. Cowgill and E. W. Sinnott (Yale University), M. L. Fincke (Oregon State College), L. S. Palmer (University of Minnesota), R. Reder (Oklahoma Agricultural Experiment Station), J. H. L. Truscott (Ontario Agricultural College), W. A. Gortner (Cornell University), A. H. Smith (Wayne University), P. F. Zscheile (Purdue University), D. J. Hennessy (Fordham University), L. E. Holt, Jr. (Johns Hopkins University), E. G. Halliday (University of Chicago), D. K. Tressler (New York State Agricultural Experiment Station), C. R. Dawson and others (Columbia University), N. L. Noecker (University of Notre Dame), and W. C. Sherman (Alabama Polytechnic Institute). The observations of Dr. Zscheile's and Dr. Burkholder's groups were particularly significant in relation to the genetic variations in the content of vitamins A, B and C in tomatoes and other vegetables.

Fortunately, the food canning industry, through the National Canners Association, supported and reported considerable research on the nutritive value of representative products. Their support of a fifteen year study in cooperation with W. H. Eddy at Columbia University gave particularly useful background with respect to vitamins that could be assayed at that time. Such animal feeding assays, however, were time-consuming, expensive and generally gave only approximate data. As the war period developed, an intensive coordinated program was organized with seven universities, assisted by an industry committee consisting of E. J. Cameron

A Good Idea

(chairman), E. D. Clark, L. E. Clifcorn, J. R. Esty and R. W. Pilcher. This group continuously reported current and earlier data to C. A. Elvehjem, chairman of the Committee on Food Composition of the Food and Nutrition Board, so the entire national program could function effectively.

Information of this nature was frequently evaluated and published by the Department of Agriculture and the military agencies in current journals. These values provided a guide for civilian populations and military personnel, and they included information regarding foods subjected to varying conditions of processing, packaging, shipment, storage and final serving. These data were subsequently compiled as the U.S.D.A. Handbook No. 8 which is the most widely used reference on food composition, as generally represented on the American market.

The early emphasis on food composition is reflected in the list of publications with acknowledgements to the Foundation during 1942-1949. In contrast to 36 publications on food composition during the 1942-1947 period, there were only 2 during 1948-1949.

Although this emphasis on research support by the Foundation was much more technological than normally desirable, the urgency of the war situation and resultant methodologic improvement justified it. As other funds for research of this type became available or the work was completed, the program was adjusted to more basic and long range studies in nutrition. Studies of an applied nature often contribute much to understanding of basic phenomena. For example, grants to C. R. Dawson at Columbia University resulted in substantial progress in studies of the copper-containing enzymes in plant foods that catalyze the destruction of vitamin C on exposure to air, in addition to studies of nutrient losses during dehydration.

V. H. Cheldelin and H. P. Sarett at Oregon State College conducted a study of the vitamin content of restaurant cooked food and a special investigation of hams and bacon as prepared for overseas shipment. It was observed then and many times since, that delays while holding cooked food before table service unfortunately cause greater loss in nutritional value than is generally recognized. They also made improvements in methods of analysis for vitamins in the B group and studied the functional role of the newly identified vitamin, pantothenic acid. After further academic experience with Dr. Grace A. Goldsmith of Tulane University, Dr. Sarett became Director of Nutrition and Biochemistry at the Mead Johnson Research Center.

M. L. Fincke at Oregon State College and E. G. Halliday at the University of Chicago also studied the general problem of nutrient losses in cooking. This aspect of home and institutional food management still presents a serious problem. Restaurant food services are all too often characterized by cooking in large vessels and prolonged exposure to air while holding at high temperatures for potential service. Under such conditions several of the vitamins are destroyed significantly in parallel with a continuing loss in flavor, color and protein quality. For example, such excellent products as fresh or frozen green peas and broccoli frequently suffer great losses of ascorbic acid and of thiamin by over-cooking before being served, both in homes and in restaurants. During our studies in New York we checked food from plates as served in a hospital using a central-service system for several buildings. Daily meals without citrus products with a calculated vitamin C content of nearly 100 milligrams were found to contain 10 to 15 milligrams. Vernon Stouffer, when in personal charge of his restaurant chain, exerted a striking de-

The First Decade

gree of national leadership on this score by insisting on small, closed-vessel cooking, electrically timed as near as possible to guest arrivals and with a minimum holding interval before reaching the table.

A grant to Ruth Reder at the Oklahoma Experiment Station permitted her to assemble and promptly publish data from a large cooperative study on food composition, representing different agricultural areas and different practices. There was no indication of lowered nutritive value as a result of the use of chemical fertilizers, but much evidence of composition differences among different varieties and according to differences in preparation.

From the studies by G. R. Cowgill, P. R. Burkhold and others at Yale University, J. H. L. Truscott at Ontario Agricultural College, and P. F. Zscheile and collaborators at Purdue University it was clear that among the commonly used vegetables and fruits there were wide variations in vitamin content on a genetic basis, but relatively small differences other than in yield per acre when grown on different soils. Among tomatoes, for example, very large differences could be identified on a genetic basis in relation to their content of vitamin A (as carotenes) and vitamin C. It proved to be quite difficult, however, genetically to combine a high vitamin content with other essential characteristics for marketing, such as yield, color, shape, uniformity, flavor, texture, and resistance to disease. However, with adequate time, industrial and agricultural plant breeders and nutritionists have accomplished such combinations through scientific breeding with nutritional needs as an objective.

Quality of Military Rations and Processing Techniques

A Canadian Air Force group discovered that their personnel had a lower body store of vitamin C than anticipated, but investigation showed that potatoes, an important vitamin C-containing food, were mostly served as mashed potatoes—and when air was whipped into them while hot the vitamin was lost. A medical officer was said to report: "Another case of too much hot air in the kitchen." Incidentally one should note that substantial improvements in food service and nutritive values were achieved by placing experienced home economists and dietetians in charge. This action was not based on social theory to advance women's rights; it was to protect rugged men from the dietetic frailties of regular line corporals and sergeants.

A practice of dispensing small packets of salt to workmen in very hot environments where there was intense perspiration had been widely adopted. When this practice was subjected to careful test, however, there was a distinctly higher "fall out" and severe nausea among those given extra salt. The salt actually created an added body demand for water and an intensified thirst, nausea and general debility. Instead, a far better practice was to add a small amount of salt to the cooked food in advance of such exposure—and to emphasize the need for drinking more water. The implication of this principle for athletes is evident, but not yet sufficiently appreciated.

Although intensive research and great care were devoted to providing improved rations for the military forces, and much progress was made before and during the war, most people are surprised to know that only the A ration (regular base camp ration within the United States, including fresh market products) and the B ration (regular base ration in other countries where reliable fresh produce was used to supplement the packaged rations) would sustain normal growth in albino rats. The C ration (field) or the K ration (packaged dry) did not meet that test, although they served well for short periods.

Failure to support growth of young rats does *not* disqualify a ration designed to maintain adult man for a limited period—the proportionate requirements for growth and maintenance, the nutrient density of the diet, and quantitative differences between requirements of different species may account for the limited applicability of such criteria. These and other limitations of animal experiments in appraisal of human dietaries were critically and responsibly examined at a conference in which I participated on March 13, 1947, a conference sponsored by the Williams Waterman Fund for the Combat of Dietary Diseases. The current practice within the armed forces, however, represents a distinct improvement by identifying each type of packaged ration with a stated time limitation for its intended use as a single food source.

To meet military requirements, particularly, but civilian demands also, there was intense interest in food dehydration procedures which assured maximum retention of nutritive quality, stability in storage, and food acceptance qualities such as flavor, color, ease of rehydration and freedom from infestation. Blanching in hot water or steam to stop enzymic changes and thus stabilize foods and to accomplish other advantages was a general practice. Freeze-drying was not well established at that time. There was considerable excitement, however, about the prospect of stabilizing foods, dry or fresh, by irradiation with beta or gamma rays. Both of these technological applications required intense research that normally would have been conducted within the industry and government agencies without major demands on the universities or private foundations. However, the potential military advantages resulted in governmental support to a wide range of coordinated research in many laboratories.

Superficially, there appeared to be a great potential advantage in the short time required for sterilization of foods by radiation. Some enthusiasts carried transparent-wrapped packages of irradiated raw meat in their pockets to illustrate how feasible it was to apply the radiation technique. But, as viewed by biochemists, there were many obvious risks. Toxic products might be formed, flavor changes might result, residual radioactivity might be induced, or essential nutrients might be destroyed.

In parallel with intensive studies by many others, our group at Columbia University, including Elmer Gaden in chemical engineering, observed that both vitamin C and vitamin A were rapidly destroyed within the estimated range of practical radiation. From observations during the tests, David Barr proposed a functional role for the intermediate formation of a free-radical form of vitamin C, and this was found to exist both in irradiated food products and in biological functions of the vitamin. It was soon evident that extensive oxidative changes were induced in most food commodities when radiation was sufficient to establish safe keeping qualities. The destruction of vitamin K was one of the last nutrient changes identified as responsible for failure of an irradiated diet to support normal growth in animals. The essential role of vitamin K in normal blood clotting made this finding of obvious interest to military personnel.

Despite several years of liberal support from the Atomic Energy Commission and the Quartermaster General's Office, and broad cooperation within the food industry, irradiation sterilization of foods has not proved feasible as a major sterilization technique. Irradiation is however, useful as a method of sprout control and pasteuriza-

The First Decade

tion. Heating, refrigeration and dehydration, accompanied by strict sanitation, remain the only major means of food preservation.

Recent success with "microwave" cooking has introduced a new technology that seems likely to expand greatly in its applications when sterilization is not essential. In many instances, of course, additions of salt, sugar, acids, spices, antioxidants and other chemical agents play important roles, as they have since primitive man discovered their value even before bacteria were known. The enormous changes in time-saving technology, packaging, sanitation, safety, quality standards and uniformity have been a boon to society in many ways, but these changes have also introduced varied problems as well as genuine services for the consumer. Reliance on fresh meats, milk, seeds, fruits, roots and leafy vegatables is steadily less evident in the grocery store, and people massed in cities increasingly view farms and fresh foods only at high speed from the sky or a thruway.

Studies of Metabolism Under Stress

At the University of Minnesota, Ancel Keys, A. Henschel, H. L. Taylor, J. M. Brozek, O. Mickelsen and others received assistance from The Nutrition Foundation for studies of the functional changes coincident with human starvation, nutritional deficiencies, exposure to desert conditions, and intense physical work under stress. These studies were among the most comprehensive university studies in this kind of research in the United States during the war period and culminated in the classic two-volume report "Human Starvation" published in 1950 by the University of Minnesota Press.

T. E. Friedemann and A. C. Ivy at Northwestern University received Nutrition Foundation support to assist them in studies of nutrition in relation to stress during sustained hard physical work and in relation to aviation feeding. Carefully controlled tests through a period of 15 months indicated that the requirements for thiamin and riboflavin (vitamins B_1 and B_2) did not rise appreciably above the intake that had been recommended for moderate work schedules.

A New National and International Resource: The Food and Nutrition Board

As the threat of active involvement in World War II became imminent, government agencies, the food industry, the health professions (especially the Council on Foods and Nutrition of the American Medical Association and the National Academy of Sciences-National Research Council) manifested great concern for nutrition research and its immediate applications. The country was shocked by the report from examinations of draftees that 25 per cent showed evidence of present or past malnutrition. The spontaneous focal point for scientists was the National Academy of Sciences, created by President Lincoln during the Civil War and greatly expanded by President Wilson in 1916, in preparation for World War I, to include a National Research Council. A new stirring was underway.

The public kick-off point was a National Nutrition Conference for Defense, called by President Roosevelt, May 26, 1941, in Washington, D.C. Nine hundred delegates were selected to represent the government, industry, labor, universities, and the major professions concerned with foods and nutrition. It was evident that agricultural, medical, military and academic personnel could best coordinate much of their nutrition research, planning and advisory services within the National Research Coun-

A Good Idea

cil. This central organization, upon recommendation of the Council on National Defense, appointed a special committee to deal broadly with food and nutrition problems. It advanced quickly from a committee status with 21 members in 1940 to a major responsibility as the Food and Nutrition Board in 1941.

When the original Committee was being organized within the Council, one of the physicians with a long career in clinical practice complained that "There is no time for research! We must give the Surgeon General answers immediately!" whereupon he wrote on the blackboard a list of foods that aviators should not eat, and beside it a list of foods to be officially approved. His confidence cooled when his associates pointed out that some of the foods appeared in both lists. (He was not appointed to the Committee.)

The Board was authorized to receive and act on appropriate grants from government or private agencies while working with a very limited administrative budget. To facilitate its work on an assured independent basis, three foundations, the Milbank Fund, the Williams-Waterman Fund of the Research Corporation and The Nutrition Foundation responded to the request by the president of the National Research Council, Dr. R. G. Harrison (Yale University), to contribute $5,000 each annually in support of staff requirements. President Harrison emphasized that membership on the Board should not be limited to government personnel who might be under pressure of line-policies, but that scientists should represent the public at large in expressing their personal judgments. It would have been folly not to have had as members of the Board representation of outstanding scientists in industry, such as C. N. Frey and H. E. Robinson who had extensive experience in both nutrition research and food technology. This practice was continued in later years, with highly qualified scientists such as H. E. O. Heineman, R. E. Nesheim, C. H. Krieger and H. Howard.

All members of the Scientific Advisory Committee of The Nutrition Foundation, including the Scientific Director, served on the Board or as members of its working committees. Several members, including the Director, served also as consultants to the Surgeons General of the Army and the Air Force and the Quartermaster General.

The Food and Nutrition Board assumed an active role in international activities including frequent guest representatives from Canada, Australia, the United Kingdom, France, Norway, Latin America and South Africa. Sir John Boyd Orr, later Director General of the United Nations Food and Agriculture Organization, was a frequent visitor and special guest of Dr. Boudreau, who was well acquainted with European personnel as a result of earlier service with the League of Nations. Colonel Paul Howe was the key liaison officer with the Office of the Surgeon General of the Army, and Colonel Paul Logan served in a similar relationship with the Quartermaster General of the Army. The Board had excellent cooperation with both men, but the sharp personal exchanges at Board meetings between Colonels Howe and Logan sometimes led to the quip, "Battle of the two armies."

When the Committee on Foods and Nutrition was first organized in 1940, the 21 members appointed were: John D. Black, Henry Borsook, Frank G. Boudreau, George R. Cowgill, Joseph S. Davis, Martha M. Elliot, Conrad A. Elvehjem, Icie Macy Hoobler, Phillip C. Jeans, Norman Jolliffe, C. Glen King, L. A. Maynard, James S. McLester, Helen Mitchell, S. C. Prescott, Lydia J. Roberts, William C.

The First Decade

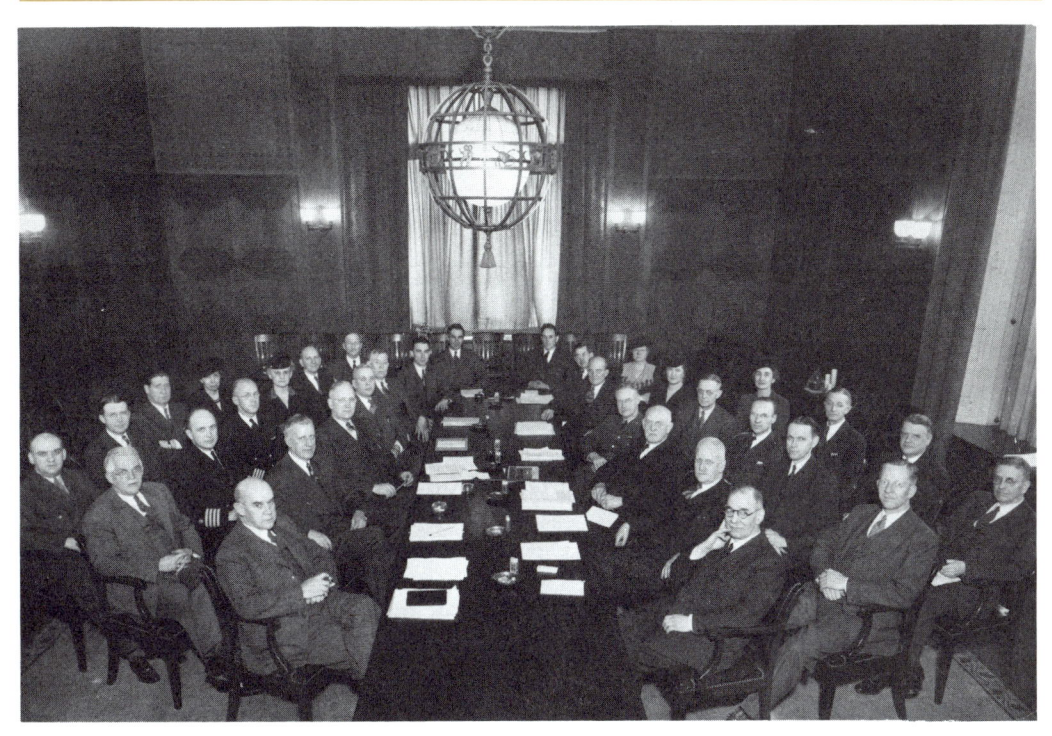

Meeting of the Food and Nutrition Board, National Academy of Sciences—National Research Council, 1943.

Left, at table front to back: *Frank G. Boudreau, Chairman; Russell M. Wilder, John D. Black, George R. Cowgill, E. V. McCollum, H. E. Longenecker, Frank Gunderson.* Right, at table front to back: *H. C. Sherman, S. C. Prescott, John. R. Murlin, F. F. Tisdall, R. R. Williams, L. A. Maynard, J. M. Cassels.* Left middle row front to back: *Robert Griggs, W. H. Sebrell, Jr, Joseph S. Davis, Helen Mitchell, C. N. Frey.* Right middle row, front to back: *E. M. Nelson, C. A. Elvehjem, L. B. Pett, P. C. Jeans, Icie Macy Hoobler, Martha M. Eliot.* Left back row, front to back: *H. D. Kruse, John B. Youmans, Norman Jolliffe, Louise Stanley.* Right back row, front to back: *W. C. Rose, Franklin C. Bing, V. P. Syndenstricker, Hazel K. Stiebling.* Members not in photograph: *Henry Borsook, A. Baird Hastings, Paul E. Howe, C. G. King, W. E. Krauss, James S. McLester, Lydia J. Roberts, G. Cullen Thomas, M. L. Wilson*

Rose, C. Cullen Thomas, Russell M. Wilder (first chairman), Robert R. Williams and John B. Youmans.

Of the 21 members appointed in 1940 there were eight biochemists, seven physicians, two home economists, two agricultural economists, one food company executive and one food technologist. Eight of the members were appointed to the first Scientific Advisory Committee of The Nutrition Foundation.

Additional Board members were appointed in 1941: Franklin C. Bing, Paul E. Howe, E. V. McCollum, John R. Murlin, E. M. Nelson, W. H. Sebrell, Jr., H. C. Sherman, Louise Stanley and Frederick F. Tisdall.

An early major contribution by the Board was to establish and obtain wide recognition of desired standards of food intake, termed "Recommended Dietary Allowances." The term "Recommended Dietary Allowance" (RDA) indicates a nutrient intake that permits optimum health

A Good Idea

in nearly all persons within a specific category of age, sex and circumstances. It includes a lifespan concept of health and an individual's capacity to function as a citizen, mentally, physically and emotionally. The new term was to replace the Food and Drug Administration Minimum Daily Requirement, below which there would be an obvious deficiency disease such as rickets or scurvy.

Clinical evidence of malnutrition that received emphasis in relation to the war effort was the occasional occurrence of three deficiency syndromes characterized respectively by mild neuritis, and peculiar eye and tongue signs of pellagra. These were associated with deficiencies of vitamins in the B-complex: B_1 (thiamin), B_2 (riboflavin) and niacin, respectively. Deficiencies of iron were also recognized as a common cause of anemia. Three nutritional diseases that had been very common in earlier years, rickets, goiter and infant scurvy, had been largely but not completely controlled by the introduction of vitamin D fortified milk, and iodized salt and early feeding of juices, especially citrus fruits, tomatoes and vegetables to infants. Fluoridation of water supplies was being initiated with excellent results in areas where the fluoride content was too low to permit optimum tooth development and resistance to decay. These effective measures were not universally applied. The government's policy had been weak in leaving the above advances on a voluntary basis and, accordingly, allowing a large sector of the population to be unprotected—as it is today!

Recognition of the effectiveness of such measures, however, raised the question —instead of relying on an educational program and requiring that grains be less refined, would it be more practical, less difficult for public and military adjustments, and nutritionally favorable to the war effort, to adopt an "enrichment" program in which three vitamins (thiamin, riboflavin, niacin) and iron would be added to wheat flour? This would provide an automatic distribution of significant quantities to nearly everyone at low cost. Vitamin B_2 was not included because the nature and extent of human deficiency and magnitude of requirement were not known. Furthermore, it was not likely to be available promptly at a reasonable cost. After intense study of the many considerations involved, the Food and Nutrition Board in concert with the Council on Foods and Nutrition of the American Medical Association recommended adoption of the enrichment program which was put into effect as War Order Number One, on recommendation of Dr. Thomas Parran, Surgeon General of the Public Health Service. By the time a senior staff member in the Public Health Service and I delivered a draft copy of the War Order No. 1 to General Parran for his signature, we had a lasting appreciation of the background that may be required for even so short a communication!

There followed a subsequent reduction in the incidence of the diseases mentioned. However, there is no way to be certain how much of the gain was a result of education, economic improvement and motivation induced by the war emergency, compared with the enrichment benefit. Certainly there was a widely increased consumption of the respective nutrients, comparable in some degree with the increase resulting from the fortification of table salt with iodide and whole milk with vitamin D in combating goiter and rickets. Dr. R. R. Williams estimated that 560,000 pounds of the anti-pellagra vitamin were introduced into bread each year. European countries followed an alternate pathway, however, of restricting the production of highly refined wheat flour—e.g., not less than

The First Decade

about 82% of the whole grain, compared with about 70% or less in patent flour.

When considering problems of the above nature it was clearly desirable to have the advice of highly qualified individuals with extensive experience and expertise in agriculture, public health, and food technology. Persons with practical experience were needed in addition to scientists with outstanding competence in nutrition research. Appointments to the Food and Nutrition Board have accordingly recognized the need for such representation, but a large majority of the members hold academic positions in nutrition, biochemistry, medicine, food technology and agricultural economics. It was an honor-with-work to serve on the executive committee of the Board from its beginning until several years after my retirement.

The work of Board members and committees has been outstanding for competence and integrity, with steadily increasing service to the public, nationally and internationally. In accordance with the general policy of the Academy, a sense of service has been their only compensation, except for full-time staff personnel. The record of accomplishment of the Board and its many Committees is well summarized in the Twenty-fifth Anniversary History of the Board. (See *Appendix G.*)

Among the early major activities of Board Committees were those dealing with (a) food composition and (b) military rations, both chaired by Dr. Elvehjem. A committee on food protection, chaired initially by Dr. Longenecker and later by Dr. Darby, was established to deal with risks from food additives, food contaminants and many related problems that required extensive study and publications. A committee on procurement of critical materials and assignment of strategic personnel, called the M-Day Committee, another on nutrition surveys, and a third on international programs were chaired at different periods by myself. Dr. Boudreau chaired a committee on the nutrition of industrial workers in addition to providing very effective administrative leadership as chairman of the Board in succession to Dr. Wilder. His associate, H. D. Kruse, served as chairman of a committee on techniques for identifying specific kinds of malnutrition.

The high incidence of tooth decay as a major cause of rejection from military service and a major challenge in relation to public health led to a committee in that area and a comprehensive monograph was prepared by Gerald J. Cox, a pioneer in dental research.

Dr. R. R. Williams, Chairman of the Committee on Cereals, gave strong leadership to the study of flour and bread enrichment and subsequent enrichment of corn meal and rice. The Committee on Protein Foods, chaired by W. C. Rose, was in continuous action.

The Board also played a valuable role in basic research as illustrated by its Advisory Committee to the Elgin State Hospital where studies guided by M. K. Horwitt were conducted in relation to human vitamin requirements, beginning in 1942.

There were frequent and urgent requests for reports on matters of government policy with respect to foods and nutrition, such as greater use of non-fat milk products, including powdered milk. The recommendation to include about four per cent by weight of powdered skim milk in bread was helpful educationally and as a practical contribution to improved nutrition, but this was not made a requirement. A favorable report on the nutritive value of margarine, compared to butter, when fortified with vitamins A and D was important from an educational, nutritional and economic viewpoint.

Perhaps the most amusing experience at

A Good Idea

Board meetings was to hear brief, intense debates on whether to recommend the inclusion of rum in life-raft emergency rations. No serious reason to do so could be cited except the insistence that the British did that and "they have had more experience at sea than anyone else." Just as it seemed possible that those in favor of rum might win the argument, word arrived that the British had discontinued the practice.

A Five-Year Resume

A summary of accomplishments of The Nutrition Foundation during the 1942-1946 period as reflected in publications with acknowledgement of its support (page 38) may be summarized as follows:

1. Research in direct relation to the war effort, including close collaboration with military and civilian agencies, particularly in relation to food composition, human and animal nutrient requirements, and food intake to meet special needs under stress (e.g., intense physical work, wound healing, blood loss, exposure to high altitudes, intense heat or cold, or severe dehydration).

2. Studies to establish adult human protein requirement in terms of essential amino acids; additional studies indicating superior utilization of whole proteins compared with the purified amino acids; and improved methods of amino acid analysis.

3. The new vitamin, folic acid, had been identified and was shown to protect man and several species of animals from anemia. In man it was effective against tropical sprue, megaloblastic anemia of infants, and pernicious anemia of pregnancy. The essential nutrient could be determined microbiologically and was shown to be labile to destruction during food preparation, processing and storage.

4. More complete knowledge was developed in relation to the composition of human milk compared with cows' milk for infant feeding and the nutritional requirements of mothers during gestation and lactation.

5. Much clearer insight was gained concerning the enzymes (catalysts) and hormones that function in normal utilization of sugars and fats and hence in the management of diabetes and other sugar- and fat-related diseases.

6. Vitamin intake levels were evaluated during long periods, finding that beneficial health effects occur at levels well above those required to prevent obvious signs of disease—and that large excesses are injurious.

7. Dominant factors in tooth decay in experimental animals were studied, including preventive measures and food and nutrition practices that are important in that relationship.

8. Substantial assistance was given in developing clearly identified strong centers of nutrition, including both teaching and research, in three of the leading schools of medicine and public health (Vanderbilt University, Harvard University, and Tulane University).

9. New methods of appraising nutritional status were developed, furnishing more reliable and specific guides to identification of nutritional deficiencies or imbalances.

10. Many advances occurred in methods of measuring vitamins, amino acids and fatty acids in foods and in other biological materials.

The First Decade

11. Chemical reactions characterizing the functions of six vitamins and nine amino acids were sufficiently identified to advance medical concepts of their relationship to health.

12. Radioactive iron was introduced as a technique for study of iron availability from foods, in hemodynamics and in relation to different types of anemia.

13. Efficient utilization of calcium from the mineral, gypsum, and legumes such as soybeans had been demonstrated.

14. A superior reference standard for vitamin A had been developed to facilitate studies of comparative food values and government regulatory practices.

15. Human and animal studies of protein quality were advanced in relation to risks of liver and kidney injury. Observations that were important in relation to the widely distributed complex lipid, lecithin, showed the relationships centered on the amino acid, methionine, and the lecithin ingredient, choline.

16. In studies with albino rats, food selection was found not to be determined dependably in relation to nutritional need. In some instances, as with vitamin B_1, the nutrient was identified and consumed rather well, but with others, such as pure protein (casein) or the mineral element, magnesium, some animals did not select enough to prevent death when the nutrient was offered among others in similar cups.

17. Several types of fatty acids had been evaluated for safety and utilization.

18. Approximately two hundred graduate students and young post-doctorate scientists received advanced training in nutrition and food science on appointments supported by the Foundation.

19. A new journal, NUTRITION REVIEWS, had been established to assist professionally trained personnel, writers and students to keep critically informed concerning worldwide progress in the science of nutrition.

20. The Food and Nutrition Board, well established nationally, was taking first steps in parallel with the American Institute of Nutrition toward a worldwide organization of nutrition scientists to be affiliated with the United Nations.

In these endeavors the Foundation was indebted for assistance and support from its Board of Trustees, the Scientific Advisory Committee, the Food Industries Advisory Committee and representatives of the government and international agencies. Supporting membership in the Foundation had grown from the original 15 to 54 on June 30, 1947.

Education—Channels and Challenges

Scientific Publications

In long-term perspective the most important contribution to education by the Foundation may have been the support of research and advanced training of personnel in graduate schools and medical centers. However, there was an urgent need to establish a more direct educational service, guided by the best qualified leadership, to reach a broader public.

As a first major step, NUTRITION REVIEWS was distributed at one-half cost in the United States and Canada at $3.00/year and fairly widely internationally at $3.50/year. The Josiah Macy Jr. Foundation supported

A Good Idea

Subjects of Research Publications
with Acknowledgements to The Nutrition Foundation
During the Period 1942-1947

I. Nutrient Requirements for General Health:	
During gestation, lactation and child development	39
Vitamins	30
Proteins and amino acids	19
Minerals	2
Carbohydrates, fats and total calories	4
Special environments (altitude, temperature, humidity, intense work)	12
II. Biological Functions and Quantitative Analysis:	
Vitamins	72
Amino acids and proteins	64
Carbohydrates, fats and total calories	35
Minerals	12
Nucleic acids (genetics and enzymes)	11
III. Special Aspects of Health:	
Anemias	23
Surveys—detection and identification of human deficiency diseases	16
Dental health	9
Liver injury	5
Cancer	5
Food selection in response to need	6
Risk of toxicity	7
IV. Food Composition:	
(Fresh, frozen, dehydrated, cooked, canned, storage)	36

More than one specific area of subject matter is generally included in a single paper, but each publication is listed within the group having dominant interest at that time. The first group of grants (thirty-six) was approved May 20, 1942.

---

the costs of direct mailing to military personnel with the Surgeon General's office during the war period. For a number of years The Nutrition Foundation supported printing and distributing a Spanish edition in cooperation with "La Prensa Medica Mexicana" in Mexico City. A further subsidy was required to permit a subscription cost of $3.00/year.

In Brazil, a Portuguese language edition of NUTRITION REVIEWS was available for several years. The demand for Spanish and Portuguese editions became less as Latin American personnel became increasingly familiar with English and increased their professional activities in nutrition. Scientists from several Latin American countries organized in 1965 the Sociedad Latinoamericana de Nutricion; the official publication of this society is a substantial, high quality journal, ARCHIVOS LATINOAMERICANOS DE NUTRICION. This publication accepts research and educational papers in Spanish, Portuguese, English or French, according to the author's preference. Nearly all papers include a brief summary in English. Cooperation with the United Nations agencies (WHO, FAO, UNICEF) and the International Union of Nutritional Sciences became increasingly helpful as the Latin American countries developed their resources.

The First Decade

In cooperation with Professor A. W. Thomas at Columbia University arrangements were made for publication by the Macmillan Company of all of Professor Sherman's research papers in a single volume. Professor Sherman contributed greatly to early knowledge of the distribution of vitamins in foods, the bioassay of vitamins, and the concept of attainment of higher levels of health and longevity through greater-than-minimal nutrient intake. For example, a diet based primarily on one-third milk solids and two-thirds whole wheat permitted higher levels of health in terms of survival and offspring of rats than a diet based on one-sixth milk solids and five-sixths whole wheat. And an intake of vitamin A four times greater than required to prevent signs of deficiency permitted a significant advantage in life span and surviving offspring.

Advances in the science of nutrition illustrate a number of points that are of interest in human relations. Perhaps the most impressive experience is to discover the great similarity in the operating mechanisms within each individual cell. A single specific discovery tends to throw light on the functions of other systems that had not been evident. A newly discovered essential mineral such as zinc or copper for a rat, chicken or oyster is likely to be a new key to understanding some aspects in the life of all other living organisms. Yet there are detailed differences, and the discovery of these can be fascinating as they are fitted into the mysteries of man and his best adaptation to each environment.

General Publications

Early, the Foundation directly or by recommending qualified authorities, cooperated with Gaynor Maddox in the preparation of brief but accurate interview reports on nutrition for the Scripps-Howard press. Such advisory educational assistance by the Foundation is now routinely extended to many communicators in all channels of the mass media—newspapers and periodicals, writers, radio, television and lecturers.

We were pleased when Dr. Stare initiated a regular press service column, thus providing timely and authoritative reports on nutrition for the public. All income from his column is given to Harvard University to support graduate training and research in nutrition.

To reach more directly to a layman's level, a 4-page leaflet, CURRENT RESEARCH IN THE SCIENCE OF NUTRITION, was distributed free on a request basis to teachers and to U.S. Department of Agriculture extension personnel. The articles were often based on progress reported in NUTRITION REVIEWS. The number of requests soon became so large that distribution had to be put on a partial cost, subscription basis.

In cooperation with Dr. Stare a 69-page booklet, GUIDE FOR COMMUNITY NUTRITIONISTS, was prepared and printed for general distribution. Another booklet, ACTIVITIES IN NUTRITION EDUCATION FOR KINDERGARTEN THROUGH SIXTH GRADE, (44 pp.) and a simpler leaflet, GOALS FOR NUTRITION EDUCATION FOR ELEMENTARY AND SECONDARY SCHOOLS, were also made available.

An Annual Report by the Scientific Director listed all grants made during the year, names of personnel affiliated with the Foundation, and a summary (about 80 pages) of research progress and educational activities. Two special booklets were prepared by the Scientific Director for distribution on request: (a) RESEARCH AND THE SCIENCE OF NUTRITION (62 pp., 1946), and (b) RESEARCH PAPERS AND LIST OF PUBLICATIONS (66 pp., 1949).

A monograph, NUTRITION IN RELATION TO CANCER, was prepared jointly with the New York Academy of Sciences and the

A Good Idea

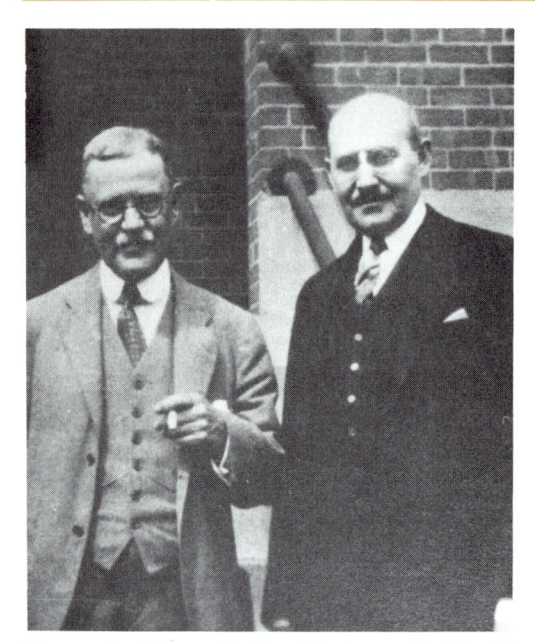

Thomas B. Osborne (left) and Lafayette B. Mendel (right), pioneers in nutrition research, collaborated in a long series of studies dating from 1911 on the nutritive value of vegetable proteins. Their fruitful basic contributions are recognized in the Osborne-Mendel Award supported by The Nutrition Foundation and selected by the American Institute of Nutrition.

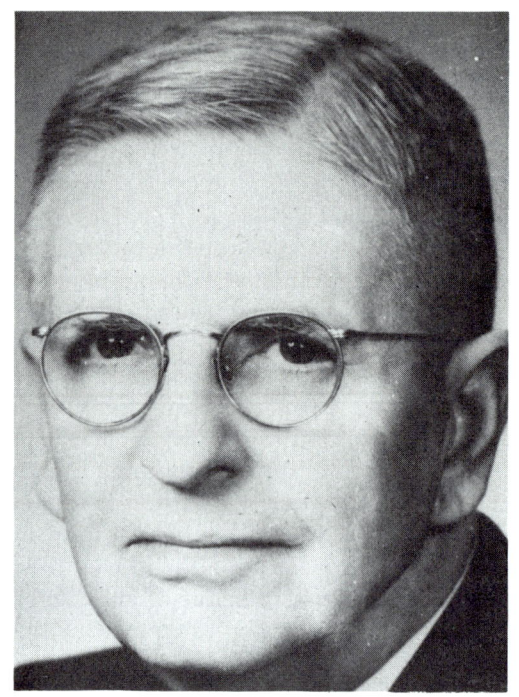

W. C. Rose, University of Illinois, first recipient of the Osborne-Mendel Award. Dr. Rose was a former student of Professor Mendel at Yale University and made classical studies that defined the requirements of man for the essential amino acids.

Committee on Growth of the National Academy of Sciences.

Press releases were occasionally made concerning reports of meetings of the Board of Trustees or awards at scientific meetings. One of the most effective channels via the press was through interviews with professional writers or by feature writing on request from editors of established magazines.

Awards

A new special educational feature introduced in 1948-49 was the support by The Nutrition Foundation of four national awards selected and administered by scientific societies closely related to food and nutrition. Each award included an honorarium of $1,000 and a certificate from the society responsible for the selection. The awards were named in honor of pioneers in research and education whose contributions illustrated the ideals and conceptual imagination that characterizes the four respective areas of professional specialization represented by the societies.

The *Thomas B. Osborne and Lafayette B. Mendel Award,* administered by the American Institute of Nutrition, was named in recognition of the pioneering accomplishments of these two professors at Yale University. Dr. Osborne was primarily an agricultural chemist in the Connecticut Experiment Station while Dr. Mendel taught biochemistry in the School of Medicine of Yale University. Each enjoyed the other's point of view and critical judgment.

The First Decade

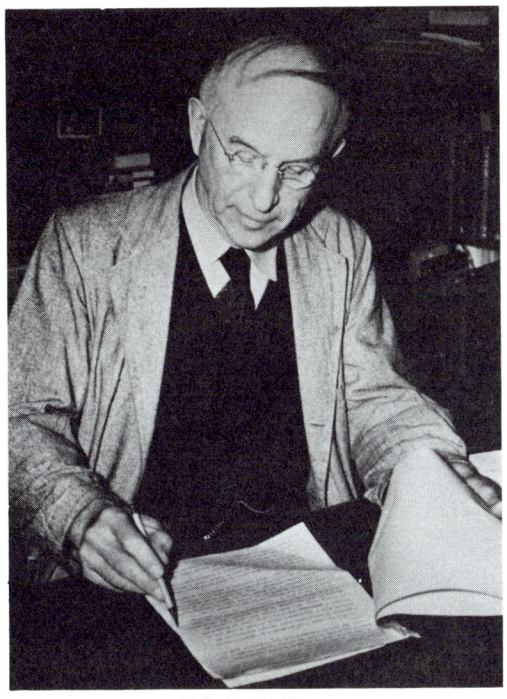

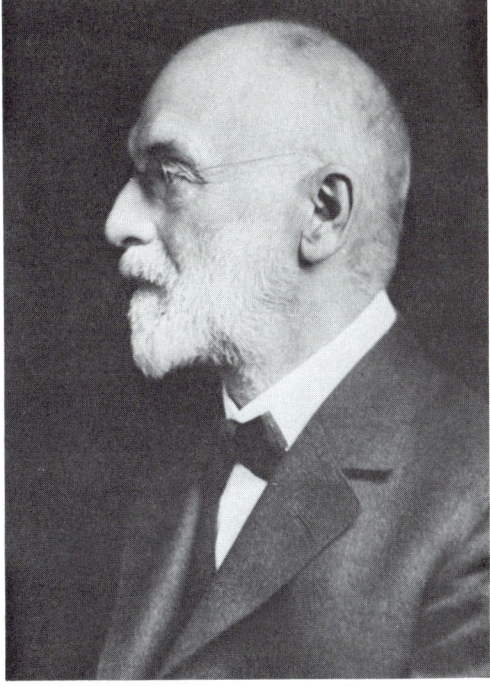

Edwin B. Hart

Stephen M. Babcock

The Babcock-Hart Award, supported by The Nutrition Foundation and selected by the Institute of Food Technologists, is named for the two founders of the continuing dynasty of nutrition and food scientists at the University of Wisconsin.

Their research, particularly during the 1910-1920 period, on the amino acid content and nutritive quality of proteins from wheat and other foods provided a classical chapter in the history of nutrition. This collaboration was followed by demonstrating the existence of "fat-soluble vitamin A" and "water-soluble vitamin B."

It was especially appropriate and heart-warming to see Professor W. C. Rose—a former student of Professor Mendel—receive the first Osborne and Mendel Award in recognition of his own contributions to our knowledge of the requirements for protein in terms of the specific amino acids and the discovery of an essential amino acid, threonine. Like Mendel, he is a meticulous writer, brilliant lecturer and inspiring teacher—sensitive, but generous, and insistent on high standards.

The *Babcock-Hart Award* administered by the Institute of Food Technologists was named for Professor Stephen M. Babcock of Cornell University and Professor E. B. Hart of the University of Wisconsin, both of whom contributed greatly to research on the nutritional values and technology of milk and its products. Both men also developed strong centers of research and education in food and nutrition. They were intensely interested and productive in relation to agricultural research and applications of chemistry in livestock technology, with an emphasis on milk. In view of the price premium on the fat content for making cream and butter, a simple mechanical separation of the fat by spinning in a

A Good Idea

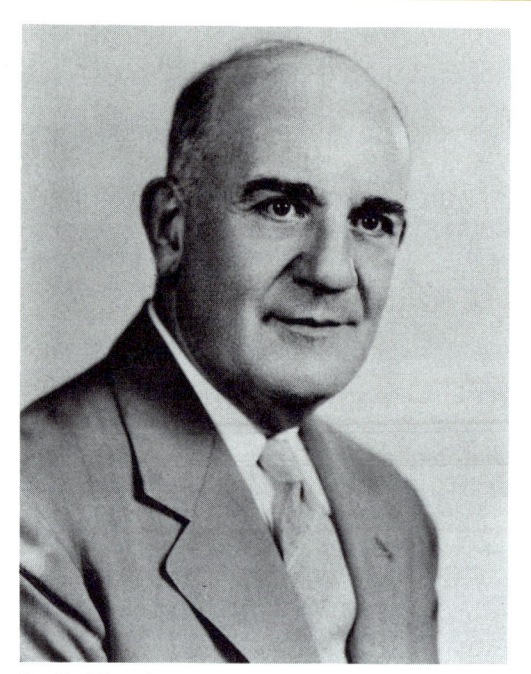

F. C. Blanck—First recipient of the Babcock-Hart Award

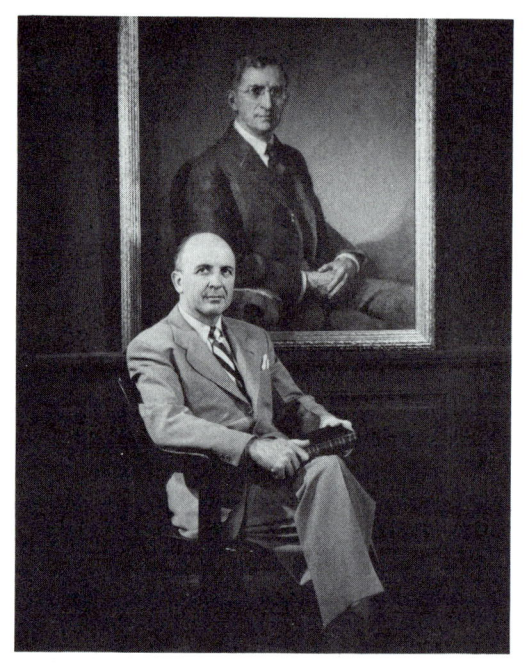

W. H. Sebrell, Jr., under the portrait of Joseph Goldberger

Dr. Sebrell, as a young U.S. Public Health Service officer, worked with Joseph Goldberger, the distinguished epidemiologist who established the deficiency etiology of pellagra. In this photograph, taken at the time that Dr. Sebrell received the American Medical Association's Goldberger Award in Clinical Nutrition (supported by The Nutrition Foundation), he is seated in Goldberger's old office chair and holds a bound copy of the Public Health Reports that contain Goldberger's classical papers on pellagra.

centrifuge after adding sulfuric acid was standardized and promoted by Professor Babcock as a test which carries his name.

Professor Hart, in contrast, is most noted for his research with students on the nutritive value of milk and the nutritional requirements of cattle and other animals. His research jointly with Dr. Elvehjem and others was particularly notable in showing that iron could not function normally in preventing anemia in rats or pigs unless there was an accompanying adequate intake of copper. Extension of the work demonstrated the essential nature also of manganese and zinc. He was one of the first to discover that dairy cows could utilize the low-cost, simple compound, urea, to synthesize body protein, thus decreasing the amount of protein needed from grain or pasturage. The conversion of urea to amino acids is accomplished by the microorganisms in the cow's intestinal tract (rumen).

The *Joseph Goldberger Award in Clinical Nutrition*, administered by the American Medical Association and its Council on Foods and Nutrition, was named in honor of the outstanding physician who as a member of the U.S. Public Health Service directed intensive studies of pellagra, a disease then endemic in many rural areas of our southern states and in other countries where maize or sorghum constitutes the major food source. He succeeded in demonstrating that the disease was essentially nutritional in origin and could be

The First Decade

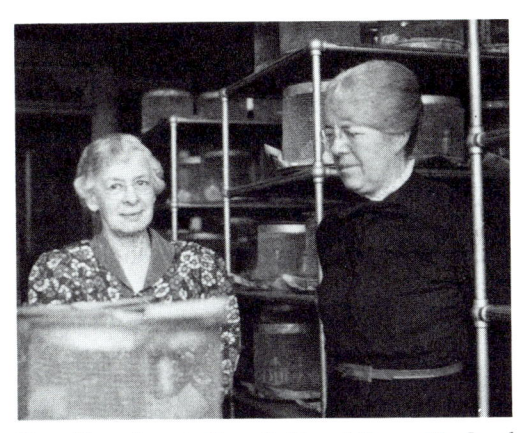

Drs. Mary Swartz Rose (left) and Grace MacLeod in the animal laboratory, Columbia University's Teachers College. The Mary Swartz Rose Award of the American Dietetic Association is supported by The Nutrition Foundation and is made to an outstanding dietitian who is pursuing a doctoral degree in nutrition. The recipient is selected by the American Dietetic Association.

prevented or cured by a diet containing a reasonable content of good quality protein food such as meat, milk or yeast. During the pre-depression years of the 1920's, about 200,000 cases of pellagra occurred in the United States annually.

Although pellagra had long been recognized as a particular form of disease, it was commonly thought to be caused by infection or a toxic material in the diet. Dr. Goldberger, a microbiologist, was assigned in 1914 by the U.S. Public Health Service to study its cause and treatment. He early observed that the disease was not transmitted to others by close association in living or working, and hence was not likely to be caused by infection. He even went so far as to feed test samples of excreta from pellagra patients to volunteers (1916) and observed no transmission of the disease. On feeding pellagra-producing diets to dogs, however, a condition ("canine black-tongue") analogous to pellagra was produced. This established the dog as an experimental animal useful in pellagra research. Goldberger recognized the involvement of a water soluble vitamin factor which he termed the P-P Factor (Pellagra-Preventive Factor). When Dr. Elvehjem and coworkers finally isolated nicotinamide from liver and demonstrated its cure of black tongue in dogs, the demonstration of a cure in treating pellagra patients followed quickly in 1936-1937 by several workers. This discovery also paved the way for recognizing that the amino acid tryptophan in good quality proteins can serve as a normal source of niacin in food supplies, since the liver converts tryptophan to niacin.

The *Mary Swartz Rose Award* is administered by the American Dietetic Association (ADA) in recognition of her remarkable career as a stimulating teacher and research associate in Teacher's College, Columbia University. She and other members of her staff were closely associated with Professor Henry C. Sherman in the Department of Chemistry. The ADA, with a generous spirit and keen understanding of the purpose of the award, chose to use it for support of graduate student fellowships to enable promising young dietetians to complete their training toward a Ph.D. degree in nutrition. The success of this program has been particularly gratifying in terms of the research and educational careers of those selected for the award.

Dr. Rose's texts on nutrition became standards in many universities and were continued in successive revisions by her associates after her death. The graduate students who studied with her toward a Ph.D. degree in the combined program with Dr. Sherman far exceeded those from any other university in nutrition professorships and leading positions in government agencies and industry. Actually, Teacher's College was originally named from a project of training teachers in an intensive program of developing vegetable

A Good Idea

gardens for children's food improvement in New York City. The man who served as President of the organization sponsoring this project was the service-minded professor of philosophy at Columbia University, Nicholas Murray Butler, who later became President of the University.

The recipients of these four awards are listed in Appendix F.

International Union of Nutritional Sciences

In the spring of 1946, the British Nutrition Society with assistance from the Royal Society extended invitations to a conference in London, primarily to review nutritional experiences in different countries during the war. Representatives from many of the European countries gave interesting reports of their respective experiences. Dr. F. B. Morrison (Cornell University) and I were appointed to represent the United States and Canada (by courtesy, as Dr. C. H. Best, originally appointed, could not attend). Since we had been in a relatively favorable position to keep in touch with journal publications during the war, Dr. Morrison was asked to review progress that had been made in feeding farm animals and I was invited to review progress in human nutrition and basic research.

The beloved Professor Joseph Barcroft of Cambridge University, chairman of the conference, succeeded in maintaining a

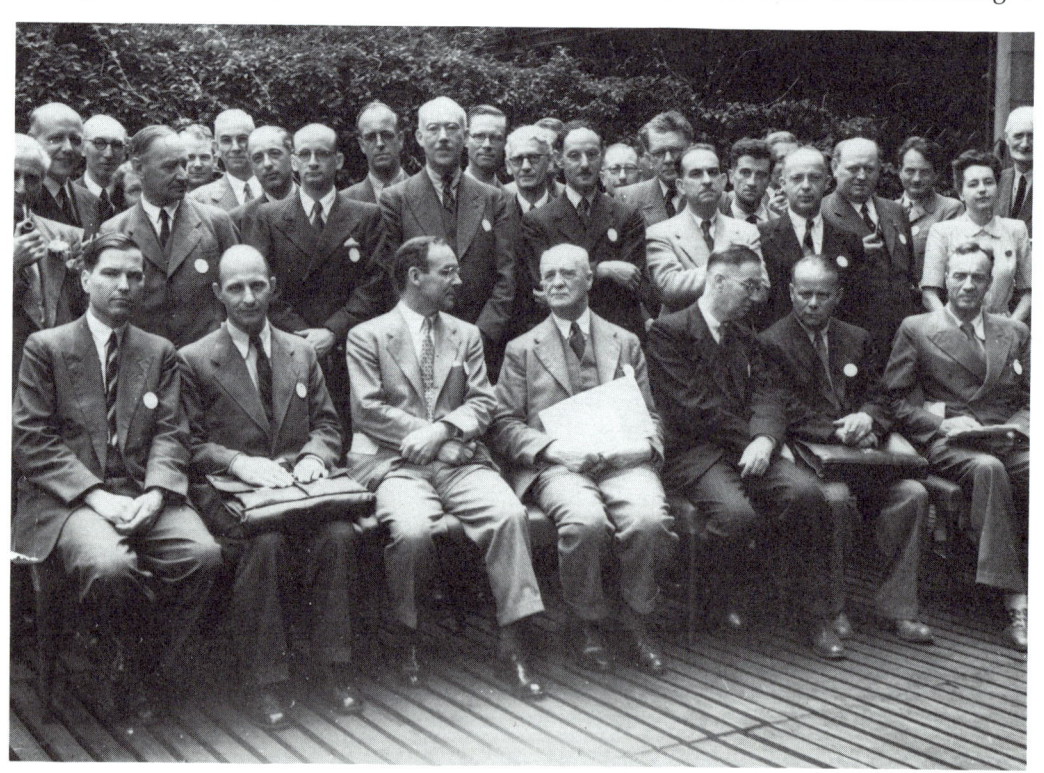

European Conference, The Nutrition Society and the British Council, London, July, 1946.
Sitting, left to right: *Torben, With, Pijanowski, King, Barcroft, Jansen, Tikka, Demole.* Standing, left to right: *Bacharach, van Eekelen, Guerden, Cruickshank, Verzar, Natvig, Morrison, Jahr, Vartiovaara, van Veen, Brouwer, Brunius, Fridericia, Harris, Kon, Breirem, Abrahamson, Simmonet, Tremolieres, Steensberg, Paluch, Jacquot, Hansen, Mrs. Day, Hammond.*

The First Decade

warm, friendly atmosphere among the delegates. Toward the end of the week a formal proposal was made that we establish a permanent international organization to sponsor continued activities among nutritional scientists. Then the atmosphere got sticky. Several participants refused to vote either way. A series of motions went sour and faces showed the tension. Finally, a whispered "We are not authorized to vote, officially" gave me a clue to address the chair with a proposal that "the Chairman might instruct the secretary of our host society to record that there was a consensus of opinion at the meeting, that it was desirable to plan for continued activity on an international basis, and that if an appropriate opportunity occurred there might be affiliation with the United Nations." There were favorable comments, no objections and apparently unanimous support. Tensions relaxed and the meeting was followed during ensuing years by organization of the International Union of Nutritional Sciences with Leslie J. Harris (Cambridge) as its first Secretary, and an established official liaison with the Food and Agriculture Organization of the United Nations. The Nutrition Foundation paid the travel expenses to enable an official United States delegate to attend the following international congresses held in Western Europe. It also contributed support for planning the Fifth International Congress on Nutrition, held in Washington, D.C. in 1960.

Nutrition Fact Finding

Nutrition is Essentially a Quantitative Science. Why?

One of the most baffling problems in nutrition is to identify degrees of deficiency, excess or imbalance that may result in a health risk when experienced over a period of weeks, months or years, but may not show overt evidence of a disease that is specific for any one nutrient. Thirst from want of water and hunger from want of calories generally became obvious within a matter of hours, but the symptoms resulting from a slight lack or excess of essential amino acids, fatty acids, minerals or vitamins are often too difficult to identify even for a physician.

The choice of foods by the average layman is largely a matter of habit. He chooses foods that appeal to him, taste good, are attractive in appearance, convenient, and within his attainable range of cost. Education is generally helpful in making selections, but often this influence is limited to broad types of food and vague indications of quantity. Records of market foods distributed within a community or to a family can indicate food consumption trends for a population group, but this information does not furnish an adequate guide in relation to individuals. Even within family groups there are often wide individual differences in eating habits.

As specific nutrients were identified and could be measured accurately in very small quantities by biochemists, a new approach to the study of intermediate degrees of malnutrition became possible. Direct analysis of two or three drops of blood obtained from the fingertip or earlobe could quantify the level of a nutrient and often permit determination of the coexistent degree of nutritional abnormality. In many instances changes in the pattern of blood cells or enzymes could also be an index to sufficiency of a nutrient, such as vitamin B_{12}, iron, or vitamins B_1 and D. The potential benefit to the public resulting from use of such techniques in medical practice and in surveys of population groups was recognized, and grants were made by the Foundation to support the necessary research.

Dr. O. A. Bessey and Dr. O. H. Lowry at

A Good Idea

Harvard University and with the New York City Health Council, had a leading role in the development of analyses that were well adapted to school and community surveys of nutritional status, including vitamin A, carotene, riboflavin, vitamin C, hemoglobin, iron, total protein, and the rickets-related enzyme, phosphatase. These methods, requiring only a few drops of fingertip or earlobe blood, marked a major turning point in identifying the specific nature and degree of nutritional deficiencies. They were quickly adapted to clinical use in hospitals, schools and field surveys of civilian or military populations. Costs per test for supplies were relatively small. These procedures were the prototype of a large number of widely used clinical methods considered today as indispensible diagnostic tests. Both of these leaders in diagnostic methodology continued to have outstanding careers: Dr. O. A. Bessey at the University of Illinois, and the University of Texas, in military service, in public health and in environmental research; Dr. Lowry, professor of pharmacology at Washington University, became a world leader in developing methods of microanalysis — even to the extent of studying quantitatively the metabolism of *a single living cell*. His work was recognized by election to the National Academy of Sciences.

In surveys of school populations in New York City, Bessey and Lowry identified the degree and extent of malnutrition among the school children in different sections of the city and related their findings to social environments, economic status, and age groups. An important correlation was the frequency with which mild or marked anemia was associated with different types of nutritional deficiencies. The correlation indicated a tendency for inadequate quantities of available iron to be derived from the diet. In a subsequent investigation they demonstrated that the anemia was correctable by simple medication with iron, thereby making a strong case for increasing the intake of this nutrient through enrichment. These workers also provided evidence for the efficacy of iron enrichment of flour in Newfoundland through measuring the changes in hemoglobin levels of school children that occurred after the institution of flour enrichment.

Different nutrients vary in the time required to deplete the concentration in tissues, blood or urine. The availability of methods for quantitative measure has greatly advanced the science of nutrition and its applications in relation to public health, industrial and home food practices, and education of the public. Faddists, fakers, ruthless advertisers and misled individuals who spread foolish propaganda are, at least in part, restrained by quantitative records that are specific and reliable when interpreted by well-trained scientists.

In a specific section of the Philippines, Helen B. Burch and J. Salcedo demonstrated that an initial program of rice enrichment with added thiamin, niacin and iron substantially increased the public consumption of these three nutrients in parallel with a sharply decreased incidence of anemia and the deficiency disease beri-beri. In contrast, vitamin C, carotene and riboflavin consumption and blood levels remained low, indicating an inadequate consumption of vegetables, fruits and milk or meat. Such assessments would not be possible without adequate methodology.

Toxic Excesses of Vitamins A and D

Dr. A. F. Morgan, Dr. H. Becks and their associates at the University of California reported on injuries to dogs caused either by vitamin D in massive single doses or by continued moderately excessive intakes.

The First Decade

Dr. S. B. Wolbach and Dr. D. M. Hegsted at Harvard University conducted a study of the toxic effects of excessive intakes of vitamin A and vitamin D, in addition to studies of tissue injury by vitamin deficiency. These early studies supported by The Nutrition Foundation have often been confirmed and repeatedly extended by observation of human injury from excessive intakes of these two fat-soluble vitamins. Recognition of such relationships would greatly improve the education of many laymen who do not realize that for *all* essential nutrients there are three quantitative levels:

1. Insufficient for optimum health;
2. An intake range that is optimal for health during each stage of development and changing circumstances of living; and
3. An excess that causes injury within hours or years, depending on the quantity.

This principle applies to *all* nutrients, from vitamin A to table salt and water, but unfortunately the public has but a very limited understanding of how fundamental these three relationships are—including the most widely damaging of nutritional excesses, the intake of total calories. Indeed, the action of the Food and Drug Administration limiting the quantity of vitamins that can be incorporated in "over the counter" items is a desirable action for protection of the public based upon this scientific knowledge. This concept of harmful excess is also essential to protection against harmfully high intakes of nutrients through unwise uncontrolled enrichment practices such as resulted in the outbreak of hypercalcemia in infants in England as a consequence of permitting excesses of vitamin D in a variety of foods.

It is well to remember that ten of the mineral elements most recently found to be essential for normal animal development were studied for several decades chiefly because in the small quantities studied they were injurious to health; intake level (2) for these nutrients had not then been discovered. There are still serious debates regarding the intake quantities of some nutrients (iron and calcium, for example) at which one passes from a desirable intake level (2) to an excessive intake level (3).

The Nutrition Foundation in cooperation with the American Public Health Association, the Milbank Fund and the Research Corporation, undertook a special study to find more effective ways of developing nutrition education and services within local and state-related health agencies. A widely used monograph was published as a result of the conference.

Another example of excessive intakes occurred because of claims that feeding large amounts of glutamic acid to retarded children would often improve their intelligence had been made in the technical literature and in extensive sales promotion. Some drugstores were selling and promoting large quantities of this substance. The thesis was based, apparently, on evidence that this amino acid, though not essential for human nutrition, could be metabolized in the brain. Since there was reason to doubt the beneficial claims on such an important issue, two highly qualified groups were supported in making an evaluation—one at Stanford University and another at the University of Pittsburgh. Both groups after careful study reported evidence that the claims were not valid.

Food Selection in Relation to Need

There is a persistent fetish that the body's appetite or sense of taste can serve as a reasonable guide in determining what the body needs. In primitive times evolution may have developed a partial guide in this respect. Those who did not select the right foods would be less likely to survive. However, tests with specific nutrients conducted by Dr. E. M. Scott at the University of Pittsburgh showed clearly that albino rats were very inefficient in selecting needed specific nutrients. In some cases, as with vitamins B_1 and B_2, the animals succeeded fairly well in selecting adequate quantities, but for others the failures were strikingly obvious. There was a marked failure in ability to select a pure protein to meet needs. Some animals starved to death for lack of good quality protein although highly purified casein was available in the feed cups. The same was true with respect to magnesium—death by wrong choice. However, in later tests with diets of mixed foodstuffs, rats selected those with good protein quality fairly well. Was it the good protein or the protein's companions?

It may be observed that the socio-cultural and economic factors influence man's choices of food so greatly that any primitive intuitive appetite is not likely to be very effective—hence the need to understand the psychologic and cultural factors that determine man's current acceptance and utilization of foods. Only in recent years have scientists widely realized the importance of consideration of these determinants of food attitudes in our programs of nutrition education.

Early Medical School Examples of Nutrition Teaching

Dr. A. B. Hastings, who had a major responsibility in the National Academy of Sciences during the war, continued for many years to advance the graduate and post-doctoral training in biochemistry at Harvard University, including the development of a strong new type of program in nutrition at the University. Dr. A. O. Bessey and Dr. O. H. Lowry assisted in biochemical and nutrition research and teaching in cooperation with other departments in the medical center. After a short time, however, they were invited to develop a new, strong program, as chief and associate, respectively, of the division of physiology and nutrition at the New York Public Health Research Institute. F. J. Stare, who had earned his Ph.D. degree with Dr. Elvehjem at the University of Wisconsin and his M.D. at Washington University (St. Louis) was appointed to a professorial position and head of the first official Department of Nutrition established in a medical school, sponsored jointly by the Harvard School of Medicine and School of Public Health.

The teaching of nutrition in medical schools of the United States and Canada varied greatly from institution to institution at that time, both as to departmental support and interest. A significant effect of The Nutrition Foundation's early and continuing support for a few medical schools was the reinforcement of faculty interest in the subject of nutrition. For example, at Vanderbilt University, where a continuous required course in nutrition has been in the medical curriculum since the 1930s, a Division of Nutrition, directed by Dr. W. J. Darby, was created in 1944. This Division, with its expanded research and teaching program, was in large measure made possible through the tripartite support provided by a grant from The Nutrition Foundation, The Rockefeller Foundation and the Tennessee State Department of Public Health. Similar interests developed at Tulane University under the leadership of Dr. Grace Goldsmith.

Some other medical schools and schools of public health developed programs of research and teaching in nutrition, but in many instances the tendency was to leave the teaching and research in nutrition to individuals classified in other departments, without a well identified, coordinated and supported program concerned

The First Decade

directly with nutrition. In the light of continuing experience, however, a trend has developed to identify the needs and opportunities for strong programs, specifically identified in nutrition and reaching out in cooperation with other disciplines such as biochemistry, physiology, medicine, pediatrics, community medicine, obstetrics, surgery, pathology and dental health. Cooperation in programming is also important in relation to schools of nursing, public health, home economics and food science or technology. The physician's viewpoint can be sharpened by such experience. In addition, he provides a most important professional service in reaching the public and holding their confidence. Fortunately, in 1976 the trend in this direction is developing steadily, stimulated and strengthened by the program of The Nutrition Foundation and other collaborating organizations — especially the Council on Foods and Nutrition of the American Medical Association, the American College of Physicians, and other foundations.

A New Vitamin

When the Nutrition Foundation was organized, there were several reports indicating that at least one more vitamin remained to be isolated and chemically identified. Like most vitamins, the active material was associated with such foodstuffs as green leaves, seeds, fish and particularly liver. Evidence for its essentiality came from studies with many species — bacteria, chickens, fish, rats, guinea pigs and monkeys. There was little information as to its chemical nature or its role in human nutrition. Five of the early grants from the Foundation accelerated research on the problem and progress was surprisingly rapid. The "monkey business" paid off first.

The several university and industrial scientists working on the problem did not know how many active products were in the materials tested. Paul L. Day at the University of Arkansas was vigorously pursuing the new factor, using monkeys as the test animal and studying its effect on blood cell development as the indicator of activity. His group had described an anemia and leucopenia in the monkey as a specific tissue injury that could be followed as a quantitative response to the factor and they proposed the name "vitamin M" for the active principle that prevented the hematologic changes in the monkey. Concentrates prepared from liver could cure the specific deficiency in monkeys and differentiated this activity from that which controlled "pernicious anemia" (and was later shown to be vitamin B_{12}).

After Dr. Day and his co-workers suggested the name vitamin M for the active factor, it was variously termed vitamin B_c, "factor U," L. casei factor, folic acid, fermentation factor, etc. The term "folic acid," indicative of its wide occurrence in leafy foods, became the most used designation.

The period 1944-1946 was especially exciting as small quantities of the pure material were isolated, the chemical nature identified and finally synthesis was accomplished. The pinnacle of excitement was the testing of the pure materials in human anemias.

Three grantees of The Nutrition Foundation were in the forefront of the studies in man. Dr. Grace Goldsmith at Tulane University observed the response of a patient with nutritional macrocytic anemia; Dr. W. J. Darby and co-workers at Vanderbilt University reported the first cases of sprue that responded to the newly synthesized folic acid ("pteroylglutamic acid"); and Dr. Tom Spies found that a variety of "macrocytic anemias," including pernicious anemia, responded hematologically. Only after the initial excitement abated did it

A Good Idea

become widely recognized clinically that this new vitamin was not the missing factor that provides replacement therapy for true pernicious anemia, but that it was the principal vitamin that was curative in sprue (commonly found in tropical and subtropical areas), megaloblastic anemia of infants, so-called pernicious anemia of pregnancy, and most of the cases of nutritional macrocytic anemia in the U.S.—all characterized by large red blood cells. The confusion with the antipernicious anemia factor resulted from the hemopoietic effect of the large doses of the vitamin initially employed and from the ignoring of earlier experimental evidence by Day *et al.* that this vitamin was not identical with the "extrinsic factor."

The wide importance of the new hemopoietic vitamins and the requirements of diverse species warranted considerable investment by the Foundation in support of research. Among the highlights of such progress, assisted by The Nutrition Foundation, was the development by Vincent Allfrey and L. J. Teply of Columbia of a new chemical method of analysis, and demonstration by W. H. Prusoff of its role in the synthesis of nucleic acid by bacteria. Dr. Teply subsequently exhibited exceptional worldwide leadership in nutrition as the chief advisor on nutrition for UNICEF and, in cooperation with WHO and FAO, as a contributor to the program of the Protein Advisory Group (PAG). Drs. Allfrey and Prusoff have become Professors at the Rockefeller University and Yale University, respectively. Studies of the folic acid deficiency anemia in chicks by M. S. Scott were supported at Cornell University, and in swine by T. J. Cunha and others at Washington State College.

Requirements of Other Vitamins

With the aid of a grant from The Nutrition Foundation, Dr. Elmer Severinghaus at the University of Wisconsin developed additional evidence regarding the human requirement for thiamin, vitamin C and niacin, in studies with volunteer prisoners. The data supported the concept of establishing "recommended dietary allowances" at levels distinctly above the minimal quantities required to prevent an obvious disease—quantities that were commonly acceptable as feeding standards in Europe and long had been used officially by some U.S. government agencies, in the so-called "minimum daily requirements."

Studies of B-Complex Vitamins at Duke University

Beginning in 1942, Dr. W. A. Perlzweig, Professor of Biochemistry at Duke University Medical School, received support from The Nutrition Foundation and developed an outstanding program of research on the metabolism of the amino acid tryptophan, its metabolic conversion to niacin, and related products. These studies contributed to understanding the prevention and management of human pellagra.

However, an incidental experience reported orally created a sudden strain on Dr. Perlzweig's sense of humor and possible tragedy in relation to practical nutrition. One forenoon he was called from his laboratory by a medical associate to examine a patient in the dental clinic. She had a typical case of scurvy, including swollen bleeding gums caused by vitamin C deficiency—and with a shock Dr. Perlzweig recognized his own long-time faithful cook! What could have happened? She had served his breakfast that very morning and merely mentioned that she planned to see the dentist later in the day. She had complete freedom to choose her food from the family supply which regularly included fresh vegetables and citrus fruits. Answer: (1) She wanted to be ready to serve his dinner promptly whenever he reached

The First Decade

home (time unpredictable) so the dinner was regularly put on to cook before taking her afternoon siesta, and the prolonged cooking destroyed most of the vitamin C (2) She did not like "sour foods," so avoided the ever-present oranges, lemons, grapefruit and tomatoes.

The nutrition group at Duke University at that time constituted one of the major centers of the nation. In addition to Dr. Perlzweig, his students and associates who contributed to the knowledge of metabolites of niacin and the usefulness of these in assessing nutriture, there were leaders in nutrition in several other departments. Dr. W. J. Dann in physiology was a leader in the identification of the role of nicotinic acid in nutrition; he had also devised the Dann-Evelyn photometric method for determining vitamin A in human blood. He was joined by a young post-doctorate from the University of Illinois, a student of Dr. Herbert Carter in Professor W. C. Rose's department, Dr. Philip Handler. Dr. Handler received assistance from The Nutrition Foundation in conducting basic studies of the anti-pellagra vitamin and investigating kidney function in response to stress from changes in the acid-base balance, liver function and hormone balances. He subsequently becameCed Dr. Perlzweig's successor as Chairman of the Department of Biochemistry. His continued career in research and education led to his present dynamic leadership as President of the National Academy of Sciences. He is a Public Trustee of the Nutrition Foundation.

Distinguished clinicians at Duke engaged in nutritional research at that time included Dr. Frederick Haines, Professor and Chairman of the Department of Medicine, a recognized expert on sprue and intestinal malabsorption; Dr. Julian Ruffin, a gastroenterologist in the Department of Medicine; and Dr. David T. Smith, a microbiologist and parasitologist. The latter two collaborated in classical studies of pellagra and Dr. Ruffin pursued clinical investigations on malabsorption and the efficacy of vitamin supplements, and counseled on military problems in nutrition during and following World War II.

During this period Dr. Susan G. Smith, wife of David T. Smith, described specific lesions of the lip due to vitamin B_6 deficiency in man. The Rockefeller Foundation placed one of its staff members at the University, Dr. D. F. Milam, to develop a program in Public Health Nutrition and nutrition surveys. The Rockefeller Foundation also sent as a Fellow into this milieu Dr. William J. Darby as a young physician with a Ph.D. in biochemistry. His studies there included biochemical and clinical assessment of nutriture, basic principles in public health, tissue metabolism of amino acids in vitamin C deficiency, and clinical experiences concerning sprue, pellagra, and malabsorption. This experience provided valuable background for his later career, culminating in his election to the National Academy of Sciences and his present post as President of The Nutrition Foundation.

Fat Soluble Vitamins E and A

Karl Mason and L. J. Filer, Jr., at the University of Rochester and Ade T. Milhorat at Cornell University received grants in support of research on the functions of vitamin E, particularly in relation to smooth muscle function and changes in fat composition. Despite many misleading claims relative to this vitamin, work by critical scientists such as Drs. Mason and Filer has led to recognition of it as an important nutrient in human and animal diets. Dr. Filer is now Professor of Pediatrics at the University of Iowa and Chairman of the Food and Nutrition Board at the National Research Council.

In view of uncertainty regarding the op-

A Good Idea

timum human intake of vitamin A, Professor Sherman at Columbia University was provided support for a long-term evaluation of different levels of intake by albino rats. His study on a life-span basis demonstrated a statistically significant benefit in length of life and survival of offspring from intakes up to about four times the amount required for protection from obvious signs of deficiency.

Dr. J. Warkany of the University of Cincinnati received support for notable investigations in which a low maternal intake of vitamin A in albino rats was shown to be a critical factor in the development of malformations in the offspring of rats that were fed barely enough to protect them from obvious deficiencies and to carry through a period of pregnancy and lactation. A striking effect of these marginal deficiencies was the incidence of deformities of the eye and skeletal structures in the offspring. The care and thoroughness with which Dr. Warkany's work was conducted constitutes an important chapter in this aspect of nutrition. It served as an experimental model for later study of fetal effects of maternal deficiency of many nutrients such as riboflavin, zinc, amino acids, and others, and as a stimulus to human investigations of maternal nutrition as a significant factor in fetal quality and defects.

It is widely held that in many of the developing countries, including sections of India, Latin America, Africa and Southeast Asia, vitamin A deficiencies rank close to protein deficiencies in importance in terms of injury to child health. In parts of eastern India and Indonesia, for example, where blindness in small children is perhaps the highest in the world, pediatricians hold that about one-half of the blindness is caused by vitamin A deficiency.

To illustrate the continuity of Foundation efforts in research, education and applied knowledge, it may be noted that during 1973-1975 it has cooperated in holding workshops on vitamin A deficiency and blindness with the American Foundation for the Overseas Blind and in preparing educational materials for international use. NUTRITION REVIEWS for June 1974 included an excellent instructive lead article on Vitamin A Deficiency, Xerophthalmia and Blindness, illustrated by superbly detailed color plates of lesions photographed by Professor H. A. P. C. Oomen.

Some of the yellow oil-soluble carotenoid pigments in plants were known to protect man and animals from vitamin A deficiency, but little was known of the location or mechanism of the conversion of these pigments to the colorless, active vitamin as it appears in the liver and other tissues. H. J. Deuel and J. W. Mehl at the University of Southern California were given support for extensive studies which demonstrated that the conversion occurred mainly within the intestinal wall. N. B. Guerrant at Pennsylvania State College was assisted in organizing a program to establish a national reference standard for evaluation of vitamin A in foods and animal feeds. This standard was based on the pure vitamin and its measurement by chemical analysis instead of the earlier standard based on the active precursor, beta-carotene. The precursor had an uncertain degree of conversion to the vitamin, and hence was not an ideal reference standard. In addition, the beta-carotene was usually associated with other yellow carotenes as it occurred in foods, and these products varied from zero to about one-half of the activity of beta-carotene.

Vitamin B_6

Although Paul György had shared in the isolation and studied the nutritional role of vitamin B_6, a major advance in discovering how this nutrient functions in living organisms was made by I. C. Gunsalus and W.

W. Umbreit while assisted by a Nutrition Foundation grant to Cornell University. They advanced our understanding of the vitamin's role as a catalyst in amino acid synthesis and in the metabolism of microorganisms. It is a pleasure to note that Dr. Gunsalus shortly thereafter became Professor of Biochemistry at the University of Illinois, succeeding Dr. W. C. Rose, and Dr. Umbreit became Professor and Chairman of the Department of Bacteriology at Rutgers University.

Dr. Stare and his associates, M. Brin and R. E. Olson, at Harvard University demonstrated the importance of vitamin B_6 functions (transaminase reactions) in heart muscle. Related enzyme systems that control amino acid metabolism were also charted by C. A. Elvehjem and others at the University of Wisconsin. These studies served to clarify many of the interrelationships of amino acids, vitamin B_6 and niacin.

Vitamin C

All carefully studied higher plants and animals require vitamin C in their tissues for normal metabolism. Most species synthesize ascorbic acid according to need, but a few species of animals, like man, monkeys, guinea pigs, certain birds and fish have genetically lost one of the enzymes (L-gulonolactone dehydrogenase) required for its synthesis. Hence, without a food source of the vitamin they develop scurvy and die. When radio-carbon (^{14}C) became available, my associates at Columbia University prepared glucose with radio carbons in known positions and fed it to rats (not subject to scurvy). The vitamin C synthesized by the rats had the labeled carbon in the same specific position as in the administered glucose, thus proving its origin from glucose and providing an indication of the reactions involved in its synthesis. In comparable tests, guinea pigs did not form the vitamin but instead, a compound (glucuronic acid) that corresponds with that formed in human metabolism. The synthesized glucose and labeled vitamin as prepared in the laboratory also permitted precise studies of its distribution in tissues and the products of its metabolism. Particularly active in the work were J. J. Burns, now Vice President of Hoffmann-La Roche Co., E. H. Mosbach, A. P. Doerchuk, J. F. Douglas, H. H. Horowitz, S. S. Jackel and L. L. Solomon.

Repeated claims were made in the scientific and lay literature from one of the universities that there was a new vitamin associated with vitamin C, functioning as an "anti-stiffness factor," required in the diets of guinea pigs to protect the animals from stiffness in the leg joints as a special form of "arthritis." The claims were challenged after reading the reports and visiting the laboratory to observe the care of the experimental animals. Dr. L. A. Maynard at Cornell University was given support to investigate the situation and test our hypothesis that the condition was caused by a poor balance of minerals, particularly calcium and magnesium. Such proved to be the case. Similarly, persistent claims that a new vitamin ("Vitamin P") was essentially associated with vitamin C in preventing the hemorrhages characteristic of scurvy, were corrected by studies supported at the University of Wisconsin and at the Cornell College of Medicine.

Proteins and Amino Acids

The outstanding work of W. C. Rose supported by the Foundation has been noted previously. His classical investigations on human and rat requirements for amino acids included the demonstration that these protein fragments were utilized more efficiently when consumed as whole proteins and with a generous supply of calories than when fed as a mixture of

A Good Idea

amino acids. His basic findings had many useful implications, one of which has been in the design of an effective source of amino acids for intravenous nutrition of surgical and pediatric patients who cannot be nourished by the gastrointestinal route.

No other scientist has a record comparable to that of Dr. Rose in identifying and establishing the quantitative requirement for so many essential nutrients. His work on amino acids stands as a classic in the history of nutrition and for the benefit of man. His summary table of amino acid requirements of man is worthy of reproduction and illustrates his meticulous manner of reporting.

Although Dr. Rose's work was always notable for great care in the design, supervision and interpretation of data, he has told of one very brief period of distraction. During a rat feeding test that had been yielding very consistent data, a few surprising individual variations in growth response appeared. Rechecking every detail in the experiment furnished no explanation. He had full confidence in his students. But one evening on returning to the laboratory both the mystery and the problem were solved—a night-shift Janitor had a small son that on rare occasions when his mother was away came with his father. The child was observed amusing himself by feeding a few tidbits to one of his newly discovered "pets"!

Among Professor Rose's many outstanding graduate students whose support came

Summary of Amino Acid Requirements of Man
W.C. Rose, R.L. Wixom, H.B. Lockhart and G.F. Lambert, J. Biol. Chem. 217 p. 992 (1955).

All values were determined with diets containing the eight essential amino acids and sufficient extra nitrogen to permit the synthesis of the non-essentials.

Amino acid	No. of quantitative experiments	Range of requirements observed	Value proposed *tentatively* as minimum	Value which is definitely a *safe* intake	No. of subjects maintained in N balance on safe intakes or less
		gm. per day	gm. per day	gm. per day	
L-Tryptophan	3*	0.15–0.25	0.25	0.50	42
L-Phenylalanine	6	0.80–1.10†	1.10	2.20	32
L-Lysine	6	0.40–0.80	0.80	1.60	37‡
L-Threonine	3§	0.30–0.50	0.50	1.00	29
L-Methionine	6	0.80–1.10°	1.10	2.20	23
L-Leucine	5	0.50–1.10	1.10	2.20	18
L-Isoleucine	4	0.65–0.70	0.70	1.40	17
L-Valine	5	0.40–0.80	0.80	1.60	33

*Fifteen other young men were maintained in nitrogen balance on daily intakes of 0.20 gm., though their exact minimal needs were not established. Of the forty-two subjects maintained on the *safe* level of intake, thirty-three received 0.30 gm. daily or less.

†These values were obtained with diets which were devoid of tyrosine. In two experiments, the presence of tyrosine in the food was shown to spare the phenylalanine requirement to the extent of 70 to 75 percent.

‡Ten of these individuals received daily intakes of 0.80 gm. or less.

§In addition to these three subjects, four young men received rations containing 0.60 gm. of L-threonine daily and sixteen others received doses of 0.80 gm. daily. No attempt was made to determine the exact minimal requirements of these twenty individuals, but all were in positive balance on the doses indicated.

°These values were determined with cystine-free diets. In three experiments, the presence of cystine was found to exert a sparing effect of 80 to 89 percent upon the minimal methionine needs of the subjects.

The First Decade

from Nutrition Foundation grants it is rewarding particularly to identify Dr. W. J. Haines, now Vice President and Director of Research of the Johnson & Johnson Company; Dr. J. E. Johnson, Vice President and Director of Research of the Dow Chemical Company; and Dr. M. J. Coon, Head of the Department of Biochemistry in the School of Medicine at the University of Michigan.

Supplementing the basic studies of Dr. Rose, J. R. Murlin at the University of Rochester and H. E. Carter, University of Illinois, received support for the evaluation of the protein quality of soybeans and yeast, respectively, including supplementation of these by specific amino acids in human diets.

Important studies of the amino acid requirements of infants and small children and observations on the physiological effects of amino acid deficiency were made by Dr. L. Emmett Holt, Jr., Professor of Pediatrics at the Johns Hopkins University and later at New York University. He and his associates, especially A. S. Albanese and S. E. Snyderman, found that the requirements of the growing infant differ moderately, both qualitatively and quantitatively from those reported for the maintenance requirements of young adults. The infant, for example, may require the amino acid histidine, but the adult apparently does not.

Extensive contributions to knowledge of the amino acid requirements of chicks resulted from work at the University of California in Berkeley by Drs. Almquist, Grau and their associates. The general pattern of requirements resembled those of the human and rat, but there were distinct differences. The chick has an appreciable requirement for the simplest amino acid, glycine; man can synthesize it in abundance—and hence does not require it in his diet.

At the University of California in Los Angeles, Dr. Max Dunn and his associates made outstanding advances in the use of bacteria and other microorganisms for measuring specific nutrients, including the amino acids and vitamins, at a time when direct chemical analyses were unsatisfactory. Microbiological tests developed with support from the Foundation were rapid, more accurate and less expensive than the available chemical procedures.

Dr. du Vigneaud's studies of choline, methionine, cystine and cysteine and the classical genetic investigations of Dr. Beadle and his associates at Stanford University have been discussed. It is worthy of noting that both at Stanford University and later at the California Institute of Technology a high proportion of the graduate students associated with Dr. Beadle later achieved outstanding careers. These include, for example, H. K. Mitchell and N. H. Horowitz, who became members of the National Academy of Sciences while professors at Cal Tech; H. S. Loring became Professor of Biochemistry of Stanford University; and W. D. McElroy, now Chancellor of the University of California in San Diego, formerly Professor of Biology and Director of the McCollum-Pratt Institute at Johns Hopkins University, and during 1969 to 1971 Director of the National Science Foundation.

Most investigations of choline, such as those of du Vigneaud, were primarily concerned with its essential functions and nutritive value, including its important role in liver, kidney and nerve metabolism. Others, including Dr. Hodge at the University of Rochester, studied its toxicity when supplied in excess either orally or by injection.

Similarly, the extensive studies of the role of amino acids in nutrition, at Johns Hopkins University and later at New York

University by L. E. Holt, A. A. Albanese, V. Irby, H. P. Sarett and their associates gave emphasis to analytic methods, tissue injury and metabolic changes induced by both deficiencies and excesses of individual amino acids. In the natural proteins of plants and animals, the amino acids have a structure designated as the L-series. When heated in solution they may change partially to a D-series, some members of which have less nutritional value. Hence studies included both the D-series of amino acids and the dominant L-series contained in food proteins. Members of the D-series occur in bacterial cells and in a few other important biological products such as antibiotics. Synthetic amino acids usually have equal quantities of the D- and L- forms. Dr. Sarett, initially a student of Dr. Perlzweig at Duke University received further experience with Dr. V. Cheldelin on a Nutrition Foundation grant to Oregon State College, later worked with Dr. Grace Goldsmith at Tulane University, and currently is Vice President for Nutrition Science with the Mead Johnson Company.

Carbohydrates, Fats and Total Calories

During the 1940-1950 period nutritionists, biochemists and physicians became increasingly concerned with the nutritional significance and biosynthesis of fatty materials (lipids) and their relationships to health. Increasing evidence related several degenerative diseases, such as atherosclerosis and diabetes, to an increased content of cholesterol in the blood and an excess of body fat. Relationships between essential and non-essential fatty acids were also in the foreground with respect to health, public education and food technology. The content of cholesterol and saturated fats in milk, eggs and meat was regarded by many as in conflict with the high nutritional rating for protein, vitamins and minerals of these choice foods traditionally held as nutritionally most desirable. Fish, chicken, margarine and oils from many seeds like soya, corn, sesame and cottonseed came into special favor with many consumers because of their high content of polyunsaturated fatty acids, lower content of saturated fats and low cholesterol content. Facts concerning their use and biological effects had to be assessed for the public as well as for scientists and industry. "Fat was in the fire" of controversy. The Nutrition Foundation had a responsibility to assist highly competent and independent scientists obtain objective answers to many questions that were posed.

Knowledge about the physiology of glucose and the relationships of hormones and enzymes associated with diabetes and furnishing energy was substantially advanced by the research of Dr. Carl Cori and Dr. Gerti Cori. This remarkable husband and wife team received grants in support of their work as partners at Washington University. In 1947 they shared the Nobel Prize for their work in this area. They studied the metabolism of several common organic acids, especially acetic acid (the acid characteristic of vinegar) which contains only two carbon atoms derived from the six carbons in the glucose molecule. By a remarkable coincidence, within a short time this two-carbon acetate fragment furnished a major key to understanding many nutritional interrelationships of carbohydrates, fatty acids, cholesterol, and vitamins. The unfolding of this story was an exciting period in nutritional biochemistry to which Foundation grantees contributed significantly.

Dr. F. A. Lipmann, one of the outstanding scientists to enter the United States from Germany, had located at Harvard University where the Foundation assisted in support of his research. He developed clear evidence that the relatively new

The First Decade

vitamin, pantothenic acid, is a part of a catalyst, coenzyme A, which controls many of the reactions by which fatty materials are metabolized, and particularly in the metabolism of acetate groups. Dr. Mark Hegsted shared in the work. Dr. Lipmann's discoveries were recognized by his selection as a Nobel Laureate in 1953. He later received an appointment at the Rockefeller University where he continued his basic research.

In the Biochemistry Department of Columbia University, Dr. Hans Clarke assembled a group of scientific associates with intensive interests in the metabolic mechanisms of sugars and fats. These included Rudolph Schönheimer, another German émigré whose pioneering studies using stable isotopes destroyed the classic concept of sharp boundaries between a static and more active exogenous series of metabolic pathways. His concepts greatly advanced the understanding of metabolism and nutrition. Notable among his associates were David Rittenber, H. DeWitt Stetten, Jr., Sarah Rattner, David Shemin and Konrad Bloch. The latter made a particularly exciting discovery relative to carbohydrate-cholesterol interrelationships; he found that the two-carbon fragment, acetic acid, readily available from glucose, was utilized in the body to produce cholesterol. This perplexing lipid is essential to the structure of each living cell, but in excess it had already become associated with such diseases as diabetes, atherosclerosis and heart disease. This discovery by Dr. Bloch pointed sharply to the probability that risks associated with too much cholesterol were linked with an excess of carbohydrate, above the caloric need. In other words, it suggested that the normal mechanism of cholesterol synthesis might overproduce from excessive carbohydrate. It also added to the significance of Dr. Lipmann's and Dr. Hegsted's discovery of the role of pantothenic acid and the research on glucose by Carl and Gerti Cori at Washington University. Dr. Bloch became the fourth of these scientists to receive a Nobel Award for their research contributions. In addition, all four were outstanding leaders in training younger scientists.

Grants from the Foundation to support basic research on carbohydrate metabolism included support for A. Baird Hastings at Harvard whose studies in glucose metabolism included labeling each carbon atom of the six in the molecule and thereby identifying their metabolic patterns. Associated with Dr. Hastings and Dr. Stare in the group at Harvard were Myron Brin, G. V. Mann, Robert E. Olson, J. Mayer and W. W. Westerfeld, all of whom later became productive research scientists and university professors.

Other grantees who did excellent work in this field were H. A. Lardy, University of Wisconsin; E. H. Stotz, University of Rochester; E. P. Kennedy and A. L. Lehninger, University of Chicago; and P. D. Boyer and R. T. Holman, University of Minnesota. All were highly productive in research and established outstanding records for training young scientists. The exact topics of research by these and other grantees are illustrated in the appended references.

Mineral Metabolism

Studies of iron absorption and metabolism in relation to anemia by Paul F. Hahn at Vanderbilt University, F. A. Johnston at the University of Chicago, and by D. M. Hegsted and C. A. Finch at Harvard University were supported by the Foundation. The results helped to lay the basic groundwork for current nutritional planning relative to meeting the iron requirements of the population through food selection and enrichment. In 1973 Dr. Finch received the American Medical Association's Joseph

Goldberger Award in Clinical Nutrition.

Support was provided also for research on the metabolism of calcium, magnesium, sodium and potassium at the University of Illinois, the University of Wisconsin, Cornell University, Johns Hopkins University and Harvard University.

At the University of Florida, G. K. Davis was assisted in extensive studies of trace mineral relationships in soil, plants and animals. The interplay of molybdenum, copper and iron was particularly interesting. As the trend toward soil acidity increased, the availability of copper for plant growth increased, but for molybdenum it decreased, hence creating a risk of deficiency. A shift toward soil alkalinity reversed the availability of the two elements. If copper were insufficiently available to the plant, the yield would be low and the low copper content would not permit animals fed on the feedstuff to utilize iron efficiently. Hence they would become anemic. The importance of trace elements in human nutrition has been strongly underscored in recent years, thus highlighting the importance of these earlier investigations.

Studies in Relation to Cancer

Potential relationships between nutrient intake and development of cancer were explored by C. P. Rhoads and G. W. Brown at the Sloan-Kettering Institute. They were primarily interested in a possible defense against known cancer-producing agents as indicated by specific changes in cell structure. Small degrees of protection by the use of riboflavin in experimental animals were found, but major differences were not observed. At the Alabama Institute of Technology, now Auburn University, R. W. Engel and D. H. Copeland observed an increased resistance to cancer-like changes resulting from exposure to a specific agent (S-acetylaminofluorene) when rats were fed a complete diet, compared with a deficient diet. The same laboratory observed cancer-like changes in the livers of rats subjected to a chronic deficiency of choline, but the work was interrupted by military enlistment. Unfortunately not enough information in this general field has been developed to clarify the potential significance of initial changes.

Food Practices During Gestation and Lactation and Their Effect on Child Health

Harold C. Stuart and Bertha Burke at Harvard University pioneered in studies of the food practices of mothers and the relationships to their own health and that of the infants. They were later joined by Clement Smith in evaluating their extensive data. The reports indicated that an infant's prospect of having excellent health was four times greater when the mother's diet was good or excellent instead of poor or very poor. The observations were chiefly among low or intermediate income personnel in the Boston area and indicated a high correlation between poor food habits of the mothers and their own health and the incidence of prematurity and illness among their offspring. In a special follow-up study of the health of children born in Holland during severe food deprivation during World War II, Dr. Smith did not find evidence of appreciable permanent damage.

At the Toronto General Hospital, F. F. Tisdall, J. H. Ebbs and W. A. Scott studied the effects of diet supplements during pregnancy for three groups of women (380 total) within a relatively low income range. One group with poor food habits received supplementary food of good nutritional value and a comparable control group continued without change. A third group was following reasonably good food practices and was assisted by an educational pro-

The First Decade

gram. The group whose diets were improved by supplementation and those that continued on good or improved diets with extra education showed better health records than the mothers and infants in the continued-poor-diet group; there were lower death rates and fewer stillbirths, miscarriages or premature births.

In the post-war years there was sufficient progress from education and improved economic conditions among the city population in Toronto to result in no dramatic health gain from distribution of special food supplies to school children or directly to their homes.

Other studies of these questions supported by The Nutrition Foundation were directed by Dr. Icie Macy Hoobler in Detroit, Dr. Nevin Scrimshaw in Rochester, and Dr. William J. Darby in Nashville. These investigations included much larger groups of mothers and infants, and the results generally were in agreement that the detectable relationships between clinical indices of maternal and infant health and nutriture were not apparent above a level of nutrition widely attained by middle income populations in the United States. These findings give added confidence that our intake standards—the Recommended Dietary Allowances—do in fact represent practically attainable levels consistent with good health during the reproductive process.

At the University of Colorado a long-term study under the guidance of Dr. A. A. Washburn was supported on a different basis. The population studied was in a relatively high cultural and middle class economic range and was in frequent communication with the research staff. The study was conducted in great detail in relation to food consumption and to physical and educational development, emotional behavior, changing growth rates, incidence of infection, and mild forms of anemia. Food practices were at a higher level than would be likely to induce any typical deficiency disease—such broadly-based studies of child development, including food practices and health, should assist greatly in the design of more valid standards of growth and development.

Pediatricians and others often have need for reliable reference standards or normal skeletal development. Substantial aid was furnished to Dr. N. L. Hoerr and Miss Idell Pyle at Western Reserve University for completing the RED GRAPH CHARTS initiated by T. Wingate Todd. X-ray prints of skeletal development of the hands, for example, can be remarkably accurate in estimating physiologic age or degree of retarded development in structure and composition. The Foundation supported a similar study by Dr. Hoobler at the Children's Fund of Michigan. The continuing need for better reference standards is still appreciated but the commitments of time and resources required to amass the requisite data discourages most investigators from undertaking the necessary long-term data-gathering and statistical processes.

Comments of Evaluation

In writing to Dr. Compton about the Foundation after ten years of observation as Public Members respectively of the Board of Trustees and the Scientific Advisory Committee, Dr. Parran, Dr. Carmichael and Dr. Nelson expressed their views as follows:

> As a result of your Foundation's activities a large body of scientific knowledge has been developed, many sorely needed scientific personnel have been trained, and through the NUTRITION REVIEWS workers in this field throughout the world have been given ready access to recent scientific accomplishments.
>
> In my view, industry as well as government

A Good Idea

and private philanthropy has an indispensable role to play in the advancement of knowledge. Joint coordinated action, such as is illustrated by the program of The Nutrition Foundation, has proven to be a most effective method to accomplish this purpose. The conception underlying the Foundation has been fully proven to be sound in actual practice.

Thomas Parran, Dean,
Graduate School of Public Health,
University of Pittsburgh (formerly
Surgeon General, U.S. Public Health Service)

We have had many examples in the past of accumulation of wealth and an unselfish donation of many to sponsor worthy causes, but the setting aside of a part of their earnings by members of the food industry for fundamental studies in nutrition sets an example that inspires confidence in the American way of doing things that gives me real satisfaction . . . Extending the opportunities for research in nutrition brings about many developments. The corralling of new and useful knowledge has its impact on agricultural and commercial practices and leads to betterment in our mode of living through an understanding of how to use, in the most practical way, what is available for food for man and domestic animals. Because the food industry is supporting this work it will keep in touch with those discoveries that lead to new and useful practices that can be applied. Progress in the food industry can only come from research of some kind and the progress that is buttressed by research in nutrition is as sound as science itself. The training of scientists to carry on the work is just as important as any research that is being carried on today and the Foundation contributes greatly to such training.

E. M. Nelson
Chief, Division of Nutrition
Federal Security Agency
Food and Drug Administration

The Foundation has made a significant contribution to a more rational use of foods and this, in turn, has laid the foundation for improved health and welfare of all the people . . .

The Nutrition Foundation is a monument to the vision, foresight and public spirit of the leaders of the food industry which I believe to be not only of great value to the industry itself, but of great significance to future progress. It offers an unparalleled opportunity to all food companies to share in a pioneering enterprise which has a truly great potential.

Oliver C. Carmichael, President
The Carnegie Foundation for the
Advancement of Teaching

Summary of Appropriations for Grants-in-Aid

From July 1, 1942 to June 30, 1952

Area I. Human Requirements of Individual Nutrients

Proteins and amino acids	$ 98,800.00
Fats	10,600.00
Vitamins	54,200.00
Minerals	22,200.00
Bone formation	7,500.00
Total, Area I	$193,300.00

Area II. Origin, Function and Measurement of Individual Nutrients

Proteins and amino acids	$335,600.00
Nucleo-proteins and nucleic acids	10,800.00
Carbohydrates	162,800.00
Fats	110,400.00
Minerals	38,900.00

The First Decade

Vitamins	495,750.00
Hormones	15,000.00
Antibiotics	14,000.00
Milk sugar	4,000.00
Total, Area II	$1,187,250.00

Area III. Maternal and Infant Nutrition

Maternal nutrition during reproductive cycle	$ 31,000.00
Nutrients of human milk and cow's milk	19,500.00
Maternal nutrition in relation to infant health	117,000.00
Nutrition of children to maturity	68,000.00
Maternal and infant nutrition in primates	14,000.00
Nutrition and lactation	12,200.00
Congenital malformations	23,600.00
Total, Area III	$285,300.00

Area IV. Public Health Problems in Nutrition

Anemia	$ 73,950.00
Bone formation	21,500.00
Calcium utilization	17,400.00
Cancer	71,400.00
Dental caries	112,500.00
Detection of nutritional deficiencies	47,500.00
Diabetes	50,000.00
Heart and vascular system	86,600.00
Infection	10,800.00
Learning ability	850.00
Liver function	115,800.00
Nutrition and chemotherapy	2,650.00
Nutrition and public health	104,000.00
Nutrition and well-being in animals	14,000.00
Rheumatic fever	8,000.00
Self-selection and appetite	12,500.00
Total, Area IV	$749,450.00

Area V. Education

Administrative practices of state and local nutrition services	$ 3,000.00
Community nutrition education	20,365.00
Conservation of nutrient losses	2,000.00
Food and Nutrition Board, N.R.C. (post-war)	42,500.00
Nutrition education in schools	26,567.00
Post-graduate fellowship fund	17,500.00
Research conferences	29,387.72
Publications:	
Nutrition Reviews	
Current research leaflet	
Monographs	
Related publications	171,814.16
Awards	24,000.00
Total, Area V	$337,133.88

Total Appropriations from July 1, 1942 to June 30, 1952

Basic Research	$2,415,300.00
Educational Projects	337,133.88
Total	$2,752,433.88*

*During World War II an additional $177,790.00 was appropriated for study directly related to the War Emergency.

2

The Second Decade:
Research, Education, Service

MEMBERSHIP growth and support of the Foundation continued into the second decade without major changes in objectives, procedures or personnel. However, ages were creeping up and forced important changes in personnel. Mr. Ole Salthe's death, September 10, 1952, was followed by the appointment of Dr. Horace L. Sipple as Executive Secretary. Dr. Sipple's background included post-doctoral research at the University of Pittsburgh and Cambridge University in England, several years of research in the food industry, and experience in a private foundation in support of research grants and education.

Dr. Compton's death, June 22, 1954, meant replacement of leadership that had been superb in every respect. In addition to his being President of the Massachusetts Institute of Technology and a great scientist called upon by the national government for a vast amount of service, he took a genuine pride in his association with the research, education and public service that leaders in the food industry had established and sustained in accord with his ideals.

Consistently courteous, cheerful, imaginative and forthright in manner, the vigor of his living was forecast during his undergraduate days at Wooster College when he became their all-time football star by winning a hard-fought game with a final drop-kick field goal from the 40 yard line. When his friends mentioned this remarkable feat, his smiling reply was likely to be "The wind was with our team that day."

Dr. Oliver C. Carmichael, then President of the University of Alabama, was elected to succeed Dr. Compton. Mr. Cason Callaway had retired from the vice-chairmanship the previous year and had been succeeded by Dr. Carmichael.

Mr. Morris Sayre retired as Treasurer and was succeeded by Mr. Ernest W. Reid, with continued service by their very competent associate, Holly Callender as Assistant Treasurer. Dr. Franklyn Bliss Snyder, President of Northwestern University, was elected Vice President of the Board.

The following year a third loss befell the Foundation in the death of Mr. George Sloan on May 20, 1955. He took great pride

A Good Idea

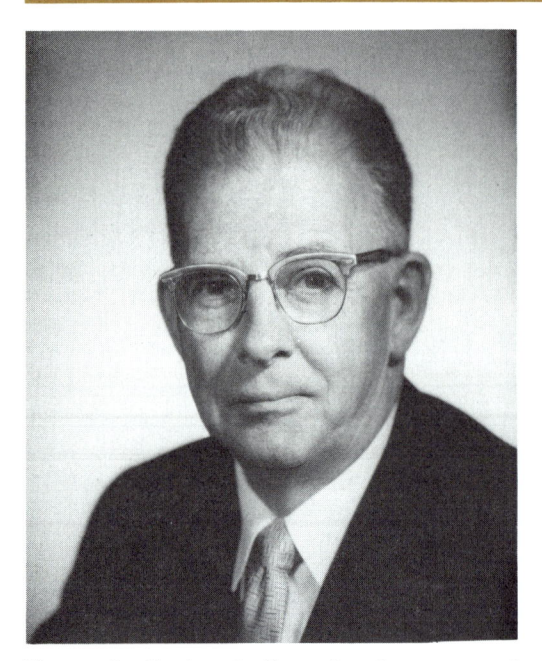

Horace L. Sipple—As Executive Secretary and Treasurer of The Nutrition Foundation over a 20-year period from 1952, Dr. Sipple contributed to all areas of the Foundation's program.

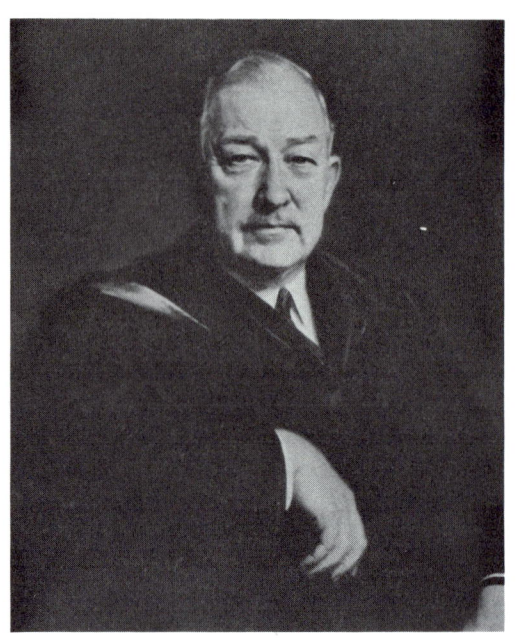

Oliver C. Carmichael—Dr. Carmichael, President of the University of Alabama, succeeded Dr. Compton as Chairman of the Board of Trustees in 1954.

in the growth, objectives and work of the Foundation. His gifts of friendship and ideals of public responsibility by industry made his service with Dr. Compton, the Board of Trustees, and the staff, always constructive. He held a major parallel position as Commissioner of Commerce for New York City and had just been elected President of the International Chamber of Commerce. He also served as President of the Metropolitan Opera Association.

Dr. Carmichael retired as Chairman of the Board in 1956 and we had the good fortune to persuade James R. Killian, Jr., who had succeeded Dr. Compton as President of MIT, to accept the position. Dr. Killian continued to bring to the Foundation those ideals and leadership exemplified by Dr. Compton.

Among the leaders from the food industry whose noteworthy service furthered the program of The Nutrition Foundation were John Holmes of Swift & Company; Charles Mortimer of General Foods; and H. J. Heinz, II of the H. J. Heinz Company, who served terms as President. From 1962, when I became full time President and Scientific Director, strong support and guidance was provided by the successive Chairmen of the Board of Directors: Daniel F. Gerber, President of Gerber Products; W. B. Murphy, President of Campbell Soup Company; A. N. McFarlane, Chairman of Corn Products Company; Lyle C. Roll, President of the Kellogg Company; and James W. Evans, President of American Maize Products Company. Dr. Sipple was advanced to serve as both Executive Secretary and Treasurer of the Foundation.

In 1961 I was elected President and Scientific Director and continued as a member ex-officio of the Board of Directors and the Board of Trustees. The research

The Second Decade

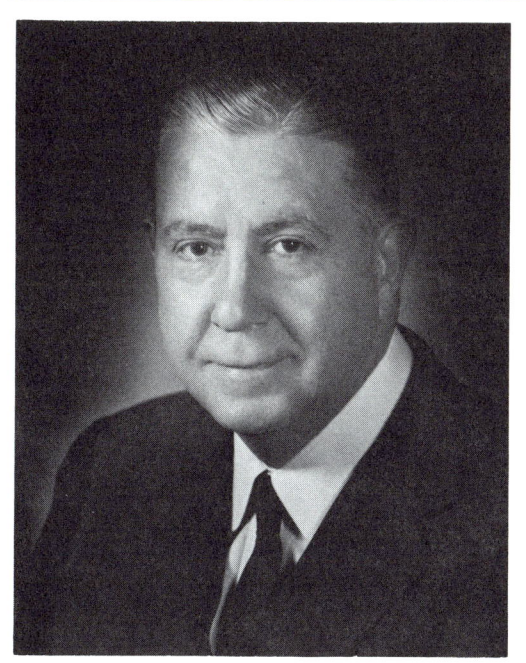

James R. Killian, Jr.—Dr. Killian, President of M.I.T., accepted the Chairmanship of the Board of Trustees in 1956.

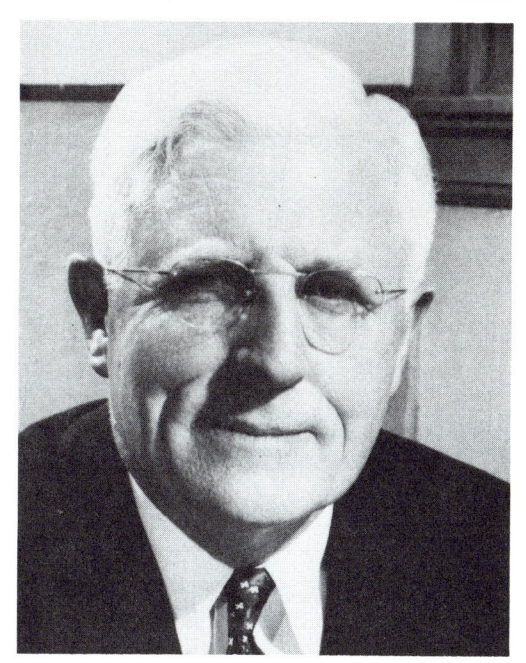

John Holmes—President of Swift and Company, served as President of The Nutrition Foundation, 1956-1957.

and educational programs were adjusted to meet changing emphases, particularly to bring to the public greater practical information concerning foods and their relationship to health, and to recognize the continuing need for support of the most competent young nutrition scientists during their graduate and postdoctorate years.

The Spread of the Good Idea

Other National Foundations

Nutrition scientists and food technologists in Europe often expressed admiration for the action taken by the food industry in establishing The Nutrition Foundation. This was true irrespective of their employment in universities, industry or government agencies. They were particularly impressed when assured of the spirit shown in providing funds to accelerate research on the nutritional problems related to plant or animal fats, cholesterol and health considerations that obviously related to controversies over specific food items such as butter versus margarine. Member companies with operations in Europe encouraged similar action there as a matter of responsibility to the public.

Mr. H. J. Heinz II took the initiative in arranging appointments for me with executives and their scientific advisers in London and later in Stockholm that led to establishing the British Nutrition Foundation and the Swedish Nutrition Foundation, patterned in spirit and in general structure on our experience. A Nutrition Foundation in the Philippines, similar in purpose but with a different structure, was established largely on the basis of R. R. Williams' and J. S. Salcedo's leadership and initial financial support from the Research Corporation.

A Good Idea

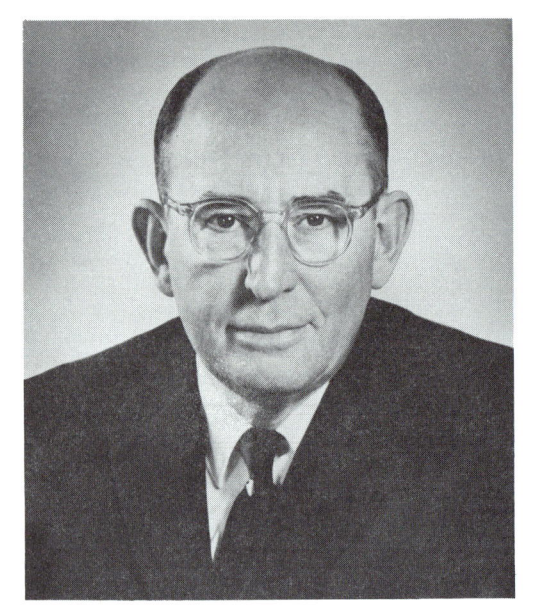

Charles G. Mortimer

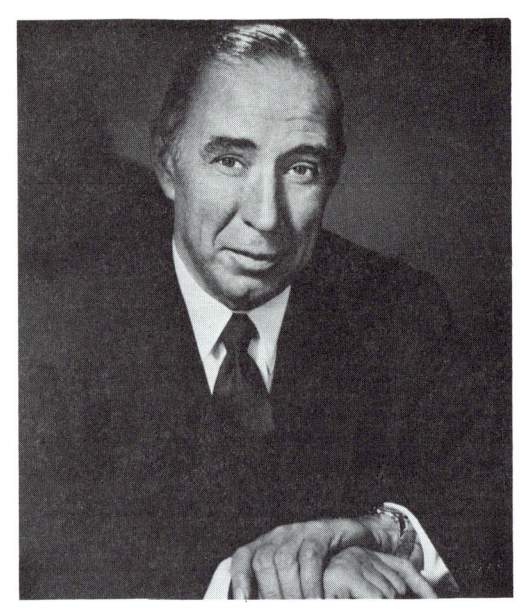

Daniel Gerber

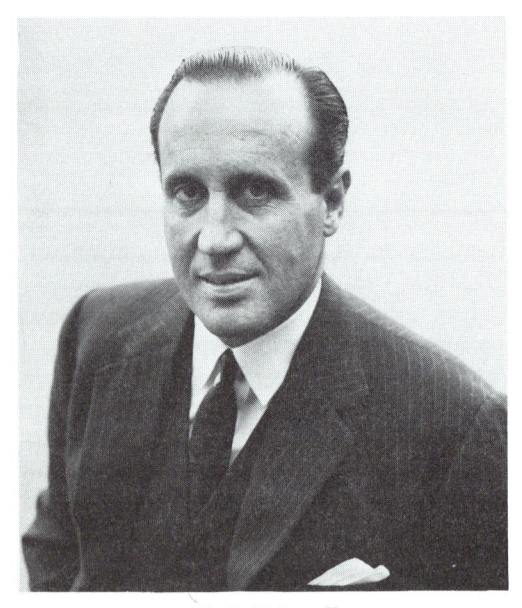

H. J. Heinz, II

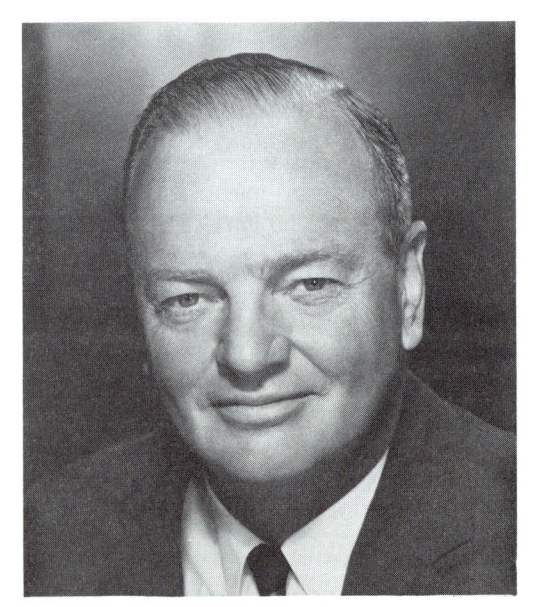

W. B. Murphy

During the latter half of the 1950's and early 1960's the Presidency and Vice Presidency of The Nutrition Foundation rotated among members of the Board of Trustees. The outstanding executives who served as President during that period were: Mr. John Holmes of Swift & Company; Mr. Charles G. Mortimer of General Foods; and Mr. H. J. Heinz, II of H. J. Heinz Company. Mr. Daniel Gerber of Gerber Products and Mr. W. B. Murphy of Campbell Soup were the early Chairmen of the Board of Directors. In 1969-1971 Mr. Murphy chaired the Trustee's Committee on Programming and Staffing.

The Second Decade

International Union of Nutritional Sciences

The International Union of Nutritional Sciences (IUNS) had grown substantially in terms of international congresses, held at three-year intervals since the formal organization was established, as suggested at the London meeting in 1946, followed by formal action at a London meeting in 1948. However, there had been very little organizational activity during the periods between congresses, except through the offices of the President, Dr. E. J. Bigwood in Belgium and the Secretary, Dr. L. J. Harris at Cambridge University. Many of the active scientists recognized this situation and urged action to meet the need for a more vigorous and continuous program.

As a member of the National Academy of Sciences and the Society of Biological Chemists, I was aware of the very constructive work being done by the international unions in chemistry, biology, physics, biochemistry, physiology and other sciences. Soon after Sir David Cuthbertson, Director of the Rowett Institute in Scotland, was elected President of the IUNS at the general assembly meeting in Paris (1957) he asked me to serve as a committee-of-one to prepare recommendations for a revision of the By-Laws along with recommendations for changes in the structure and activities of the organization.

Edmund Rowan in the Foreign Sec-

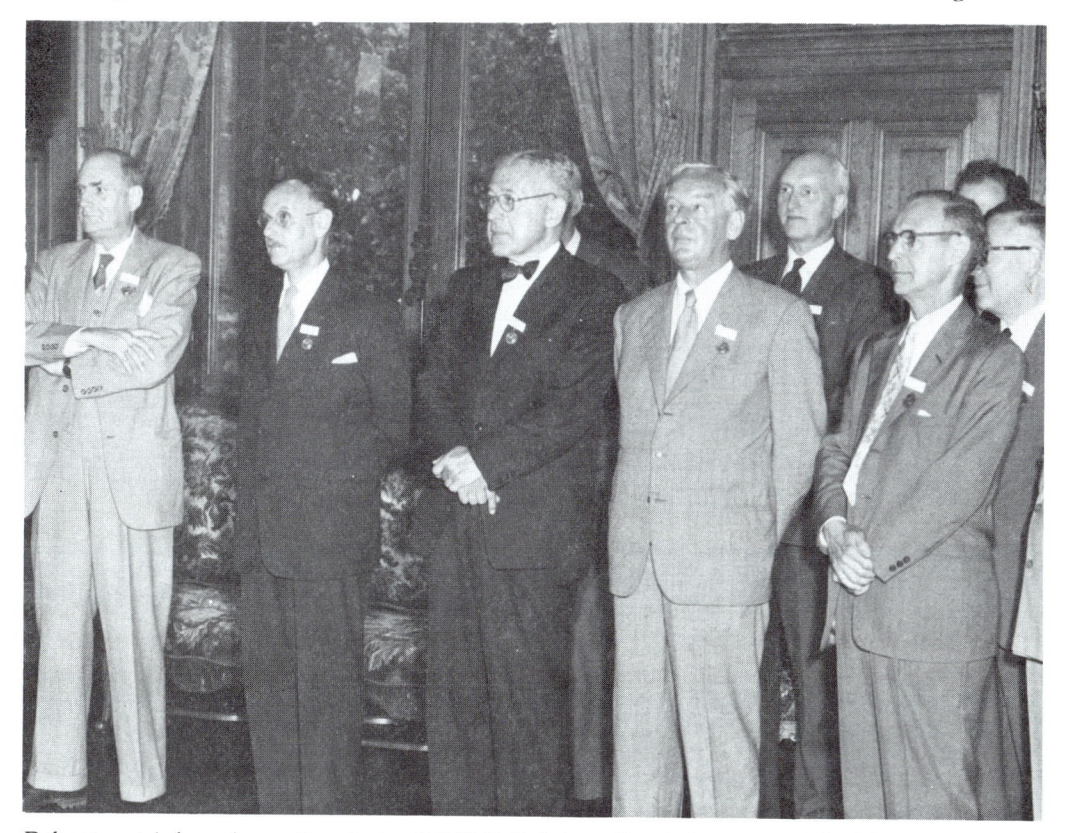

Delegates at informal reception during IUNS Sixth International Congress on Nutrition, Paris, 1963. Left to right: E. J. Bigwood, Leslie J. Harris, Paul György, W. R. Aykroyd, Sir David Cuthbertson, C. G. King.

retary's office at the National Academy of Sciences was most helpful and generous of his time and advice in preparing a report that would reflect the experience and best practices among other international unions. The recommendations were adopted practically *in toto* at the next General Assembly of the IUNS (1960) in Hamburg, and the traditional fate of a committee chairman followed—my election as President of the IUNS, with an implied: "Now make it work!"

Grants from The Nutrition Foundation and the Research Corporation made it possible for me as a Lecturer at the Institute of Nutritional Sciences, School of Public Health, Columbia University, to have essential secretarial and office facilities.

A Council and appropriate officers were proposed within the IUNS to provide broader and more efficient administration. Increased and regular dues were proposed on a scale related to resources available within the national societies.

Working commissions and committees were proposed to study and report on:

I   Nomenclature, Procedures and Standards — A. Frazer, Chairman
   1. Committee on Nomenclature — T. Moore, Chairman
   2. Committee on Protein-Calorie Malnutrition — C. Gopalan, Chairman
   3. Committee on 9th International Congress — S. Zubiran, Chairman
   4. Committee on Food Standards — J. A. Campbell, Chairman
   5. Committee on Recommended Dietary Allowances — W. H. Sebrell, Chairman
   6. Committee on Therapeutic Diets — H. Gounelle, Chairman
   7. Committee on Biological and Clinical Evaluation of Protein Foods — N. S. Scrimshaw, Chairman

II Operational Programs — A. E. Schaefer, Chairman
   1. Committee on the International Biological Program — O. L. Kline, Chairman
   2. Committee on Nutritional Surveys — A. E. Schaefer, Chairman
   3. Committee on Publications — D. L. Duncan, Chairman

III Human Development with Special Reference to the Preschool Child — P. György, Chairman
   1. Physical Development — F. Falkner, Chairman
   2. Functional Development — M. Behar, Chairman
   3. Ecological Factors and Practical Management — D. B. Jelliffe, Chairman

IV Genetic Patterns of Special Nutritional Importance — W. S. Hartroft, Chairman
   1. Diabetes and Cardiovascular Diseases — J. Christopher, Chairman
   2. Endemic Goiter — V. Ramalingaswami, Chairman
   3. Nutritional Anemias — H. Lehman, Chairman

V   Nutrition Education and Training — C. Den Hartog, Chairman
   1. Schools of Medicine — E. Kodicek, Chairman
   2. Schools of Agriculture — A. Bacigalupo, Chairman
   3. Schools of Food Science and Technology — B. Schweigert, Chairman
   4. Schools of Home Economics, Nutrition and Dietetics — E. Empen, Chairman
   5. Schools of Public Health — F. J. Stare, Chairman
   6. Schools of Dentistry — N. L. Eeg-Larsen, Chairman
   7. Schools of Veterinary Science — A. T. Phillipson, Chairman
   8. Graduate Degrees — G. Briggs, Chairman
   9. Schools of Pharmacy — F. Fidanza, Chairman
   10. Education of the Public — L. J. Teply, Chairman

VI Nutrition of Agricultural Animals and Fish — K. L. Blaxter, Chairman (Six committees organized later)

Each committee had an international representation of 6 to 8 members and

The Second Decade

specific assignments for study and reporting in one or more journals with a worldwide circulation, at least one of which would be in the English language, and available for publication in other languages if desired. Most of the committees and commissions have published one or more formal reports based on their studies, except some of those in commission VI which were delayed in activation. However, the committee on the nutritional requirements of fish was particularly active in its work and publications and two others within commission VI published official reports.

Publication of a directory outlining the development of the IUNS and, with the addresses of its active participants, served to facilitate its work and make its significance more readily evident to others.

Developments of this nature in addition to the congresses made it possible for the IUNS to be of greater service and to accelerate both pure and applied research in the science of nutrition. The increased activity also favored the prospect of acceptance as a member of the International Council of Scientific Unions (ICSU), with a representative serving on the ICSU Executive Committee. ICSU provides the major channel through which scientists over the world have a direct liaison with the United Nations Educational, Scientific and Cultural Organization (UNESCO) through their respective international unions. Sixteen international unions had been accepted into membership at that time.

Support of Basic Scientific Advances

Carbohydrates, Fats and Energy

Recognition was steadily growing that cholesterol and some individual fatty acids could be important food constituents in relation to health. These lipids were long recognized as normal constituents of tissues and their synthesis and biochemical functions were subjects of intense research. Their broader nutritional importance was not being examined. Increasingly it was suggested that total dietary fat and specific fat ingredients were associated with major chronic diseases and high death rates in the age range 45 to 65 years, when people should be in their prime for leadership and responsibility. Leaders in the health professions and many laymen realized that the vaunted lengthening of the average life span in the United States, Canada and Western Europe during the last half century had resulted chiefly from improvements during childhood—due to the sanitation of water and milk supplies, early vaccinations, improved infant foods to supplement—but hopefully not to replace—breast feeding, and better drugs to fight infections.

Beyond 45 years of age, little progress had been made in extending life expectancy. Cigarette smoking was being identified as an important contributor to chronic suffering and death from cancer and emphysema, but not the only risk factor. Evidence was pointing strongly to other such factors as excess body fat, too much cholesterol, a special need for polyunsaturated fatty acids, lowered physical fitness resulting from greatly decreased physical work or exercise, and diseases of blood vessels, heart, liver, kidneys, pancreas and brain, in addition to cancer. Examination of tissues of young men killed in the war were reported to reveal a surprisingly high incidence of early changes indicative of future atherosclerosis.

During this era of increasing national affluence most people were free to consume as much food as they liked, including high-calorie, flavorsome fats and sweetstuffs. From infancy to old age excess body fat and diseases associated with it became of public health concern. Severe deficiency diseases such as pellagra, rickets, goiter and scurvy had given way to moderate or slight deficiencies that were potentially significant but not immediate causes of death. Cerebral strokes, heart attacks, hardening of the arteries, liver diseases, kidney failure, diabetes and cancer were the chief killers. There was intense concern about cholesterol and the general area of animal versus plant sources of fats and oils.

Members of the Food Industries Advisory Committee suggested that if the Foundation officers and trustees would welcome the responsibility, they would attempt to raise at least a million dollars above their regular membership payment to support research in this area of the "degenerative" and "metabolic" diseases and the potential role played by food practices, so that they could effectively serve the public in their provision of products and information to best serve the health needs of the nation. They strongly preferred action on this basis instead of a narrow basis of encouraging each company to push for research in which they might have an immediate economic interest. This viewpoint was deeply appreciated, personally, and was heartily welcomed by university personnel, government agencies, the public and the Foundation's Board of Trustees because it avoided any question of bias, lethargy or criticism in planning or reporting on the work urgently needed. The broadly diverse support base of The Nutrition Foundation and its organization assured that the research supported should be objective and in the best of scientific tradition and not self-serving. I knew these men well and was completely confident of their sincerity. The fund did pass the million dollar mark and added substantially to the research and educational program of the Foundation and the nation. Anticipating favorable action, the Scientific Advisory Committee had planned carefully for its most efficient use.

Government agencies were under pressure to regulate in some degree the practices in advertising and labeling, as illustrated on a micro-scale by the baker in Connecticut who put a small bit of vegetable oil in his cake and advertised it with the slogan, "Eat our cake and protect your heart!"

The evidence had long been clear that some, but not all of the simple glyceride types of fats could be derived from starch, common sugars and amino acids, but there were many gaps in the picture of how the intermediate changes occurred and what the relationships might be to slowly developing diseases. The rate of gathering new knowledge of the biosynthesis of complex fats, cholesterol, bile acids and several hormones would not have been possible before the availability of "tagged" atoms of the radioactive or "heavy" isotopes of the elements—especially carbon, hydrogen, oxygen, nitrogen, sulfur and phosphorus.

Starches and Sugars

Much of the basis of today's understanding of diseases related to carbohydrate and sugar metabolism, including diabetes and many "inborn errors of metabolism," was developed during this decade by workers receiving support from The Nutrition Foundation. Using the tagged atoms, Dr. Carl Cori and his associates at Washington University succeeded in separating from living cancer cells, enzyme systems that form a viscous material (hyaluronic acid) that is characteristic of mucous membranes, body fluids, immunizing material and cell surfaces. Similar compounds are currently, in 1976, of intense interest in relation to brain functions, cancer and immunity. Two units in the product were

The Second Decade

derived from glucose and aided in elucidating the total structure. This research group also identified a number of enzymes of key importance in carbohydrate metabolism: one in animal tissue that functions in the formation of glycogen ("animal starch"), another from yeast that controls the formation of an important derivative of glucose, acetyl-glucosamine, and new enzymes that function with vitamin B_6 in the regulation of glucose metabolism, including polymerization of glucose to form chitin, of common occurrence as a covering protective material in the shell of many insects and crustaceans, such as lobsters. Dr. Cori usefully reviewed the role of glucose in normal and diabetic rats and his wife, Dr. Gerti Cori, in a brilliant series of studies, identified the nature of a peculiar genetic disease in which a glucose polymer, analogous to normal glycogen, is formed with an abnormal structure. Dr. P. A. Sant'Agnese at the Columbia Medical Center published a review of five diseases that are characterized by abnormal sugar metabolism that result from genetic peculiarities in a specific enzyme.

H. O. L. Fischer at the University of California synthesized the 4-carbon sugar, D-erythrose, and demonstrated that its phosphate ester was a normal intermediate in the metabolism of glucose in muscle. A similar synthesis and proof of function was shown for a 3-carbon sugar, D-glyceraldehyde. He and H. H. Baer made further contributions by the study and synthesis of a 3-amino sugar present in several antibiotics.

From the University of California (UCLA), J. Brown reported on the biological activity of the glucose derivative, 2-deoxyglucose. This is a constituent of the nucleic acid (DNA) involved in the genetics of all forms of life and constitutes a necessary part of all cell nuclei. Brown also reported that persons prone to obesity nearly always had about twice the concentration of free fatty acids in their blood, compared with normal persons, twelve hours after fasting.

George W. Thorn and A. E. Renold at Harvard reported new evidence on liver and pancreas functions when specific drugs were used in the management of diabetes and continued their studies of the interrelationships of fatty tissue, liver functions and hormones secreted by the pancreas, adrenal and pituitary glands. Both men are now among the world's leading medical scientists in research and education in relation to endocrinology and diabetes.

A. L. Lehninger at Johns Hopkins University traced the sequence of reactions of glucose in forming a series of acids, including ascorbic acid (vitamin C). He was particularly interested in the processes within specific cellular structures (mitochondria) and the role of the hormones, thyroxine and adrenaline, in energy-yielding reactions during the metabolism of sugar fragments.

V. H. Cheldelin at Oregon State College studied the bacterial metabolism of sugars as a means of detecting reaction systems not yet clarified in animal tissues, including intermediate steps in the formation of oxalic acid (a major ingredient in kidney stones) and glutamic acid.

George M. Guest of Cincinnati, although primarily concerned with diabetes, reported observations on a disabling genetic disease, galactosemia, in which the infant cannot utilize the galactose from milk sugar (lactose). As a result, unless milk sugar is replaced promptly by another sugar there is a risk of rapid failure in nerve functions, blindness due to cataract formation, and early death.

H. C. Knowles published in 1960 a resume of observations at the University of Cincinnati, initiated by Dr. Guest and con-

A Good Idea

tinued for many years, in which the dietary management of diabetic children was on a relatively liberal basis and monitored chiefly by observations on fat metabolism instead of sugar, and by very careful examinations of the eyes as an index of tissue injury. It is well known that blindness often develops among diabetics due to injury to either the lens of the eye (cataract) or to damage of the retina.

R. Bentley at the University of Pittsburgh reported on the comparative metabolism of glucose in heart muscle, including analogous reactions in a mold where the steps could be more readily identified.

Fats Become Exciting

The body's continuous expenditure of energy is chiefly dependent on the oxidation of glucose, supplied as starch or sugars, and the oxidation of fatty acids supplied from oils and fats. In addition, amino acids from proteins are partially converted to glucose or fatty acids and normally supply about 10 to 20 per cent of the total calories.

High quality protein foods such as meat, fish, eggs and milk have a high priority in food planning because of their excellent amino acid content, their high content of vitamins and essential minerals, and their attractive flavor. Their market cost in proportion to their yield of calories, however, is generally great.

The body has a great capacity to adapt to differences in the proportion of calories furnished by fats, carbohydrates and protein, but health is seriously jeopardized by a long continued excess or deficiency of total energy intake. On a weight basis fats contribute a caloric yield 2¼ times that of carbohydrates or proteins. Hence they are critically important in controlling the total caloric intake. (The respective values are usually expressed as 9, 4, 4 kilocalories per gram.) Fats also are important as carriers of fat-soluble vitamins A, D, E and K, and at least one fatty acid, linoleic acid, has long been known to be an essential nutrient. Two other fatty acids, linolenic and arachidonic, can be derived from linoleic acid and if supplied in food they spare the needed quantity of linoleic acid.

Arachidonic acid had recently been recognized as of very special importance as the *essential starting substance* to form within the body a series of about 16 important hormones, the prostaglandins. Among these newly identified hormones are regulators of the central nervous system, smooth muscle functions, blood pressure, sex glands, adrenal glands, lungs, membrane permeability, and the release of fatty acids from their storage in adipose tissue. Several of these functions have been identified in man and in experimental animals—and currently, this is one of the most active fields of biological and medical research.

Vitamin B_6 is essential for the conversion of linoleic acid to arachidonic acid, and B_6 deficient animals often store less than 10% of their normal content of essential fatty acids.

The remarkable capacity of the body to adapt its caloric balance and complex functions for survival is illustrated by the extreme of the primitive Eskimo whose diet of fresh, fat meat and fish provides extremely little carbohydrate. This contrasts with common tropical diets which consist chiefly of rice, corn, sorghum or root crops, and fruit, with extremely limited supplements of protein foods or fat. Another striking contrast is provided by a relaxed man spending most of the day dreaming or reading in a hammock or comfortable chair and expending about 2,000 calories per day as compared with a logging camp worker of similar age and weight who may expend 6,000 calories per

The Second Decade

day. Apparently, however, there would be relatively little difference in their vitamin and mineral requirement.

New Biochemical Aspects of Fats in Nutrition

New aspects of the biochemistry of fat metabolism were developed as a consequence of the enhanced interests in the nutritional significance of lipids (fatty material). A. H. Lehninger at Johns Hopkins, E. P. Kennedy and K. Bloch at Harvard and E. H. Stotz at the University of Rochester were particularly active in this area. The scope of interest excited is illustrated by invitations for these grantees to discuss their developments before scholarly groups. For example, Dr. Lehninger was invited to present a review of the reaction systems at a special symposium organized at the National Academy of Sciences and another in the Harvey Lecture Series. He published new data (a) on the conversion of cholesterol to sterol hormones of the adrenals, (b) on the oxidation of fatty acids by the cytochrome system (copper and iron-containing enzymes) and (c) on other studies in which vitamin-containing enzymes were the catalysts. A further series of papers clarified some of the reactions of energy-yielding systems from sugars, fatty acids and amino acids, and reactions by which fatty acids are formed or utilized in heart, liver, kidney, brain and muscle tissues. The respiratory factors in the intracellular particles (mitochondria) were studied extensively, including the sulfur-linked systems and water balances.

At the University of Chicago, and later at Harvard where he succeeded Dr. Hastings as head of biochemistry, E. P. Kennedy was particularly interested in the biological formation of complex fats such as lecithin and other phospholipids in brain, liver and kidney tissue. The research was extended to include comparative studies with bacteriological systems. His studies contributed to understanding of the transport of fats in the bloodstream, lipid passage through membranes, blood clot regulation and fatty deposits in the arteries.

Assistance was also given to the New York City area studies relative to diet and cardiovascular health conducted by Drs. Norman Jolliffe, George Christakis and their associates. Gradually there was general acceptance of the view that (1) excess storage of body fat is a serious deterrent to health, whether resulting from eating fatty foods, carbohydrates, or an excess of calories from all sources; (2) moderate consumption of cholesterol in foods normally could be adjusted by lesser synthesis within the body, but that elevated concentration in the blood above normal values (from any sources) was an indication of an increased health risk; (3) increased blood fat as measured by centrifuging and separation into specific layers could often identify an unfavorable trend; (4) specific provision should be made to include linoleic and linolenic acids in the diet and to avoid an excessive dietary ratio of the high-melting saturated fats to the polyunsaturated fats (special interest also developed in relation to the length of fatty acids, in addition to their degree of saturation); and (5) specific provision should be made for an adequate intake of the fat-soluble vitamins, A, D, E and K, although K is often supplied adequately by intestinal biosynthesis.

E. H. Ahrens, Jr. and his associates at the Rockefeller Institute developed an outstanding research program in studies of fat metabolism in adult human subjects. Known quantities of different fatty acids were fed to evaluate their effects on both the fatty acids and cholesterol in the blood stream, through long enough periods and control of energy output to provide an indication of permanent effects. They also made a critical study and adaptation of the newly developed gas-liquid chromatographic methods of separation and analysis of individual fatty compounds from extremely small quantities of blood, milk or other biological material. Their contribution to other research laboratories in this respect alone was of great assistance. They prepared a special report covering the respective details in the new, revolutionary methods of analysis and permitted it to be printed and distributed free to other investigators as a special 30 page supplement (August 1959) of NUTRITION REVIEWS. His laboratory became an important training center for other groups.

Further advances in the analysis of fats and their metabolic products, such as bile acids and cholesterol, in relation to liver function were developed extensively by Grace Goldsmith's group at Tulane University, E. H. Mosbach at Columbia University, F. J. Stare at Harvard and S. R. Lipsky at Yale University.

Electron microscopic studies by W. J. S. Still and R. M. O'Neal at Washington University indicated that the initial stage of arterial injury was marked by the penetration of fat-filled cells characteristic of those carried in the bloodstream.

As the close of the second decade of The Nutrition Foundation approached, consolidation of the new research findings began. During 1961, Grace Goldsmith, F. J. Stare, W. S. Hartroft, T. B. Van Itallie and R. E. Olson published in different journals critical reviews of current information on dietary relationships of fat metabolism to atherosclerosis, cholesterol accumulation, blood pressure and other aspects of health. Publication of the Proceedings of the Fifth International Congress on Nutrition provided a comprehensive review of worldwide research on fats and its interpretation by leading scientists. Conferences were arranged by The Nutrition Foundation each year at which the leading academic and government scientists could discuss areas of progress with members of the Food Industries Advisory Committee. The Food and Nutrition Board was assisted also in maintaining an active forum on the related problems. Thus the nutritional importance of lipids in nutrition, in food technology and in relation to health was substantially advanced by the special funds provided by industry to The Nutrition Foundation for support of basic research in universities.

Vitamins in the Second Decade

Grace Goldsmith and her associates at Tulane University were very active in vitamin research, particularly in relation to the vitamin B group. They made basic contributions to knowledge of the requirements of nicotinic acid, the conversion of tryptophan to niacin, and the availability of niacin from corn. The long-debated question of whether lime water as used by the Latin American Indians in preparing corn meal masa for tortillas increased the availability of niacin was studied more carefully in man than had been done previously. The conclusion was that the effect, if any, was small, although there was an obvious gain in both flavor and calcium intake.

The Tulane group was also in the forefront of work on the intrinsic factor in pernicious anemia. Early in their clinical studies they documented that in normal persons or patients with pernicious anemia, the quantity of vitamin B_{12} required to produce a rise in the blood concentration or urinary excretion was about 300 times greater when given orally than when given by injection. A direct test of the capacity of blood proteins to combine with the vitamin was a useful confirmatory indication of pernicious anemia. Failure of the stomach to secrete the carrier protein (intrinsic factor) necessary for absorption

The Second Decade

of the vitamin was well recognized. They contributed to the wide recognition that an excessive intake of folic acid could interfere with a diagnosis of vitamin B_{12} deficiency and thereby permit irreparable neurologic damage to occur. This was an illustration that misuse of packaged vitamins by poorly informed laymen, excessive dosage levels of over-the-counter preparations, or improper diagnosis and treatment of anemia by physicians can be injurious.

Estimates of a practical recommended dietary intake of vitamin B_{12} were investigated at Vanderbilt University by Dr. W. J. Darby and his associates. From studies of requirements of B_{12}-depleted patients with pernicious anemia, the maintenance needs of patients, the vitamin B_{12} turnover in man, and the absorption of isotopically labeled vitamins added to foods, this group concluded that normal adults can absorb at least 5 μg of B_{12} daily from a diet that contains 5-15 μg; there is an obligatory loss rate of 0.1 percent daily of the body pool; the physiologic body pool can be estimated at 2-5 mg. of B_{12}. The minimal daily requirement adequate to maintain health and normal storage levels was reasoned to be 3 to 5 μg daily. They also observed some age-related decreased ability to absorb vitamin B_{12}. Studies of the vitamin B_{12} content of diets, even relatively poor ones, indicated that such levels were attained readily when the diet contained minimal needed amount of products of animal origin, such as lean or organ meats. Their estimates of allowances were in keeping with their earlier quantitative information derived from maintenance requirements of patients with pernicious anemia.

Research by the clinical group at the University of Cincinnati with R. W. Vilter also contributed to understanding the functions and practical use of folic acid and vitamin B_{12}. Although initial changes in blood cells are similar for both vitamins, B_{12} deficiency differs in that it may lead to neurological injury. These authors reported that in normal persons 0.7 microgram of vitamin B_{12} per day was fully protective over a period of six or seven years against the signs of deficiency associated with pernicious anemia. In contrast, only three among 36 patients with apparent pernicious anemia were protected against relapse and deterioration in health when they were given folic acid alone. Nearly all of the remaining members of the test group showed recurrence of pernicious anemia in less than four years.

In summarizing their experience over several years, Dr. Vilter reported that the most frequently encountered anemia was that of iron deficiency induced by excessive blood loss instead of dietary deficiencies. He emphasized the risks involved in self-medication or reliance on superficial guidance from sales promotion sources, such as advertisements, radio talks, "health foods," television programs or door-to-door salesmen. Since a failure to absorb vitamin B_{12} taken by mouth instead of a deficiency in the diet is the cause of pernicious anemia, medical care is critically required in the diagnosis and management of each patient.

In animal tests Cecile H. Edwards at the Tuskegee Institute observed during vitamin B_{12} deficiency a rapid decrease in liver enzymes containing niacin, riboflavin and molybdenum. Studies by J. M. Buchanan demonstrated the catalytic role of B_{12} in the synthesis of the amino acid, methionine. In feeding tests with farm animals at Washington State College, J. McGinnis found that added vitamin B_{12} permitted more rapid growth when the feed was based on soybeans or casein for protein, but not when weanling pigs were reared normally with sows receiving farm rations.

The metabolic importance of B-complex

A Good Idea

vitamins in the nervous system was further reflected in studies by J. Brozek, University of Minnesota. Intermediate degrees of vitamin B₁ (thiamin) deficiency in young men were introduced under controlled conditions. The schedule was (a) one month of preliminary standardization, (b) 168 days of partial restriction, (c) 15 to 27 days of complete deprivation, and (d) a final period of 21 days when 5 milligrams of thiamin were supplied daily during recovery. An intake of 0.2 mg. of thiamin per 1,000 calories was the approximate margin at which measurable deficiency could be identified on the basis of sensory or motor functions. During acute deficiency, such evidence was observed within a few days or weeks. Depleted subjects given a supplement of 5 mg. of thiamin per day evidenced improvement in physical performance within a few days, but recovery of peripheral nerve damage was much slower. One depleted subject exhibited a peculiar walking gait, even after several months of restored vitamin intake. These observations were of special value in understanding comparable experience of our prisoners of war returning from the Pacific area.

Research on vitamin B₂ (riboflavin) in rats by O. H. Lowry and H. Burch at Washington University included measurement of normal storage of activity of specific enzymes in heart, liver, kidney and brain tissue, in relation to variation in intake. Confirmation of the relationships by clinical observations was published soon afterward from areas in Latin America where deficiencies were exceedingly common.

Other investigations of vitamin B₂ intake by children in middle class circumstances living in the Denver area were undertaken by V. A. Beal and J. J. Buskirk. Nearly all children were found to have an adequate intake of the vitamin in their regular food supply without the use of supplements. There were wide variations in the storage of the vitamin in red blood cells, however, and infants generally showed greater storage than older children.

In clinical investigations by Ancel Keys and his associates at the University of Minneapolis, hard physical work did not cause significantly increased losses of vitamin B₂ from body storage. However, during a three day period of acute starvation and hard physical work there was, under sedentary conditions, a three-fold increase in the rate of excretion and a five-fold increase within a seven day period. Exposure to high temperatures and humidity for 10 hours per day for six days caused about 50 per cent increased excretion of the vitamin.

B. S. Wostmann at Notre Dame University compared the vitamin B₁, pantothenic acid, B₆, A, carotene and B₂ requirements by rats in normal and in germ-free environments, as an indication of availability without the usual interference by intestinal microorganisms. The relative stability when foods were treated by intense irradiation was found to be in the sequence just listed.

Interesting relationships of chronic vitamin B₆ deficiency to deposits of oxalates in rat kidney stones were reported by S. B. Andrus, S. N. Gershoff and associates at Harvard University. Chronic vitamin B₆ deficiency and supplementary feeding of glycine markedly increased the rate of stone deposition in the kidneys and adjacent structures of the urinary tract. Within six weeks the test animals showed conspicuous evidence of the oxalate deposits. The workers estimated that about one-third to one-half of human kidney and urinary tract stones are of similar composition—chiefly calcium oxalate. No stone deposits occurred in the control group on

The Second Decade

the same diet plus a normal supply of the vitamin. Within seven weeks of deprivation, only one out of eight showed stone formation in the group without added glycine. There has been little direct evidence that the above relationships pertain in human experience. A study of school children in Boston indicated some correlation.

Personnel supported to study nutrition and dental disease included H. D. Moon at the University of California (San Francisco). He and his collaborators carefully investigated vitamin B_6 deficiency in relation to oral and arterial lesions in monkeys. A marked increase in the incidence of tooth decay resulted from prolonged deficiency even though the rhesus monkey is not highly sensitive to dental caries when the diet is adequate in vitamin B_6. Deformed, shortened, stunted teeth were frequently observed in deficient animals. Whether a similar relationship would hold in man was not decided; few people would be likely to have an intake as low as that studied. There is little information concerning the intake of vitamin B_6 in children. It has been observed, however, that the amount in milk that has been heated for sterilization is very low and continued intake may result in convulsive seizures. Care to protect commercial supplies has been taken by enrichment before sterilization.

G. A. Emerson and her associates at the University of California (Los Angeles) also studied the relationship of vitamin B_6 deficiency to tooth decay and atherosclerosis in monkeys. They considered an intake of 2 mg. per day necessary for normal growth and apparent health. Intakes in the range of 0.1 to 1.0 mg. per day resulted in poor growth, loss of hair, and disturbed walking gait; intakes less than 1 mg. also resulted in convulsions. L. D. Greenberg at the University of California (San Francisco) also studied the effect of restricted intake of vitamin B_6 in rhesus monkeys and found that beyond a depletion period of 16 months there was extensive tooth decay, poorly formed teeth, and gross injury to the gums.

Discovery that vitamin C was necessary for normal metabolism of the amino acid tyrosine, in guinea pigs, was followed by demonstration of a similar relationship in human infants and adults. Later, massive doses of folic acid were found partially to correct the tyrosine defect in C deficiency. Studies of the vitamin C/folic acid relationship by W. J. Darby and his associates showed that both vitamin C and folic acid influenced tyrosine metabolism in the guinea pig, but that the folate effect was probably indirect. Later work confirmed this even in a broader sense—that vitamin C is essential to formation of the protein enzyme that catalyzes the metabolism of tyrosine and numerous other biological materials, including lysine and proline in the formation of collagen.

In association with others in our group at Columbia University, J. J. Burns studied ascorbic acid metabolism in guinea pigs and rats. He prepared the vitamin labeled with radio-carbon so that its distribution and conversion to other products could be followed. Most nerve depressants and many carcinogenic agents greatly stimulate the synthesis and excretion of vitamin C, extending the early findings at the University of Pittsburgh in relation to the nerve depressants. Dr. Burns continued in this type of research and in related fields at New York University and the National Institutes of Health with an outstanding record. He is now Vice President for Research at Hoffmann-LaRoche, Inc., past-president of the American Society for Pharmacology and Experimental Therapeutics and a member of the National Academy of Sciences. The company in 1973 completed a new, completely enclosed,

A Good Idea

automatically controlled plant costing more than $65,000,000, with an annual production capacity of more than 10,000 tons of vitamin C. The effluent from the plant is purified to the quality that rainbow trout thrive in it continually. A large part of the output of ascorbic acid is consumed by the food and feed industries to improve or conserve the nutritive value, stability, color, safety and other qualities of many major products — particularly food products. This type of usage greatly exceeds the quantity used in direct marketing as a vitamin or vitamin mixture as in drug store channels, even after the claims made for huge intakes to prevent or lessen the severity of colds.

R. R. Becker, H. H. Horowitz and their associates in our Columbia laboratory proved that in rats (not subject to scurvy) ascorbic acid is normally formed from glucose, via glucuronic acid. The vitamin then serves as a regulating agent in cellular oxidation, protein synthesis, membrane functions and many other roles, including an effect on cholesterol metabolism. N. F. Barr, E. R. Gaden and others collaborated in studies of ascorbic acid oxidation during radiation as proposed for food processing, and suggested an intermediate formation of mono-dehydroascorbic acid as a free radical in the reaction. This was later proved experimentally as characteristic also of enzymic oxidations in which the vitamin has a role. Vitamins A, E and K are also very sensitive to destruction during radiation.

The oxidative loss of vitamin C in foods and other biological materials on exposure to the air results largely from catalysis by copper in (a) active combinations with proteins that are true enzymes, (b) less active, non-specific combinations of copper with protein, and (c) copper in ionic form as a dissolved salt. C. R. Dawson and his students at Columbia University clarified the contrasts in behavior of specific forms of copper containing enzymes.

Based on several years of investigation, R. E. Lee at Cornell University published findings on the reported effect of rutin, hesperidin and other flavonoids on the blood vessels and nutritive state of experimental animals (guinea pigs and rats). The flavonoid substances exerted no apparent effect on spontaneous or induced hemorrhages in rats or guinea pigs under the conditions of observation, and there was no evidence that the flavonoids influence the requirement for vitamin C or otherwise serve as vitamins. "Neither gross signs of dietary deficiency nor any peripheral vascular phenomena were found that could be explained by a lack of rutin or hesperidin in the diet, or corrected by their supplementation." This work confirmed and extended the evidence that the flavonoids are *not* essential nutrients and should not be referred to as vitamins, even though they are often promoted for sale as such. Tests at the University of Wisconsin were in agreement with this conclusion and assisted in decreasing misleading advertising and claims for such products.

An improved method of measuring vitamin K was developed by R. H. Barnes and his associates at Cornell University. One microgram of the vitamin per 100 g. body weight was found to be sufficient for complete protection of blood clotting tissue in rats.

Chemical identification of vitamin C had permitted extensive metabolic research from a biochemical viewpoint and good methods of analysis quickly followed. These were based chiefly upon its reaction with a dye in acid solution. However, improvements were made to give more precise information. An important one was by J. H. Roe at George Washington University. It included measurement of the vitamin in its normal form (ascorbic acid), in a partially oxidized form (dehydroascorbic acid), and a third (inactive) product when oxidized irreversibly, as may happen quickly in many food products.

H. A. Lardy at the University of Wisconsin studied the potential effect of an excess of thyroid gland activity in relation to vitamin C requirements and demonstrated that an excess of thyroid hormone measurably increased the requirement for the vitamin. This relationship was confirmed in our laboratory at Columbia University and was of special interest, analogous to the well known increase in vitamin B_1 requirement in hyperthyroidism.

Research on Proteins and Amino Acids

Looking into the swollen face and blind eyes of a small child broken in health and handicapped for life by a deficiency of vitamin A and good quality protein food gives a different impression than looking at a package label or a booklet on food composition. If the child is beside 50 others *in a similar condition* in a pediatric ward, the picture is remembered for a long time—it translates protein and vitamin research into human values.

The word "protein," coined originally to imply "of first importance in living organisms," is well merited. And a high nutritional rating of protein foods is doubly justified because they are nearly always excellent sources of water-soluble vitamins and essential minerals. For a total diet, however, even protein foodstuffs may have specific limitations. Milk, for example, is one of the best protein sources and it carries vitamin A, but it is low in iron and copper; lean meats are high in iron and copper, but are low in calcium and vitamin C; and eggs, with the highest score for protein quality, are high in cholesterol. All three are without fiber, which may not be essential but is widely regarded as valuable in relation to motility of the large intestine and colon. Nevertheless they are all excellent foods around which to build a good meal.

Hence, it is a good practice to center attention at each meal, or at least for two meals per day, on a main course with a high quality protein food, accompanied by a cereal, one or two vegetables and fruit, with total calories adjusted to actual need. The problem of calories then becomes primarily a matter of experience in the size of portions consumed to maintain body weight in an ideal range.

As the need to restrict the cost of food increases, a common tendency is to shift toward cereals and root crops that are high in carbohydrates and relatively low in protein and fat and that will satisfy the sense of hunger or satisfy the sheer enjoyment of eating in terms of sweet goods. Pampered children and indulgent adults display a similar tendency regardless of cost, a tendency to select large portions of high-calorie desserts, snacks on a "sweet"-only basis, only tea or coffee for "breakfast," and excessive use of high calorie drinks—soft or alcoholic—between meals. Research in nutrition is steadily furnishing needed information on protein food requirements and the interplay between proteins and all other nutrients in relation to health.

The critical importance of adequate good quality protein foods during pregnancy, lactation and early child development is very evident. Educational measures to guide the public and the food industry are urgently needed, especially in areas with high population density and low economic status. Agricultural and food policies, nationally and worldwide, are increasingly under pressure to make high quality protein foods available at minimum costs to the public. Increased efficiency in feeding animals (including fish) is an important part of the overall need to supply animal-

A Good Idea

source protein foods. Progress is encouraging in regard to genetically improved grains as illustrated especially well by The Rockefeller Foundation program and similar efforts. There is, however, an urgent need for similar programs on legumes, and these are getting underway in a promising manner. The kinds of crop improvement developed by The Rockefeller Foundation and assisted in applications by The Ford Foundation in Latin America, the Philippines, Colombia, India, Southeast Asia and Africa have been particularly successful. A substantial beginning has been made in relation to both cereals and legumes in the above areas.

Responding to urgent demands and technical guidance from the Protein Advisory Group, the United Nations organizations and finally the World Bank are undertaking support of long-range programs to build up food production to meet human needs in the most critical areas of the world. The need is urgent and will require sustained support on a large scale, and with very competent management.

Beyond the problems of protein food deficiencies in the technologically advanced countries, the urgency for progress on behalf of millions of children in less advantaged parts of the world is a powerful incentive. Research that is basic helps not only in areas where malnutrition is severe; it also guides the efficient production, processing, distribution and satisfying use of high quality foods everywhere; it assists the medical profession in the care of sick patients, infants, the aged and all with whom they counsel to safeguard health.

As a consultant to the United Nations Children's Fund and the World Health Organization and experience with the Protein Advisory Group that serves to coordinate their programs with the Food and Agriculture Organization, it was possible to coordinate The Nutrition Foundation's modest research and educational activities with other parts of the world. These opportunities were further augmented by continuous participation in the work of the International Union of Nutritional Sciences and the Food and Nutrition Board of the National Academy of Sciences-National Research Council.

A good illustration of the above type of cooperation was our appeal to the Rockefeller Foundation for a research grant via the Food and Nutrition Board to permit that Board's committee to develop jointly with the U.N. Protein Advisory Group a worldwide research program specifically directed to attack practical problems of protein deficiency among mothers and children in the developing countries where conditions were most severe. James M. Hundley, with extensive experience in clinical nutrition (now president of the American Heart Association), served full-time in coordinating the program and assisting in programs within each area. At the close of the project, an international conference chaired by W. H. Sebrell, Jr. was held in Washington, D.C. to review progress and make recommendations for continued and increased action.

During the period 1954-1956, Dr. Rose completed publication of his sixteen classical journal publications on "The Amino Acid Requirements of Man." The studies were based on young adult men, but the basic pattern could be extended to include approximate values for others under varying circumstances of age and environment.

Greatly aided and stimulated by the availability of such basic information on amino acid requirements of man and animals, the emphasis among research groups shifted toward exploration of the biological functions of the amino acids and their relationship to health. Meanwhile the techniques of amino acid analysis and the availability of isotopes of carbon, hydro-

The Second Decade

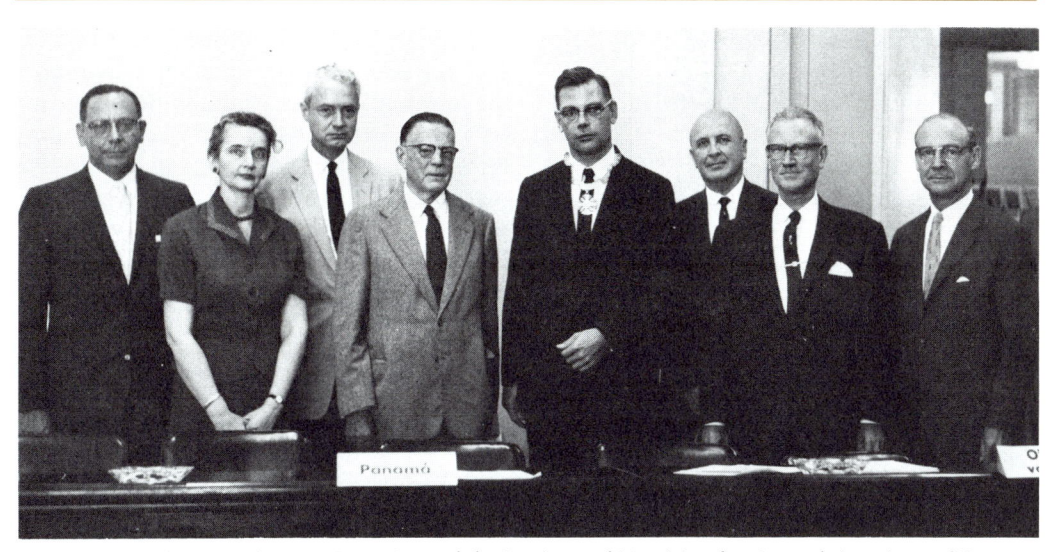

Meeting of Technical Advisory Committee of the Institute of Nutrition for Central America and Panama (INCAP, 1961).

Left to right: *Allwood Parades, Bertlyn Bosley, William J. Darby, John Gordon, Nevin S. Scrimshaw, W. H. Sebrell, Jr., Peña Cheverras, C. G. King. Dr. Scrimshaw has just received a decoration from the Government of Guatemala in recognition of his great service and leadership.*

gen, nitrogen, oxygen and sulfur had revolutionized the tools with which scientists could study the biological functions of amino acids and related proteins. These advances were also tools in solving the practical problems in food science and technology.

One of the world's most productive research and training centers in the attack on chronic and severe protein deficiency was initiated and developed in Guatemala City under the leadership of Nevin S. Scrimshaw, subsequent to advanced training at Harvard University (Ph.D) and the University of Rochester (M.D.) where his research on maternal and child health was assisted by the Foundation. His policy in Guatemala was to restrict staff appointments to young people whose home background had been in Central America. As they proved their merit in terms of capacity, integrity and quality of performance, they were supported by fellowships for advanced training in the United States.

The Institute of Nutrition of Central America and Panama (INCAP) was established in 1949 as a cooperative project for the six countries, under the administration of the Pan American Health Organization, and was given substantial assistance by the W. K. Kellogg Foundation. Funds from The Nutrition Foundation were used chiefly for fellowship support and related activities. For example, Moises Behar, with fellowship support from The Nutrition Foundation, concluded a valuable post doctorate training period in the U.S.

Deficiencies of iodine, iron, fluorine and vitamin A were common in the area, but the most severe and damaging deficiency, and the one most difficult to correct, was the lack of good quality protein foods in rural areas and villages. A high percentage of the children were passed from weaning and insufficient food to a monotonous diet based chiefly on tortillas ("pancakes" made from lime-water-soaked ground corn), supplemented by limited supplies of

A Good Idea

boiled beans. Gradually, for those who survived through periods of permanently stunted growth and development, there would be limited supplements of coffee, fruits and vegetables.

In addition to a vigorous educational program to reach professional and administrative personnel with information about conditions among low income segments of the population, research at INCAP included practical measures for improvement in the choice of foods and the use of mixtures of locally produced foods, as in the combination meal, Incaparina. Initially this product consisted of a mixture of corn meal with cottonseed meal, yeast, calcium carbonate, soybean and green leaf meal. Increased efficiency in feeding chickens and pigs was also developed to obtain animal protein foods. The emphasis on good quality legumes served as a sound basis for later and parallel work in the extensive development of Mother Craft Centers that have been remarkably successful in Haiti, the Philippines and other areas. Major support was provided by the Research Corporation, WHO, and others, including The Nutrition Foundation.

Research was very active in developing techniques of identifying degrees of protein deficiency through the complete range from mild deficiency identified by detailed blood or urine analysis, to fully developed kwashiorkor "characterized by retarded growth, edema (swelling), diarrhea, skin changes, hair changes, low blood protein and enzyme content, gross apathy, fatty or cirrhotic liver, atrophy of the intestinal wall and pancreas, lowered resistance to infection, and atrophy of glandular tissues."

The most damaging period of high death rates, irreversible injury to the brain, and permanent stunting in body growth follows the decrease in breast milk consumption, and the weaning of the child onto a diet consisting chiefly of corn meal, tapioca root, crude sugar or other food markedly low in good quality protein and other nutrients normally associated with good protein, as in meat, fish, eggs and milk—or marginally in beans, peas and nuts. Often there is a period of partial starvation in terms of calories (marasmus) as a result of decreased milk supply even earlier. A low intake of vitamin A, which is often a major problem in protein deficient areas, decreases the body's capacity to synthesize protein essential to body functions. Conversely, protein deficiency impairs the transport of vitamin A, i.e., it restricts the synthesis of the vitamin A-binding protein that carries vitamin A in the blood plasma. Special studies also included contrasts in changes induced chiefly by caloric deficiency (marasmus) with changes caused chiefly by protein deficiency (kwashiorkor). Drs. M. Behar, G. Arroyave, F. Viteri, C. Tejada and J. Mendez were among the very active collaborators in the INCAP program, and those young scientists' development was made possible by the agencies that supported INCAP.

When Dr. Scrimshaw accepted a position as head of the newly organized Department of Nutrition and Food Sciences at Massachusetts Institute of Technology in 1961, Moises Behar succeeded him as Director at INCAP. Dr. Behar is now Director of the WHO Nutrition Section at WHO headquarters in Geneva, and Dr. C. Tejada has assumed the Directorship of INCAP.

Dr. Joaquin Cravioto gave important assistance at INCAP during the period when studies were being initiated in relation to impairment of the central nervous system in small children as a result of severe protein food deficiency. Later he resumed his work in Mexico City. In this new approach to a worldwide problem of so great importance, it was gratifying to see excellent co-

The Second Decade

operation between private foundations and government agencies that recognized the need for intensive and competent investigation.

J. J. Vitale with the Harvard group in cooperation with A. Pradilla and members of his staff in Cali, Colombia, observed a frequent association of kwashiorkor and folic acid deficiency with characteristic changes in red blood cells, in the areas adjacent to Cali. Recovery was accomplished rapidly on a diet of skim milk supplemented by folic acid.

A. E. Harper of Wisconsin and others were especially active in studies of the effects of imbalances in supplying the total amino acid intake, either as pure amino acids or as furnished in proteins of different composition in foods and feeds. The relationships to total caloric intake were important as noted originally by them in relation to pellagra and the tryptophan and niacin balance. Dr. Rose's work on adult human requirements also illustrated the marked interdependence of amino acids and total caloric requirements.

When offered mixed diets on a multiple choice basis, with or without a balanced content of amino acids, rats quickly learned by appetite control to select the most favorable ratios. The time factor in showing effects on appetite control and on tissue enzyme activity is quite varied for different amino acids but it was surprising to discover that a difference is often evident within a few hours. More recent work shows that the signals start reaching the brain (and thence, the urge to eat) as soon as the ingested food reaches the small intestine. A poor balance of amino acids tends temporarily to decrease appetite.

A general conclusion was drawn from these studies that for rats, and perhaps for people, a protein intake of good quality is optimal within the range of 10 to 20 percent of total calories.

Important research closely related to the Wisconsin studies was developed by J. B. Allison at Rutgers University. In rats, a specific imbalance or deficiency became evident within a few hours in the enzyme activity of muscle, kidney and spleen tissue. The heart muscle and brain were most resistant to such changes.

Dr. Goldsmith at Tulane University completed studies that resulted in the Food and Nutrition Board recommending that 60 mg. of tryptophan should be accepted as equivalent to 1 mg. of the vitamin, niacin, in human diets.

Dr. Paul György at the University of Pennsylvania and L. E. Holt, Jr. at New York University were particularly interested in the optimum protein intake for infants and small children. This area of research is of crucial importance in relation both to regions where deficiencies are severe and in the most advantaged countries because of the rapidly increasing use of formula feeding instead of breast feeding. The protein content of human milk is superior in quality to the protein in cows' milk for infant feeding. The proportion of protein to milk fat and milk sugar is also lower in human milk. Other ingredients in human milk are beneficial in terms of intestinal flora and resistance to some diseases. Both Drs. György and Holt convincingly argued the superior nutritive value of breast milk, particularly for the first few or several months.

G. F. Wilgram at the University of Toronto concluded from extensive studies of the essential amino acid methionine and its partial conversion to choline that "normal mixed diets supply adequate amounts of choline or its precursors. The therapeutic use of extra dietary choline does not seem to be warranted on physiologic grounds." This report was a much needed warning against wasteful practices that might be promoted for the needless use of choline and the related risk of excessive intake.

J. S. Fruton at Yale University and J. L. Wood with S. L. Cooley at the University of Tennessee observed that in many instances peptide combinations of nonessential amino acids were more efficient in supplementing the essential amino acids than when fed as separate free acids. In practical feeding this relationship appeared to have considerable advantage and a favorable consideration in the appropriate use of gelatin.

Another finding of practical significance was the tendency for lysine to react with reducing sugars and similar products in foods when heated, thus reducing its nutritive value in protein foods when heated during cooking or commercial processing. Studies of this so-called Browning reaction by A. R. Patton at the Colorado Agricultural and Mechanical College included an improved method of measuring the changes that result from heating. The reaction is characteristic of the "browning" color change in toast, cakes and other cereal products—associated often (unfortunately) with improved flavor. The current personal research of Dr. C. O. Chichester, as Vice President of The Nutrition Foundation since 1972, has now much elaborated the nutritional significance of the products of the browning reaction.

At the University of California in Los Angeles, M. S. Dunn and M. H. Cammien continued their extensive research in developing sensitive, rapid and inexpensive methods of amino acid analysis, using the growth response of specific microorganisms.

As part of his research in chemical aspects of genetics, Norman Horowitz at the California Institute of Technology studied the enzyme systems related to tyrosine metabolism in plants and developed a valuable method of measuring the heat stability of enzymes in plant and animal tissues. The information is useful also in relation to food products and their stability after heat treatment.

At Massachusetts Institute of Technology, J. M. Buchanan clarified some of the chemical aspects of amino acids in forming the enzymes and nuclear structure of living cells; and R. I. Neateles reported the production of substantial yields of L-tryptophan by special mutant strains of bacteria (*Escherichia coli*). If available at low cost there would be active interest in the use of tryptophan for food improvement, analogous to the current interest in lysine.

Harold Stuart and his staff at Harvard University reported in 1961 on a longitudinal study of 125 children through ages 1 to 18 years, mostly from low or average income families in the Boston area. Among the 64 boys and 61 girls, the boys showed a gradual increase in intake of animal protein from 30.6 grams per day at age 1 to 3, to 76 grams at age 17 to 18 years. The lowest and highest individual averages respectively were 15.0 and 42.5 grams at age 1 to 2 and 30.0 to 142.5 at age 17 to 18. The mean value for girls at age 1 to 2 was 32.1 grams per day, rising to a maximum of 57 grams at age 15 to 16. Most of the values for total protein per day were within the range of 12 to 14 per cent of the total caloric intake. This record, like the studies in Denver, was regarded as favorable in comparison with earlier studies in Boston, Canada and England.

Mineral Metabolism

Calcium utilization by human adults as affected by different fatty acids was studied by H. H. Mitchell at the University of Illinois. P. H. Phillips at the University of Wisconsin demonstrated the pathology of calcium deposition in the tissues of cotton rats as induced by imbalances with magnesium and other nutrients, and H. E. Harrison at Johns Hopkins University studied the effect of phosphates and citric acid on calcium metabolism in children with rickets. Sodium, potassium and magnesium functions were also studied in relation to blood pressure regulation, kidney function, and during stress from dehydration. There is much support for the belief that magnesium deficiencies and imbalances with calcium and other electrolytes are more important than is generally recognized in human experience.

The Wisconsin and Harvard studies of fluoride intake continued to demonstrate its safe and strong protective role against tooth decay.

In studies of the trace elements in kidney tissue, G. Kalnitsky at the University of Iowa observed that the quantities of copper, zinc, manganese and magnesium were all closely interrelated in their effect on carbohydrate metabolism. A marked change in any one of the group affected the balanced role of the others.

Maternal Nutrition and Child Development

An indication of improvement in the nutritional status of the population in the area of Nashville, Tennessee, during the preceding decades was given in a 1958 report from studies at Vanderbilt University by W. J. McGanity, E. B. Bridgforth and W. J. Darby entitled "Effect of Reproductive Cycle on Nutritional Status and Requirements." It was based on a study of 2,338 white women who reported for prenatal care at the outpatient clinic. They represented families with gross annual incomes of $3,000-$12,000. Physical, chemical and dietary data were obtained once during each trimester of pregnancy and post-partum. The average nutrient intakes were found to be close to the Recommended Dietary Allowances of the National Research Council except for a moderately lower caloric intake that probably was beneficial. They reported that "No instances of clinically recognizable disease were encountered during the reproductive interlude"; and in summary, "A dietary that will provide the essentials is readily obtainable from food.sources." Seventy-three per cent of the patients did not receive special supplements nor were supplements routinely prescribed.

However, a need for more effective education of the public was indicated: "Among the few mothers whose protein intake was below 50 grams per day, or whose caloric intake was below 1,500 calories, there was a slightly higher incidence of obstetric and fetal complications." The most frequent nutritional damage—and perhaps the most serious—was obesity, with an incidence of 11.5% during the first trimester. Some vitamin C intakes were as low as 20mg/day—obviously too low to provide an adequate supply of vitamin C to their infants. Slight skin and eye lesions were regarded as too subjective and variable for interpretation. Vitamin E intake ranged from 2.9 to 33.3 mg/day, but there was no indication of correlation with health for mothers or infants. Neither was there any correlation in health between those who did or did not take supplements. The same lack of correlation with the use of supplements was evident in a large survey of mothers and their offspring in Philadelphia.

In general, the study at Nashville reflected a different picture than the study in Boston, using different techniques and representing a different environment, or the studies in Denver and Detroit where the population selected for study had a more favorable economic background.

The statistics from studies directed by Dr. Hoobler in Detroit were presented in condensed form for immediate and wide

A Good Idea

distribution as a special issue of the Journal of Nutrition. The study included continuous medical, biochemical and nutritional records of 1,064 selected maternity patients in good health from three different socio-economic groups. An especially detailed study was made of blood constituents of 427 mothers and their respective infants. The concentrations of hemoglobin and vitamin C were approximately twice as high in infants as in their respective mothers. Serum protein, vitamin A and carotene were higher in the mothers. These very careful studies indicated both the value of competent prenatal care and the widespread occurrence of faulty nutrition practices among the lower socio-economic groups.

In a series of four papers in 1962, R. L. Pike and her associates at Pennsylvania State University reported detailed studies of low and high intakes of sodium by albino rats during pregnancy. Changes occurred in electrolyte balance, body weight, food intake, water retention, and the composition of different fluids and tissues, including the brain, bone, muscle, heart, adrenals, plasma, amniotic fluid, fetal plasma and total fetus. The interpretation indicated substantial risks from either too low or excessively high intakes of salt, with an emphasis on protection of the fetus and maintaining hormone balances in addition to water and electrolyte balances.

Continued support was provided for the work of N. L. Hoerr's group at Western Reserve University in building up the first available record of cranial or skull thickness at selected points, covering the age range from 3 months to 21 years. The *rate* of increase in thickness at all points of measurement showed a decrease after about 5 years of age, but a measurable increase until about age 17. It is interesting to note how closely the age during which this rate is rapid corresponds with the period when mental injury imposed by malnutrition is at the greatest risk of becoming irreversible—highest during the first year after birth and still fairly high during the second year.

A. H. Washburn, R. W. McCammon and Virginia Beal in Denver reported meticulous records of total development, physical, mental and social, in addition to nutrition practices from early infancy to 5 years of age. The children studied were from upper middle class homes. Calcium intake rose steadily during the first year, to within the range of about 1 g/day, and then decreased to about 0.75 g, depending chiefly on milk as a source. Iron intake, depending largely on formulas or a mixed diet, rose rapidly to a peak of about 11 mg/day by the end of the first year, then decreased as the diet changed from formulas to mixed diets, when the intake dropped to about 6 mg/day. The pediatricians raised a query as to possible risk of liver injury from excessive iron in some of the formulas. During the first year, as reported in 1962, only one child in 59 consumed less than 0.5 mg of iron per kilogram body weight. Although 25 per cent of the children received supplementary iron, there was less efficiency in utilization and no evidence of advantage. They suggested that "pediatricians should be reluctant to build for internists and geriatricians a legacy of potential disorders of a type so difficult to treat . . . There is no evidence that higher hemoglobin levels provide any advantage to the infant."

A study in Boston of growth and nutrition of 67 infants from 2 to 15 months in age by R. Rueda-Williamson and H. Rose (1962) noted that median intakes of iron were higher than recommended by the National Research Council, usually by at least 50 per cent and often two or three times

The Second Decade

higher. Infant cereals with an iron content as high as 1 mg per tablespoonful apparently were responsible for the high intakes. They found no gain from the over-generous feeding.

With respect to vitamin E deficiency in infancy, K. E. Mason, who had been a pioneer in this area of research at the University of Rochester, pointed out in 1953 that all types of animals tested thus far had shown a requirement for the vitamin, but there had been no substantial evidence of a human deficiency. He expressed the view that is now generally accepted, namely, that "the designation 'anti-sterility vitamin' was unfortunate."

Recent evidence, however, has identified special circumstances when there is a need for an extra supply of vitamin E. The premature infant may present evidence of low vitamin E nutriture. Infants fed an unusual formula with a high content of polyunsaturated fatty acids not accompanied by a normal content of vitamin E have been reported to need extra vitamin E.

During this decade grants were made to assist both P. A. di Sant 'Agnese at Columbia University and H. Schwachman at Harvard University in the improvement of techniques for identifying and caring for infants and small children afflicted with cystic fibrosis. The genetic-limiting disease is characterized by a functional impairment of the mucus tissues of the body, including those that secrete digestive juices and permit duct drainage in many parts of the body. Early identification of the disease and application of measures to assist in utilization of foods as soon as possible are of critical importance in protecting the child victim who suffers from poor digestion of starches and fats and an excessive need for salt. Both physicians made valuable contributions, and Dr. di Sant 'Agnese soon became head of that division of research in the National Institutes of Health.

Vegetarians

Support was provided for a very limited and brief, but interesting, comparative study of the nutrient intake, physical examination, blood content and general health status of 26 adult "pure" vegetarians (no animal product foods), 86 lacto-ovo-vegetarians (used milk and eggs), and a "control group" of 88 non-vegetarians of comparable age and environment in California. No striking differences in nutritional status, health records, or physical condition were revealed in the study. The number of subjects was relatively small to serve as a basis for conclusions, but the indications were worthy of reporting. The study was conducted in cooperation with experienced Harvard University staff members.

Calculations of nutrient intake indicated that for most nutrients the intake had been above the (then stated) Recommended Dietary Allowances except for a few "pure" vegetarians whose protein intake had been relatively low, in the range of 56 to 83 grams per day. The non-vegetarians had a caloric intake of 300 to 900 calories per day higher than the vegetarians, and their serum cholesterol values were higher. The pure vegetarians had a body weight advantage of about 20 pounds below that of other groups. The vegetarians were not extremists in the use of rice for a main caloric source, as so many faddists recommend. **They made good use of legumes and other plant sources of fairly good quality protein and essential nutrients. Within their respective limits they were, in general, quite careful in their food practices.**

A Good Idea

Education

During the second decade of the Foundation NUTRITION REVIEWS continued to serve as an effective channel for bringing worldwide research progress to the attention of people with a moderate or high degree of scientific training. This journal also served as a valuable reference for feature writers and laymen who were interested in education but had limited scientific training. Each year a subject index was published to facilitate reviews and references for writers, students and teachers.

Another useful publication was a leaflet, "Current Research in the Science of Nutrition," distributed to teachers, technologists not trained in nutrition, writers, health officials, extension personnel and others who were interested and in close communication with the public. In addition, small leaflets and booklets were printed from time-to-time and special articles were written by invitation for journals and occasionally for the press. Participation in radio programs or press interviews was not uncommon, but was not on a scheduled basis.

There was complete agreement that much more needed to be done to meet the needs of the public and the Foundation's goal. Special grants were made to Harvard University and Columbia University to support studies of teaching practical nutrition in elementary and intermediate schools. This program had some success in improving textbook recognition of nutrition in the respective grades. One of the staff members in the study at Columbia, Dr. Mary Hill, became head of the nutrition educational services in the Department of Agriculture.

Ten annual scholarships were supported for summer training of selected medical students in nutrition in cooperation with the Council on Foods and Nutrition of the American Medical Association. These served to stimulate the interest of students and faculty alike, and the program now has been much expanded and is completely supported by the American Medical Association.

Press releases regarding the annual awards in cooperation with the American Institute of Nutrition, the American Medical Association, the Institute of Food Technologists and the American Dietetic Association were of educational and inspirational value in reaching students and the public.

There was continuous participation in the educational activities of the above four organizations and the Food and Nutrition Board, the American Public Health Association, the New York Academy of Medicine, the New York Academy of Sciences, the International Union of Nutritional Sciences, and the American Society of Biological Chemists. All of these organizations reach the public press and other channels of education with occasional items of interest in nutrition.

The American Dietetic Association, with early leadership from Muriel Wagner and others in Detroit, Michigan, developed an excellent service for reaching the public through their *Dial-a-Dietitian program* in cooperation with radio stations and the press. They maintained this volunteer service with a remarkable devotion of time and administrative care, so that anyone within the respective city areas could call a designated number in the telephone directory and obtain competent, practical, nutritional advice on a call-back basis, without charge. They made arrangements in advance with local medical societies so that the range and nature of their service would be understood, and the dietitian could suggest appropriate physicians in the community to whom individuals could be referred when their service appeared to be needed. Physicians also had an in-

The Second Decade

creased resource in identifying dietitians of special merit in working with the public. Small grants from the Foundation assisted the A.D.A. in getting a number of the programs underway and onto a self-supporting basis from local sources. Stemming from this beginning in 1958, nineteen such centers were operating in 1973, and plans were underway for increasing their cooperation with the public press and broadcasting agencies.

Meetings of scientific societies are nearly always supplemented by extensive activities of educational value in reaching the public via the press, radio and television programs in addition to their primary goal of exchanging ideas among scientists themselves. There has long been an active organization of well trained science writers who take pride in their skill of interpreting reliable progress in scientific research to the public. Officers and committeemen in the societies assist representatives of the press, radio and television services in identifying program topics and personnel that are most likely to be of interest.

Small grants were made from time to time, also, to support conferences from which monograph or journal publications became available. For large conferences such as national or international meetings our grants generally took the form of assisting committees in making efficient plans, or support for the publication of the proceedings.

The largest undertaking of the above kind was the Fifth International Congress on Nutrition. After four successful international congresses in Europe under the auspices of the International Union of Nutritional Sciences, the Fifth International Congress on Nutrition was held in Washington, D.C., September 1-7, 1960. The American Institute of Nutrition was the primary host organization, in cooperation with the National Academy of Sciences and its National Committee for Nutritional Sciences.

Grants from public foundations, including The Nutrition Foundation, supported the early planning for the Congress by officers and committees beginning in 1957. Canadian and Latin American scientists helpfully participated in developing and staging the Congress and in extending hospitality to guests from overseas. Government agencies and the food industry contributed generously in meeting the overall budget requirements. The margin of funds not expended was set aside to assist selected young scientists in attending subsequent Congresses.

The leadership of Mr. H. J. Heinz, II, assisted by Dr. H. E. Robinson, in securing financial support from the food and related industries and the outstanding work of Dr. Paul György as Chairman of the Organizing Committee were major factors in making the Congress a notable success. In addition, the excellent work by eight committee chairmen with their respective members through a period of three years made my responsibilities as president of the Congress very reasonable. Participants from 62 different countries reached a total registration of 2,300, by far the largest of any of the previous congresses.

In addition to research and review papers there were two half-day symposia on worldwide food needs and resources, including papers by the heads of U.S. government and United Nations agencies and The Rockefeller Foundation. As in all of our congresses there were well organized programs in food science and technology.

The high spot in excitement and inspiration was the surprise welcoming address by President Eisenhower who spoke in his usual warm and enthusiastic manner at the opening Plenary Session, as the previously unidentified "Representative of the United States Government." Many suspected

A Good Idea

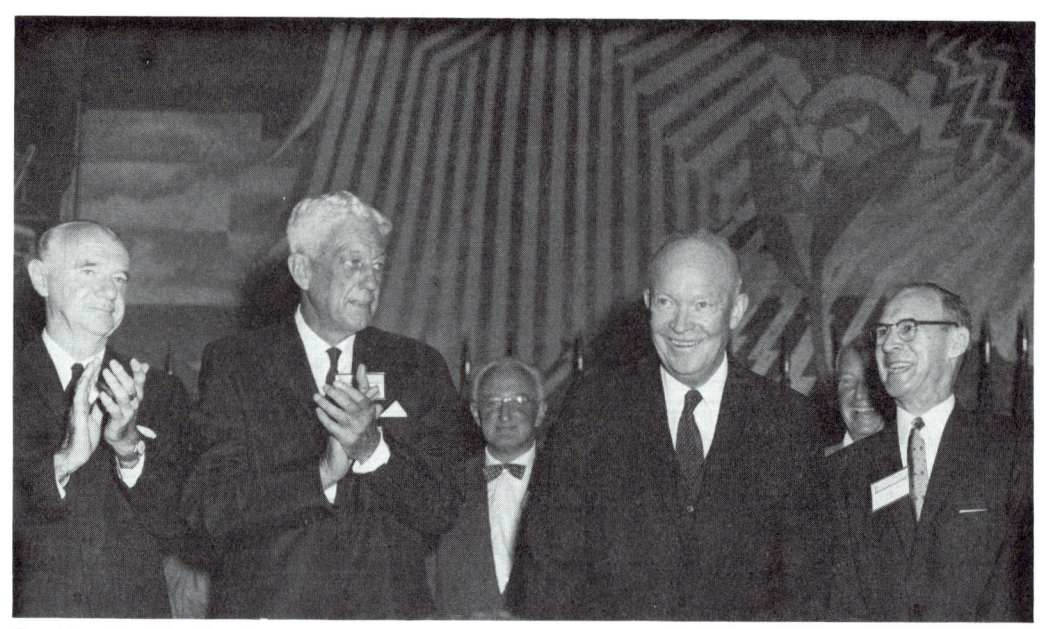

President Dwight Eisenhower opened the Fifth International Congress of Nutrition, Washington, D.C., September 1, 1960.

Left to Right: *Vincent du Vigneaud, Maurice Pate, President Eisenhower, C. G. King.* Second row center: *S. Kon.*

that the President might speak when the Marine Band was scheduled for two thrilling 15 minute numbers during the preliminary program, but having had only a moderate acquaintance with him at Columbia University, I was surprised when he said he was sure the conference would be a great success, "with a King for President." I suspected that Clare Francis, who had facilitated our initial invitation, had seen the manuscript.

Based on continuing discussions and actions taken in 1960, many of the member companies voluntarily increased their payments to the Foundation by 25 per cent for a minimum period of three years so that the educational program could be increased without detracting from the funds for research. This added fund provided an increment of $209,985 for education between January 1, 1961 and June 30, 1963.

Dr. Sipple was very helpful in developing the program, and I was confident that he would carry on after my scheduled retirement.

During 1961, the outreach in lay education in the United States and in Canada was substantially increased in the daily press, magazines and radio programs. There were more than 1,700 informational articles in newspapers. A large part of the coverage was through the voluntary and independent science writers, Alton Blakeslee, Gaynor Madox and Josephine Lowman. By June 30, 1963, the United Feature Syndicate brought the number of special newspaper articles to 3,200. As estimated by professional press standards the magazine stories reached about 40 million actual readers during the year, including *Good Housekeeping, American Weekly, Cosmopolitan, Modern Medicine, Family Circle,*

The Second Decade

Woman's Day and *Parents Magazine*. In 1962 *McCall's*, *Food Field Reporter*, *School Lunch*, *Travel Trends* and *Food Engineering* were added. More than 350 feature articles appeared that were prepared or sponsored by the Foundation. For a few years we had assistance from two staff members, and several of the intermediate sized chain stores introduced nutrition literature or personal advisory service in their stores by a home economist or dietitian.

Radio programs were presented occasionally over NBC and six hundred radio stations used a series of 13 special interviews. Two special leaflets were prepared in cooperation with the Public Affairs Committee, with a distribution of about 350,000 copies. In response to requests, I had written 26 educational articles for technical and lay journals between January 1, 1962 and June 30, 1963.

The Foundation's support of research that advances the frontier of knowledge in relation to foods and nutrition also serves education substantially by training young scientists. Through them there is a continuing educational service within the professions of medicine, public health, agricultural extension, and within the food industry. Each year about 150 to 200 graduate or post-doctorate young scientists were assisted in their educational careers by Nutrition Foundation grants.

A summary of all appropriations through the period July 1, 1942 to June 30, 1963, is given in the accompanying table. Lines of division between areas of subject matter could not be drawn sharply, however, because the goal in research was to develop new knowledge for use by all members of society. For example, a single manuscript on a new vitamin might deal significantly with its relation to protein metabolism, its requirement in feeding infants, its relation to disease among adults and its risk of loss during processing.

Scheduled Retirement

Although members of the Board of Trustees and Board of Directors had urged me to continue in office beyond July 1, 1963, I was determined not to stay beyond age 67. I had observed too many instances of administrative officers remaining in their position beyond a normal age for retirement. There was obviously an opportunity for continued growth in membership and an urgent need for the kinds of service that the Foundation could give, with great benefit to the public and to the best elements in the industry. I felt privileged to have participated in the Foundation's growth from an excellent idea and fifteen members to seventy-two members and a substantial record in support of research, education and health improvement on a national and worldwide basis and other forms of human service. Beyond retirement it has been an honor and treasured privilege to be invited to serve as a public member of the Board of Trustees.

Early in the spring of 1963, I accepted a three year appointment, to become effective on July 1, 1963, as Associate Director of the Institute of Nutrition Sciences with Dr. W. H. Sebrell, Jr., Director of the Institute of Nutrition Sciences in the School of Public Health at Columbia University, in parallel with an opportunity to serve approximately half-time as a consultant in international work with The Rockefeller Foundation and occasionally as a consultant with the United Nations agencies.

A Good Idea

Summary of Appropriations for Grants-in-Aid
July 1, 1942 to June 30, 1963

Area I. Human Requirements of Individual Nutrients ....$ 458,500.00
Area II. Origin, Function and Measurement of Nutrients and Metabolites 3,437,400.00
Area III. Maternal and Infant Nutrition 437,280.00
Area IV. Public Health Problems 1,627,550.00
Area V. Professional and Public Education 1,151,260.00
Total Appropriations from July 1, 1942 to June 30, 1963:
  Research—Areas I-IV $5,960,730.00
  Education—Area V 1,151,260.00
   Total $7,111,990.00

3

The Third Decade: The Program of the 1960s

BEGINNING July 1, 1963, Paul B. Pearson served as President and Scientific Director of the Foundation. His background included Ph.D. training in biochemistry at the University of Wisconsin, teaching and research at Montana State College, the University of California and the Agricultural and Mechanical College of Texas where he served as Dean of the Graduate School and head of the Department of Biochemistry. For nine years he then was chief of the Biology Branch of the Atomic Energy Commission, in parallel with a part-time professorship at The Johns Hopkins University, followed by five years as a member of the staff of The Ford Foundation.

Dr. Killian continued to serve as Chairman of the Board of Trustees, W. B. Murphy as Chairman of the Board of Directors, and Horace L. Sipple as both Executive Secretary and Treasurer.

Dr. Killian's sustained enthusiasm for the program was expressed in the 1963-1964 report: "Because of its unswerving dedication to the public interest and its long record of pioneering support of basic research in nutrition science, I have counted it a privilege to be associated with The Nutrition Foundation. It has had the benefit of wise scientific direction, ably supported by an able science advisory committee. It has also had the good fortune to command the sustained support of a group of companies with a high sense of public responsibility and a recognition that one of the ways to discharge this responsibility was to sponsor a non-profit foundation devoted to the advancement of science and education in its field.

"The Foundation's record of identifying and aiding young scientists who subsequently became distinguished, of augmenting our mastery of nutrition science, and of assisting in the establishment of new educational programs in this field provide ample evidence that it has met the objectives of its member companies and its Board of Trustees."

In preparation for the Foundation program in the '60s, the Trustees appointed a review committee to assess the directions and priorities that would predictably be of greatest public benefit. As was apparent,

A Good Idea

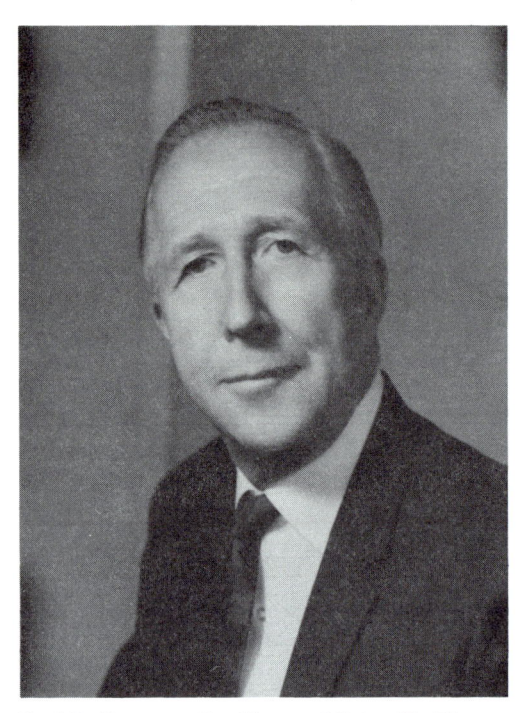

Paul B. Pearson—President and Scientific Director of The Nutrition Foundation July 1, 1963-December 31, 1971.

many changes nationally and internationally had occurred—some of which reflected the successful influences of the Foundation itself. By 1963, large sums of monies were available for support of research from the National Institutes of Health and the National Science Foundation; the Food and Nutrition Board was giving continued leadership in many nutritional matters; the United Nations organizations had active programs in food, agriculture and health; and the U.S. bilateral aid programs were beginning to be aware of their responsibilities for nutritional-planned assistance, especially as a result of the surveys and reports of joint programs evolving under the dynamic guidance of Arnold E. Schaefer, Director of the Interdepartmental Committee on Nutrition for National Defense (ICNND). The scientific literature of nutrition was growing nationally and internationally. What role should The Nutrition Foundation now take in this changed milieu?

The review committee asked William J. Darby, a long time grantee, a former Associate Editor of NUTRITION REVIEWS, and an active member of the Scientific Advisory Council to meet with the Committee. The Committee's report emphasized the important opportunities for the Foundation in furthering personnel development, innovative research, and education in professional schools and, especially in assisting the public in developing food habits that would conserve health.

To illustrate the confidence and viewpoint of leaders in the food industry, Mr. Murphy reported:

Food companies, including suppliers, distributors and processors, have recognized for many years the importance of fundamental biological research in the over-all development of the industry. The Nutrition Foundation was founded in 1941 to support basic research in the science of nutrition. There is wide recognition that advancing the knowledge of nutrition is to the benefit of mankind and also of major importance to the food industry.

The Trustees, through a committee of scientists and industry representatives, have now reevaluated the role of the Foundation in current and future developments in the science of nutrition in the light of increasing federal support of all fields of science. The Trustees reaffirmed the broad objectives of the Foundation.

The needs and opportunities of the Foundation were held to be as great today, though different, as they were one or two decades ago. Two vital needs in the field of nutrition are: (1) the encouragement of new research in fields not now supported by government or other organizations, and (2) the advancement of nutrition education and dissemination of sound information on nutrition. The relatively underdeveloped state of the nutrition sciences and the many complex and unresolved relationships of nutrition to health are of concern to the food and

The Third Decade

allied industries and will continue to be so for the indefinite future.

In essence the report of the review committee was a restatement of the initial purpose of the Foundation, followed by suggestions of adaptions in emphasis, expressed as follows: "1) To advance the science of nutrition and to further its use for the health and welfare of mankind; 2) to aid the food and allied industries in serving the public through advances in nutrition and food science; 3) to pursue these goals as a public, non-profit institution dedicated to the improvement of nutrition and health.

"The principal effort will still be in research, but the emphasis will be on creative new fields, new developments and younger people. There will also be substantial efforts to strengthen nutrition education."

It was also decided to continue the limitation of research grants to North American institutions with allowance for special circumstances when collaboration with one or more other groups might be of major significance, as in Latin America. The Foundation would continue to encourage cooperative activities with other national and international organizations.

In an effort to build up strong, relatively new research and educational programs where there was excellent leadership, occasional grants not to exceed $10,000 per year would be made on a departmental basis, with freedom to explore new avenues of research and training as envisioned by young staff personnel. Applications for this type of grant would not have to be restricted to a specific time limit but could be extended at the discretion of the Foundation.

These grants were to encourage exploratory research and were made only in situations where there was a strong, mature research leader associated with promising young scientists and in a favorable environment. The intent was to foster initiative in research in a manner that would permit the maximum expression of originality and creativity. Immediate availability of these funds served the units as a "savings account" and enabled the unit often to accumulate sufficient data to attract funds several times greater than the original grant. They also permitted a greater flexibility of use than conventional research grants, and hence were exceedingly valuable departmental resources. The absence of termination date often encouraged frugality of expenditure. Immensely popular as they proved to be, the difficulty of subsequent identification of specific research accomplishments resulted in discontinuing that type of grants.

In relation to education the report stated: "The Foundation seeks ways to strengthen nutrition education at the university level in professional schools, in secondary schools and in adult education. Preference will be given to projects that offer innovation in nutrition education and to projects that offer the opportunity to reach large segments of the population through individuals or groups who have direct contact with the public. The Foundation will be on the alert for opportunities to aid in developing new centers of excellence where it appears that an institution can be significantly aided in that respect."

A Poetic Turn

Dr. Killian continued to give outstanding service until his retirement in 1965 when he was succeeded by Herbert E. Longenecker, President of Tulane University. This was a poetic turn of events. Dr. Longenecker had been one of The Nutrition Foundation's early grantees in 1942. He had come to the University of Pittsburgh from Pennsylvania State College on a

A Good Idea

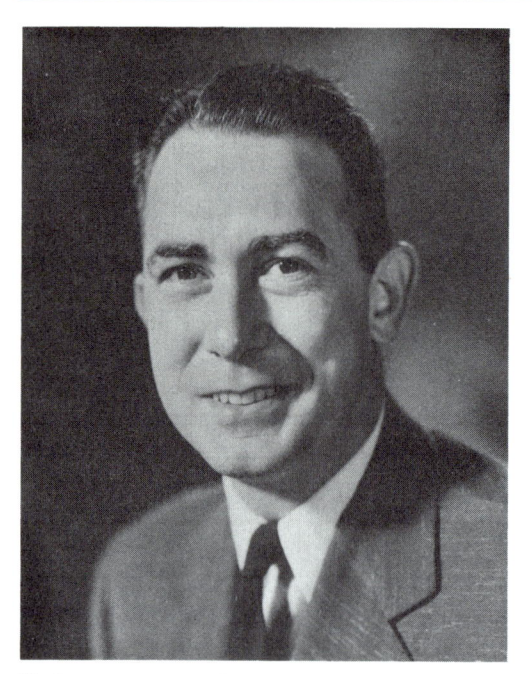

Herbert E. Longenecker—Dr. Longenecker, President of Tulane University, succeeded Dr. Killian as Chairman of the Board of Trustees of The Nutrition Foundation in 1965. His long association with the Foundation dates from 1942 when he was an early grantee.

post-doctoral fellowship appointment, supported by a grant from the Buhl Foundation in Pittsburgh. After a notable career in lipid chemistry and becoming Dean of the Graduate School there, he served as Vice President of the University of Illinois in Chicago, before going to Tulane University as President.

The 1965-1966 Report of the Foundation was a Twenty-Fifth Anniversary Report, reviewing the history of the Foundation and noting the cumulative value of work aided during the intervening years: the war period, strengthening the Food and Nutrition Board, training highly qualified young scientists through their graduate and post-doctorate years, and basic research on each of the major types of nutrients, including genetic relationships and functions in relation to health.

Education and potential applications of basic research in homes and in industry clearly added up to higher standards of living, nationally and worldwide. The support base for the Foundation was increased moderately by a higher scale of membership payments especially from the larger companies. The program pattern was not changed greatly. Trends were indicated, however, in the following respects:

1. Many of the basic research grants were renewed and new ones added in accordance with recommendations of the Scientific Advisory Committee. They covered the major classes of nutrients and their relation to health, as in heart disease, diabetes, dental caries, obesity, hypertension, anemia and protein or other specific deficiencies.

2. Provision was made for developing Centers of Excellence in universities and medical schools. Advantage was taken of this opportunity by only a limited number of institutions—the University of Missouri, Mt. Sinai Medical School, and Columbia University.

3. Dental schools received special consideration in developing research and improved teaching in relation to nutrition. This effort was initiated by supporting a nationwise Conference on Nutrition Research and Teaching in Dental Schools, held at the Massachusetts Institute of Technology.

4. Future Leaders Awards were made to provide research support on a broad basis for selected promising young scientists in their early academic careers. This action proved to be especially rewarding and has been of substantial assistance in aiding some very able young faculty members to become established as productive leaders in nutrition.

5. Press releases were distributed regularly

The Third Decade

to over 500 daily and weekly newspapers, assisted by a full-time science writer, Mr. Robert Plumb.
6. A color TV program on nutrition for elementary school children was produced and distributed for visual educational programs to reach public audiences.
7. Liaison was maintained with the Food and Nutrition Board of the National Research Council, the Nutrition Committee of the American Academy of Pediatrics, and many other scientific societies.
8. In relation to education, two areas received special consideration:
   a. In research, the processes of learning by animals and by people were studied as influenced by such factors as flavor, hunger, habit, food composition, environment and nutritional quality. Understanding these relationships was judged to be of potential value in designing effective programs for reaching both the public and industry as guides for meeting public acceptance.
   b. Specific educational programs and techniques were studied to assess their effectiveness—particularly in schools and via the mass media. A special Educational Advisory Committee was appointed to guide this and related efforts. The primary goal was to improve practices that are conducive to health.

Research in the Third Decade

Protein Foods

Research on proteins and amino acids continued to advance along several lines, but the most exciting studies were those in which the protein intake during pregnancy, infancy and early growth might be made optimal for human development. Important advances were made also in relation to the normal formation and functions of the individual amino acids in living organisms—in plants, animals or human experience. An association of protein deficiency with obvious sickness, stunted growth, and high death rates (as in kwashiorkor, with obvious skin and hair changes, edema, etc.) merits urgent attention, but still greater urgency is called for if there is an irreversible injury to the central nervous system. This situation calls for research through the entire life cycle.

In Guatemala, G. Arroyave and his associates studied the serum protein and related changes during pregnancy and lactation among urban and rural populations. The types of change observed in areas where clinical deficiencies range from slight to severe degrees are of distinct value in relation to studies in the United States and Canada where deficiencies seldom are severe enough to be recognized by a physical examination only. The work in Guatemala and Mexico had special value because it was associated with much of the pioneering study of Dr. J. Cravioto and others aided by the Foundation in developing evidence of impairment to the central nervous system, in addition to physical stunting, caused by protein food deficiency.

Studies of the amino acid requirements of men 50 to 70 years of age by W. H. Griffith, M. E. Swendsied and their associates at the University of California (Los Angeles) indicated only a slightly higher requirement than for young men about 20 years of age.

Methods for determining the nutritive quality of protein with greatest accuracy and particularly in the use of rats as standard animals were examined by D. M. Hegsted at Harvard University in cooperation with different laboratories.

F. C. Dohan at the Pennsylvania Psychiatric Institute received support for studies of whether schizophrenic-like states might be induced in individuals who are sensitive to wheat protein by consuming wheat products. It has been observed that some persons with this condition have derangements that often resemble the condition induced by gluten sensitivity.

At the University of Wisconsin A. E. Harper and his associates continued their contributions to clarifying the effects of feeding different ratios of amino acids in comparison with feeding unbalanced total proteins. Amino acid ratios have a great importance in relation to disease prevention in countries where grains and legumes must serve as major sources of protein. They are of additional practical importance in calculating the most efficient protein requirements for feeding poultry, livestock and fish on a commercial basis. An interesting observation showed that unfavorable ratios of amino acids in protein foods tend to exert a depressant effect on appetite, thus adding to the handicap in their use as related to human or animal growth.

Clinical studies of children with kwashiorkor (chiefly protein deficiency) and marasmus (chiefly caloric or total food deficiency) were conducted in Cali, Colombia, by J. J. Vitale and others, in comparison with observations on monkeys under careful control in the laboratories at Harvard. Changes in red blood cells were characteristic of the major types of deficiency that occur in human populations and were attributed to deficiencies of both protein and folic acid. These results were in striking contrast with observations in the United States, Canada and Northern Europe where the incidence of anemia is chiefly a result of iron deficiency.

Minerals

D. M. Hegsted, J. J. Vitale and their associates made an interesting observation in finding that the requirement of rats for magnesium as measured by growth response was two to four times higher when an ambient temperature of 55° F. was maintained compared with 78° F. There is considerable interest in the magnesium-calcium ratio, in part because a low intake of magnesium and a high intake of calcium tends to increase excessive deposits of calcium and complex fat in the cardiovascular tissues. This particular aspect of their work apparently has had little further study.

Observations in Peru and elsewhere in South America failed to disclose evidence of calcium deficiency despite daily intakes as low as 100 to 200 mg. This was in striking contrast to the prevailing view in the United States that 800 mg/day is a desirable intake level. In controlled tests with dogs no injury resulted from intakes as low as 0.034 per cent of the diet—roughly equivalent to common human diets in Peru.

In studies with rats, deficiencies of magnesium during a high intake of calcium and phosphate resulted in excessive calcification of the arteries, heart and kidneys. On the other hand, generous intakes of magnesium tended to result in better adjustment of blood proteins, cholesterol and bile acids. Yet it was difficult to find consistent data from human experience to support the prospect that similar relationships were of major importance in public health. Heart muscle from ducklings proved very sensitive to magnesium intake; and tests with rats consistently yielded findings suggestive of atherosclerotic lesions. In dogs, low magnesium intakes distinctly favored formation of vascular plaques and excessive calcium deposits in the vascular system. In studies of the Boston population there appeared to be occasional instances when the low magnesium-calcium ratio may be related to atherosclerosis, but the trend has not been established often enough to make it a

The Third Decade

major issue. However, one can hardly believe that it is not significant in the worldwide picture. The time factor makes it very difficult to conduct controlled human experiments, but different populations show great differences in the relationship of nutrition to aging, crippling diseases, and death rates.

Until the recent expansion in trace mineral research by the Department of Agriculture, one of the few medical research laboratories dealing broadly with the trace elements was developed by B. L. Vallee at Harvard University. It was a pleasure to encourage and assist him in that direction. Early reports from his laboratory dealt with trace element-containing enzymes and with the importance of maintaining an adequate content of magnesium in the serum of patients with zinc deficiency and of cirrhotics. A deficiency of magnesium was characterized by a diseased condition in five patients studied in detail in relation to tetany (convulsions). He and H. E. C. Wacker expanded their interest to embrace the trace elements zinc, chromium, iron, manganese, nickel and copper, all of which elements now are the subject of intense research and medical interest. Dr. Vallee is now recognized as one of the world's leaders in this area of medical and nutrition research.

G. K. Davis, T. J. Cunha and their associates at the University of Florida conducted careful studies of the interplay of molybdenum, calcium, phosphates, copper, iron sulfur and zinc, tracing the relationships in soil, plants, animal feeds and their relation to tissue enzymes. This group has also become recognized as leaders in the area of soil-feed-and-animal research.

An extensive study of animal and human nutrition in relation to the trace elements was developed by R. W. Engel and his associates at the Virginia Polytechnic Institute. Their work included special consideration of molybdenum, sulfur and phosphate in soil studies and parallel studies with trace element nutrition in children. For several years Dr. Engel has had a major responsibility for developing a national nutrition program in the Philippines, and in 1974 he received the Conrad A. Elvehjem Award from the American Institute of Nutrition.

J. M. Orten at Wayne State University reported the isolation and analysis of three major pigment carriers (porphyrins) of iron, and Dr. Hegsted cooperated with Dr. C. A. Finch at Harvard in investigations on the utilization of iron.

The importance of maintaining optimum concentrations of sodium, potassium and other electrolytes in relation to hormonal control, blood pressure, muscle function, water balance and related aspects of health was studied extensively by W. S. and P. M. Hartroft at the University of Toronto and Washington University (St. Louis). They were particularly concerned with related functions of adrenal, pancreatic and pituitary hormones.

The importance of potassium balance in the regulation of heart muscle and other tissues was studied extensively by P. D. Boyer at the University of Minnesota and J. L. Gamble at Johns Hopkins University.

Although iodine deficiency to the extent of causing goiter is no longer rampant in areas where iodized salt has been widely adopted, many parts of the world continue to have a very high incidence of goiter. Functions of the thyroid gland exerted by secretion of two iodine-containing hormones were investigated by H. A. Lardy at the University of Wisconsin in relation to energy-producing reactions to carbohydrates and fats. It would be safe and a valuable public service if all table salt offered for general service in food markets were required to be iodized. Non-iodized table salt could be available on request, or through other channels for special individuals on religious or medical grounds.

Selenium, long of interest because of its toxicity when consumed in excessive amounts in feedstuffs, became recognized as an essential nutrient of great practical importance in feeds for poultry and sheep production. It is now known to be essential for a wide spectrum of animals. Its role as an antioxidant and its interrelationship with vitamin E, the antioxidant properties of which have given rise to postulated relationships to the polyunsaturated fats, indicate its wide involvement in biological processes. L. C. Norris and M. L. Scott at Cornell University were active investigators in this field. Both selenium and vitamin E deficiencies have been involved in experimental muscular dystrophy, brain damage and enzyme changes. The requirement of selenium is small—estimated at about 0.1 part per million in a food supply when it contains vitamin E, and about 0.14 ppm. when vitamin E is not adequate. Both nutrients must be supplied to prevent muscular dystrophy.

The crucial importance of fluoride intake to permit normal tooth development and continued protection against decay was clearly demonstrated in continued research at the University of Wisconsin by P. H. Phillips and his associates, and at Harvard University by J. H. Shaw, R. F. Sognnaes and others. Calcium, phosphate and other nutrients were recognized as important physiologically, but in practical experience, deficiencies of fluoride are most crucial and most within reach of prompt and large scale prevention. A thorough study of fluoridation in England confirmed the successful experience in many communities in the United States. Continued research and experience fully support this view. By 1964, 1256 communities had adopted fluoridation of water supplies, thus affording a decreased rate of decay within a range of 50 to 70 per cent. In the face of abundant evidence, it is a pity that so many children are denied their normal human right to develop decay-resistant teeth that would afford substantial life-time protection.

Studies at the University of Wisconsin with cotton rats confirmed the special importance of nutrition early in life to establish optimum decay resistance. There was practically no difference among commonly used sugars in their tendency to induce or accelerate decay, and no apparent benefit resulted from adding 15 percent of corn oil to the diet. In oat hulls, however, there was found a complex phenolic material that afforded some protective benefit. Poorly balanced intakes of magnesium and calcium such as resulted in arterial injury also resulted in increased tooth decay in animals on a semi-purified diet. Within the range of sensitivity of the test procedure, supplements of vitamins, zinc or manganese gave no protection. The Harvard studies by Dr. Shaw, Dr. Sognnaes and others indicated that the ash from a good stock diet of mixed foods contained protective mineral material in addition to those recognized; continued research may supplement still further the well-established major requirements for fluoride, phosphate and calcium that are provided in a good diet.

Nutrition and Maternal and Child Health

Human studies of nutrition in relation to maternal and child health gave early indications of widespread injury by low intakes of good quality protein foods. Retarded physical growth was evident. Little was known, however, about the age, time or intensity relationships to the child's ability to make a complete recovery. Malfunction of the central nervous system was evident during severe deficiency, but it was difficult to ascertain the

The Third Decade

degree of permanent mental or other functional impairment. Hence, early suggestions that the changes were often irreversible demanded investigation. Among the major difficulties were:

1. Separation of nutritional effects from differences induced by environmental factors such as home or cultural background;
2. Variations in exposure of mother and child to infections that characterize populations in countries where there is a high incidence of protein-calorie malnutrition;
3. Techniques of measuring functional differences in the central nervous system of very small children were not precise nor standardized;
4. Research of this nature would be relatively expensive and would require large numbers of subjects and specialized investigators making observations through a long period;
5. It would be difficult to isolate effects of single-nutrient deprivation.

Recognizing the enormous potential significance of the problem, however, from observations on millions of people in Latin America, Africa, the Middle East, India, Southeast Asia and on a lesser scale in technologically advanced countries, the Foundation early and consistently supported carefully selected human and experimental animal research in this field and encouraged other agencies to do so. Assistance to J. Cravioto in Mexico, N. S. Scrimshaw and M. Behar in Guatemala was followed by support of studies by R. H. Barnes at Cornell University (Ithaca), M. Winick at Cornell University (N.Y.), F. Monckeberg in Chile, and F. J. Zeman at the University of California. Dr. Cravioto had underway a long-term study from birth to seven years of age on a group of 305 children living at home in the village of Tlaltizapan, Mexico. Records were kept of their nutritional practices, environment, health and development, beginning with tests each month subsequent to birth until age 3 years, and then about every 3 months. Long term support to his group has resulted in a clarification of several factors—nutritional versus social deprivation, especially, of the malnourished child.

Dr. Monckeberg has studied a total of 500 children within three sub-groups in Santiago, Chile. Group A lived in middle class homes not subjected to severe malnutrition. Group B lived in low-income homes where severe malnutrition had been common, but they were given supplementary feeding, free milk and medical care; they showed little or no malnutrition. In these two groups only 3 percent had IQs less than 80 (subnormal), while group C, comparable with group B but not given food supplements, showed a high incidence of malnutrition and 40 percent had subnormal intelligence. He reported that "In severe cases the skull grew at a slower rate, and brain growth is not only less, but there is real brain atrophy."

Dr. Monckeberg believes that the widespread similarity in IQ tests among mothers and their children occurs because frequently malnutrition in each successive generation is a result of repetition in malnutrition during infancy, and the first few years of childhood—a vicious circle that cannot be broken without major improvement in food practices. He regards this relationship as far more significant than any slight correlation based on genetic trends or the frailties in methods of testing.

Originally at Cornell University Medical College and more recently Director of the Institute of Human Nutrition, Columbia University, Dr. Myron Winick as a Future Leader Awardee developed an outstanding program in studies of nutritional effects upon cellular growth and composition, with emphasis on the central nervous system. The very early growth of body tissues is characterized by a rapid increase in the number and differentiation of cells, compared with the later enlargement of each part of the body that tends to result from increasing the size of individual cells instead of increasing the number. This trend can be identified by a difference in cell composition. Dr. Winick's research has been concerned particularly with changes in brain composition with age and as influenced by nutrition. His initial studies were with rats, but as work advanced opportunities were found for clinical observations that confirmed the evidence from animal tests. When very young rats were rendered deficient in protein and calories, the rate of cell division was retarded in essentially all tissues, including the brain. When adequate feeding was restored they again grew in physical stature, but the number of brain cells did not increase in a manner comparable to the increase in other tissues. When older animals were subjected to deprivation the distortion in brain size and composition was not so great.

In view of the continuing rapid growth of an infant's brain structures in the months after birth, the chemical evidence strongly supports findings from performance tests indicating that early severe deficiencies in good quality protein foods can cause damage to the central nervous system that is not entirely reversible. The extent of damage is likely to correspond with the time and severity of the deficiency.

The technique of studying brain tissue in terms of age and cellular composition is now being extended to other body tissues such as the liver, kidneys and glands, and to include other nutrients. Studies of placentas are also useful as an indication of the nutritional states of both mother and fetus during pregnancy and the potential risk of influence on the offspring.

After extensive studies with rats, there was an invitation to Winick to examine the tissues from children who had died from severe malnutrition before they were one year old. Three of nine children studied by chemical means had less than 40 percent of the normal number of brain cells; the others showed a marked reduction. Detailed explorations of the specific parts of rat brains showed the greatest change in relation to age and degrees of protein or caloric deficiency.

From such studies with rats and considerable observation of infants it appears that the most critical risk period for irreversible suppression of human brain growth is from before birth to one year.

A parallel study of suppression of brain development by malnutrition in rats was supported at the University of California (L.A.) by S. Zamenhof. His findings also indicate a very close relation of protein deficiency to development of specific structures of the brain and the resultant effect upon learning ability.

Evidence of impairment to emotional stability in rats by protein deficiency in early life was shown by the studies of B. Sevitsky and R. H. Barnes at Cornell University.

Comparable studies show similar relationships in other tissues, such as the fat-storing cells of adipose tissue. Fat babies, overfed in terms of total calories when infants, appear to be at greater risk of being fat as adults and accordingly jeopardized in health. This pertains even though they do lose excess fat stores if the caloric intake is sufficiently and consistently restricted. In later years would they be more susceptible to diabetes? Or atherosclerosis? These remain as unanswered questions, but there is a trend of evidence that the relationship will be verified.

The Third Decade

It will be exciting in the years ahead to find what deficiencies or excesses of other essential nutrients besides the amino acids can exert irreversible injuries to health very early in life. Deficiencies of iodine, at least, have comparable effects; very recent studies in animals indicate that zinc may, also.

R. R. Zimmermann at the University of Montana developed an interesting program in studies with baby rhesus monkeys. After exposure to protein deficiency for various periods during their first year, in comparison with a normally fed group, "The malnourished monkeys are fearful in a social situation and do not engage in play with the frequency that is characteristic of the normal animal. They spend much of their time avoiding other animals . . . (are) frightened of change and novelty . . . (and) deficient in his ability to socialize and interact with the world around . . ."

Taste Perception and "Eating" Areas of the Brain

A number of grants, closely linked with problems in nutrition education were made to discover physiological functions that in part determine what people actually eat. Social courtesies, costs, family discipline, convenience, advertising, appearance and confidence in sanitation are often major factors, but in the background, purely physiological responses associated with the central nervous system are significant. Among these, taste perception and the way one feels before, during and after eating are important.

Many physiologists and psychologists are interested in discovering the mechanisms in the body that relate the brain centers with hunger or appetite, thirst, satiety at mealtime, salt or sweet taste stimulus and response, or flavor combinations such as formed in ice cream, apple pie and chocolate bars.

In 1968, the Foundation joined with other organizations in support of an international conference on olfaction and taste, held at the Rockefeller University where Carl Pfaffman has long been active in this area of research. About 120 scientists working as physiologists, psychologists, zoologists and chemical engineers participated in the presentation and discussion of some 80 papers. Proceedings of the third such conference were published in monograph form by the Rockefeller University Press.

The three main nerve-related tissues whose functions in chemical senses were of major interest among grantees were the taste buds, an area in the base of the brain called the lateral hypothalamus, and the gastrointestinal tract—particularly the stomach and the adjacent section of the small intestine.

Dr. Pfaffman had a special interest in salt deprivation, in part because a common disease, Addison's disease, is accompanied by a craving for salt, and hence there was an opportunity to study a pure chemical role in nerve transmission. His experimental approach with animals was in testing the mechanisms of specific terminal nerve transmission from the tongue to the brain. Normal men were studied also in their responses after periods of salt deprivation.

George Wolf at the Mt. Sinai School of Medicine sought to trace the exact course of nerve transmission from the brain cells to the taste buds in relation to an appetite for salt as soon as a deficiency was developed by salt deprivation. The results indicated that instead of a major nerve channel function there are multiple nerve channels for the message transmission so that two or more must be severed to exert an effect.

M. R. Kare and Owen Maller at the University of Pennsylvania were assisted in studies of the over-all effect of palatability or "taste" as a composite of several factors,

A Good Idea

including flavor, odor, temperature, and the number of attractive foods available from which to make choices. Multiple choices from a group of attractive foods, as at a Thanksgiving dinner, tended to induce excess caloric intake by rats as well as man.

This early support to Morley Kare, like many other Nutrition Foundation grants, has been followed by a remarkable research and training development in the Monell Chemical Senses Center. Within a brief period Dr. Kare has built a staff of imaginative, productive young investigators who are internationally recognized as unique in their contributions. For example, they have devised techniques for assessing the taste discrimination of infants and newborns and have established that the preference for sweet taste is an inborn, not acquired, characteristic. This preference is present at birth. Dr. Kare is now a Public Trustee of The Nutrition Foundation, and the present President of the Foundation, Dr. Darby, is a member of the Monell Center's Board of Advisors.

In studies of voluntary regulation of food intake by normal persons at St. Luke's Hospital, Columbia University, Sami Hashim has observed the voluntary eating habits when subjects were fed a nutritionally complete liquid diet by mouth, through a plastic tube. Each push of a button by the subject delivered a mouthful and was recorded (without the subject's knowledge). This arrangement has permitted study of voluntary eating schedules —the subjects predictably preferred eating at about regular meal time. When on a work schedule they automatically consumed food enough to keep in caloric balance, even though they could not from experience appraise the number of calories eaten nor the caloric density. The opportunity to study appetite-regulated mechanisms is evident.

When obese volunteer subjects (50 to 300 pounds overweight) were served with trays having a variety of attractive foods the subjects usually ate everything on the tray—to as high as 3,500 calories per day; then if invited to join in a discussion, with a bowl of potato chips within reach, they would start nibbling on them. Under the same conditions normal subjects found the chips or snacks without appeal. When put on the liquid diet, however, the adult obese persons dropped their caloric intake about 400 calories per day; but adolescent obese patients continued at the original high calorie intake. When the liquid diet was served in cups instead of by tube, obese adults nearly doubled their caloric intake. Understanding of such food intake behavior is clearly important in preventive and therapeutic nutrition—indeed essential to improvement of patient compliance. Additional experimental studies of regulatory factors in food consumption by A. Epstein were supported at the University of Pennsylvania.

Direct studies regarding the effect on food consumption of drugs and electric "messages" recorded as impulses to and from the brain were supported at Princeton University by B. G. Hoebel and at Rockefeller University by Neal Miller. Amphetamines were of special interest because of their wide use as appetite depressants. Other drugs were used experimentally to identify effects on nerve functions in the brain, stomach and intestinal tract.

Information on the role of the intestinal tract in regulating food intake was advanced by Drs. Barnes and Levitsky at Cornell University. As food from the stomach enters the small intestine, individual nutrients and the proportions of these result in differing messages to the brain that in turn signals an increase or decrease in food intake. Continued progress in this field has indicated that at least some of these effects are controlled by hormones released from the intestinal wall and transmitted by the bloodstream to the brain, and thence by nerve impulse to effect appetite control.

Education

A temporary committee on education of the public with H. M. Cleaves, a Trustee, and R. K. Plumb, a science writer on the staff, as co-chairmen, was followed by a permanent committee consisting of independent academic personnel with Professor George M. Briggs at the University of California as Chairman. They agreed that there was an urgent need for honest and effective education of the public in relation to food practices, and that a great many people were being grossly misled by faddists and fakers through popular books, lectures, the press, radio and television programs, and organized groups without competent training in nutrition.

The leadership of Dr. Briggs and his associates at the University resulted in action on a national scale. Qualified leaders in nutrition education from universities, government agencies and independent scientific organizations joined in organizing the Society for Nutrition Education. A grant was made by The Nutrition Foundation to assist the group to prepare a prototype of a new journal. The new quarterly publication, THE JOURNAL OF NUTRITION EDUCATION, was launched, and organized national meetings were programmed. The Society received further assistance from the Foundation to enlarge the readership of the journal that is now sustained through membership dues, subscriptions, advertising and sustaining memberships of industry.

The Foundation's efforts were concentrated on developing materials, new methods of teaching nutrition, getting information on nutrition and food into the school systems, and on working with specialized groups to reach the public through the mass media. The following items illustrate the nature of actions taken during this decade:

The Foundation's highly successful publication, NUTRITION REVIEWS, continued to furnish brief reports on research advances in nutrition for guidance of professional personnel in teaching, public health, medical fields, food technology, agricultural extension service and science writers for the public press.

Primarily for low-income groups the Foundation collaborated with the Department of Agriculture in the production of 50,000 copies of a color booklet, "Food—A Key to Better Health." The booklet was circulated widely in the Extension Service, among Public Health and Welfare personnel, 4-H leaders and teachers.

A third edition of the monograph "Present Knowledge in Nutrition," prepared by the NUTRITION REVIEWS staff, had a wide distribution. A Spanish edition was produced also, with the sponsorship of the Institute of Nutrition of Central America and Panama.

Dr. Diva Sanjur, on the faculty at Cornell University, with a background of home life and experience in Panama, was given a three year grant in 1969 to study the food habits of preschool children among three low-income groups: (a) urban blacks in Buffalo, N.Y., (b) Puerto Ricans in Geneva, N.Y. and (c) rural whites in Plattsburgh, N.Y. In brief, from her experience she reported stingingly that "American scientists know a lot more about what Latin Americans eat than what black people in Buffalo, N.Y. eat." Whether or not a valid conclusion in such broad terms, it reflected a shock from her observations.

Support was continued for the Food and Nutrition Board of the National Academy

A Good Idea

of Sciences—National Research Council. Its committees had a great influence in public educational service such as evaluation of data from the National Nutrition Survey, evaluation of food protection practices and Recommended Dietary Allowances.

Specific items developed with Foundation support included:

1. A Board monograph of special value, "Maternal Nutrition and the Course of Human Pregnancy" was aided by a grant in support of its publication.
2. Conferences were supported to deal with the problem of iron deficiency which persists widely, particularly among women. Increasing the iron content of flour under the cereal enrichment program was given support.
3. Dr. Virginia Beal published reports on Breast and Formula Feeding of Infants, Termination of Night Feeding in Infancy, and Iron Nutriture from Infancy to Adolescence.
4. A publication by the Foundation entitled "Food, Science and Society" included manuscripts presented at a conference organized by Dr. Sipple in cooperation with the Institute of Food Technologists. Dr. Sipple also published a paper "New Approaches to Nutrition Education."
5. A monograph on Olfaction and Taste, edited by Carl Pfaffman, was based on the symposium sponsored jointly with the Rockefeller University.
6. Dr. Pearson published papers on Effect of Malnutrition on Learning and Behavior, Effect of Malnutrition on Development and Productivity, and International Cooperation Through Foundations to Increase Protein Resources.
7. A film, "Journey Into Nutrition," for children aged 6 to 12 years was produced with Foundation support by National Educational Television, in 1970.
8. A filmstrip, "Nutrition Education for Disadvantaged Families," was also produced with Foundation support by the Detroit American Dietetic Association Nutrition Advisory Committee, Merrill-Palmer Institute, 1970.
9. Support was provided for production of three videotapes and curriculum guides for teacher training in nutrition education: "Kindergarten Through Third Grade"; "Fourth Through Sixth Grade"; "Seventh Through Ninth Grade." These were developed by Gail Harrison, Cornell University, and distributed to teachers in New York State through the State's Bureau of School Health Education.
10. Special press releases as follows were issued:
    Protein Rich Potatoes May Benefit Many—September 1968
    Calorie Cut in American Diet Urged by Nutrition Foundation—November 1968
    Nutritional Status of Children Being Studied, Specialists Report—March 1969
    Iron and Calcium in Short Supply in American Women's Diets—June 1969
    Fluoridation Benefits Oldsters as Much as Youngsters—September 1969
    Obesity Can Trigger High Blood Presure—October 1969

In reviewing his experience as President of the Foundation, Dr. Pearson expressed particular regard for the values derived from: (1) continued basic research in the science of nutrition, (2) research in which nutrition is directly related to public health, (3) the training of young scientists as graduate students and post-doctoral fellows, and (4) educational measures to reach the public.

The Third Decade

In addition he took special note of the values developed from : (1) "Future Leaders" awards, in which selected young staff personnel, upon recommendation of their department head, were given support on a broad basis for one to three years in developing their careers without restriction to specific research subjects; (2) conferences and publications leading to improved nutrition training in schools of dentistry and medicine; (3) assistance in building "Centers of Excellence" in nutrition, illustrated by the strong dental research and educational program in nutrition at Tufts University and in the program on human development at the Institute of Human Nutrition, College of Physicians and Surgeons, Columbia University; (4) increased use of press releases as an educational medium, including a scheduled distribution program requested by over 500 daily and weekly newspapers; (5) production of a color TV program on nutrition for elementary school children—used also by many public broadcasting stations; (6) increased financial support, especially from several of the larger member companies; and (7) liaison with other nutrition foundations, as in the United Kingdom, Sweden, the Philippines and France.

Dr. Sipple participated very actively and helpfully in all areas of the Foundation's program, including activities of the Board of Trustees, the Scientific Advisory Committee, the Food Industries Advisory Committee, the Advisory Committee on Education, and the Treasurer's office. His fortunate background had included experience in basic research, followed by several years each in food technology and grants management. His loyalty to the ideals and service of the Foundation were always at a high level.

4

Reorganization for the 1970s

IN view of the pressing need to continue research support and possibly increase substantially the educational program, the Trustees decided at their meeting on November 8, 1968, to study the situation vigorously in planning for the future in terms of costs, organizational structure and related considerations. A second and related item was the approaching age retirement of both Drs. Pearson and Sipple. Plans would need to be developed in a manner to avoid, in so far as possible, disruptive delays in the on-going activities.

A third crucial item was the recognition that a program as envisaged would require much greater financial support. Inflationary trends made it obvious that costs for personnel engaged in research in the universities, together with supplies and equipment, had risen substantially since the Foundation was established. An increase in the staff of the Foundation and their support would also be essential. There was a suggestion that a part of an increased program might be shared with other organizations.

To develop guidelines, Dr. Longenecker was empowered to "form a Review Committee for the purpose of re-examining the Foundation's program and recommending future activities."

Dr. Pearson's review of the program during 1967-68 emphasized the following items:

1. An International Conference on Malnutrition, Learning and Behavior was supported and the proceedings published as a 500-page monograph.
2. Third Edition of a monograph on Present Knowledge in Nutrition was published, including translations in Japanese and Spanish.
3. Support was provided for a new publication, "The Journal of Nutrition Education," and organization of the Society for Nutrition Education.
4. There had been wide circulation of nutrition education releases to daily and weekly newspapers, house organs and labor union papers.
5. Over 100 research papers had been published by grantees in scientific journals.
6. An international conference and monograph on "Olfaction and Taste" had been sponsored jointly with the Rockefeller University.
7. An international symposium on "Food,

Science and Society" had been sponsored jointly with the University of California and the Northern California Section of the Institute of Food Technologists and the proceedings published.
8. Support was provided for reorganization of the International Union of Nutritional Sciences and its election to membership in the International Council of Scientific Unions, providing a stimulus and a key to world-wide recognition of nutrition as a major science.
9. There had occurred increased recognition in the grants program of (a) the relationship of nutrition to learning, behavior and development of the nervous system, (b) appetite, taste and dietary patterns, and (c) nutrition of the preschool-age child.

At the Board of Trustees Meeting on May 2, 1969, Dr. Longenecker announced the appointment of Herbert M. Cleaves as Chairman of a six-member committee to review the objectives, purposes and future course of the Foundation. Dr. Seitz, President of Rockefeller University and former President of the National Academy of Sciences, shared responsibility as public members of the committee with Dr. Longenecker and Dr. Pearson; James W. Evans and A. N. McFarlane represented industry. The committee, after two meetings, recommended the employment of a consultant firm to study the situation on a broad basis and make suggestions, with a special emphasis on problems of education.

Planning advanced rapidly as indicated at the Board of Trustees Meeting on May 7, 1971. The committee prepared and distributed for review a draft copy of recommendations covering (a) guidelines for the future program, (b) changes in the organizational structure, and (c) a commitment to broaden substantially the base of financial support, including increased membership payments and cooperation with other organizations such as private foundations, organized societies and government agencies, working toward similar objectives in nutrition research and education.

Program plans outlined were as follows:

1. That the Foundation maintain a leadership role with respect to the furtherance of sound nutrition. This meant involvement in organizations, meetings, statements and public events to improve public awareness and *understanding* of nutrition in relation to good health. It also meant encouraging the acceptance of sound nutrition principles in governmental, academic, industrial and consumer areas.
2. That the Foundation broaden its programs to include a strong effort to improve nutrition education at all levels—elementary schools, high schools, colleges, professional schools and universities—including trainee and personnel development and an expanded publication program.
3. That the Foundation continue its present course as a non-profit institution to advance the science of nutrition, including appropriate research grants. This research role should be expanded and strengthened.
4. That effort be made to select specific nutrition research areas as primary targets with a concentration of funds and efforts which would make possible scientific breakthroughs and other noteworthy achievements.

Several desirable changes were recommended for the organizational structure. Specific items included:

(a) replacement of the Board of Directors by an Executive Committee to assist and

Reorganization for the 1970s

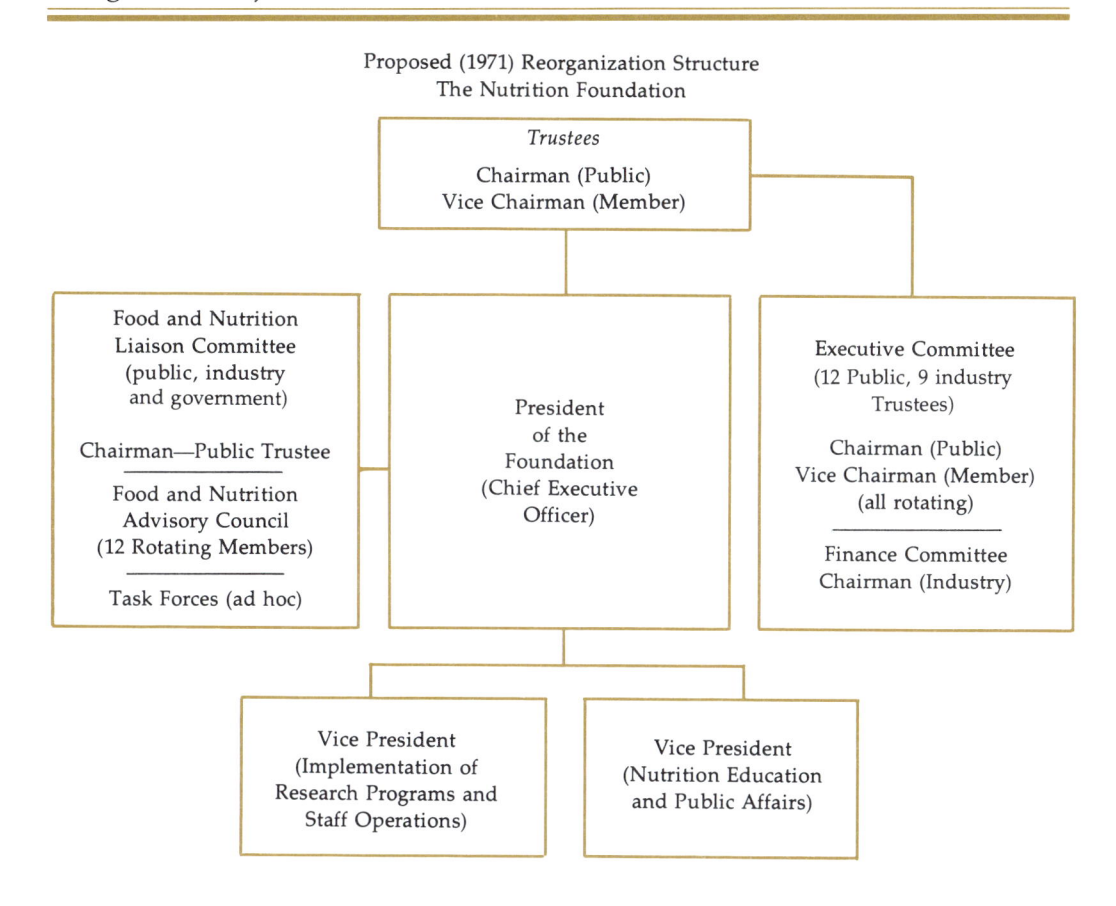

Proposed (1971) Reorganization Structure
The Nutrition Foundation

```
                    ┌─────────────────────────┐
                    │        Trustees         │
                    │   Chairman (Public)     │
                    │  Vice Chairman (Member) │
                    └─────────────────────────┘
                              │
   ┌──────────────────┐       │       ┌──────────────────────┐
   │ Food and Nutrition│      │       │ Executive Committee  │
   │ Liaison Committee │      │       │ (12 Public, 9 industry│
   │ (public, industry │      │       │      Trustees)       │
   │  and government)  │      │       │                      │
   │                   │   ┌──────┐   │  Chairman (Public)   │
   │ Chairman—Public   │   │President│ │ Vice Chairman (Member)│
   │    Trustee        │───│of the  │─│   (all rotating)     │
   │                   │   │Foundation│ │                    │
   │ Food and Nutrition│   │(Chief   │ │  Finance Committee   │
   │ Advisory Council  │   │Executive│ │  Chairman (Industry) │
   │ (12 Rotating      │   │ Officer)│ └──────────────────────┘
   │    Members)       │   └──────┘
   │                   │       │
   │ Task Forces       │       │
   │   (ad hoc)        │       │
   └──────────────────┘        │
                    ┌──────────┴──────────┐
        ┌───────────────────┐    ┌─────────────────┐
        │  Vice President   │    │ Vice President  │
        │ (Implementation of│    │(Nutrition Education│
        │ Research Programs │    │ and Public Affairs)│
        │ and Staff Operations)│ │                 │
        └───────────────────┘    └─────────────────┘
```

report to the Board of Trustees (original structure);

(b) *requirement* that the Executive Committee have a public member as Chairman (an initial practice) and that public members would have a majority representation in the total membership (12 and 9, respectively);

(c) a large Liaison Committee reporting to the President would include public, industry and government members;

(d) a Food and Nutrition Advisory Council and Task Forces appointed by the President would undertake specific assignments; and

(e) two Vice Presidents, one primarily to assist in technical and scientific aspects of the program and another to guide an increased number of publications, education of the public, public affairs and related activities.

The Food Industries Advisory Committee was replaced by a Food and Nutrition Liaison Committee, with a public trustee as Chairman, together with a representative (normally a scientist) of each Member Organization. Their primary responsibility would be to study and report on new areas of broad interest in relation to research and education.

The Food and Nutrition Advisory Council, consisting of 12 members serving in rotation, would be designated by the President, subject to approval by the Executive Committee, and charged with making recommendations in regard to grants and policy matters relating to research, education and public affairs.

A Good Idea

A Finance Committee would consist of five or more Member Trustees appointed by the Executive Committee.

A Committee, which Dr. Longenecker chaired, had prepared a pension plan for employees and present retirees comparable to practices in similar organizations that participate in the program of the Teacher's Insurance and Annuity Association. The generous inclusion of the retirees was greatly appreciated because there had been no provision during the first 10 years.

Mr. Murphy, Chairman of the Committee on Programming and Staffing, reported that Dr. Pearson and Dr. Sipple had accepted their invitation to continue in office through 1971 and that new by-laws would not go into effect until January 1, 1972.

Grants approved at the May, 1971, meeting included: (a) four Future Leader grants—at the University of Missouri, University of Iowa, Vanderbilt University and Cornell University, totaling $89,575 during the subsequent two years; (b) two grants in nutrition—to Cornell Medical College and Columbia University, totaling $29,800; and (c) four specific research grants—to New York University, University of Montana, University of Pennsylvania and University of California (Davis), totaling $81,000 through the next two years.

At Mr. Murphy's request Dr. Longenecker had appointed a special committee to follow through after the meeting on May 5th to finalize the new by-laws and to search for the new president and nominate new public and member trustees in accordance with the new by-laws. Appointed

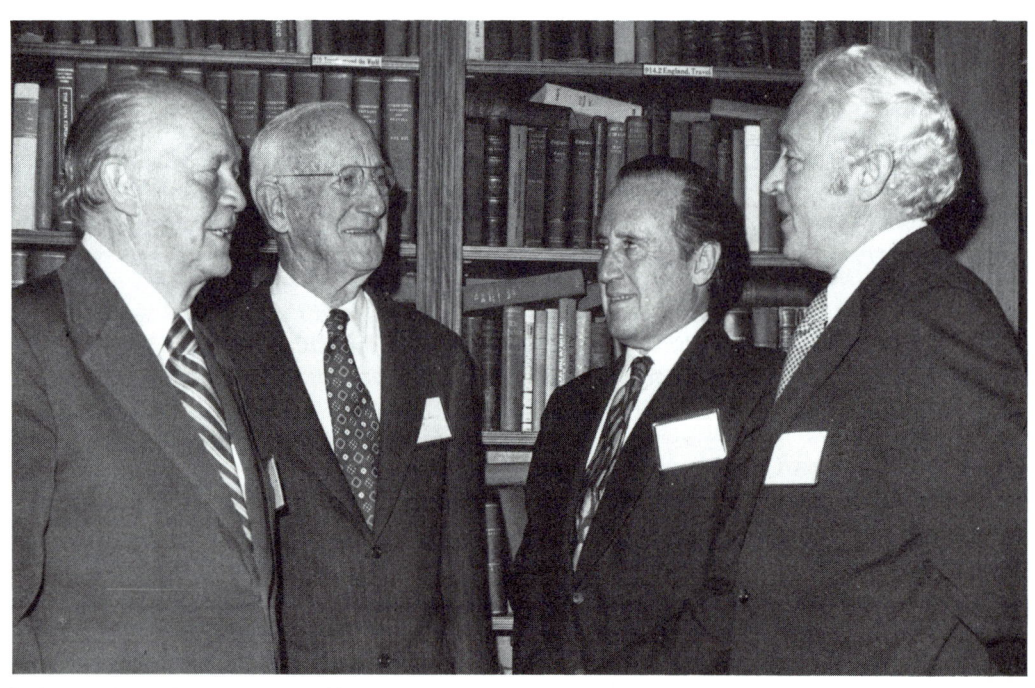

Left to right: *J. George Harrar, Clarence Francis, H. J. Heinz, II, William J. Darby.*

At the May, 1975 meeting of the Board of Trustees, Clarence Francis, whose initial interest helped launch The Nutrition Foundation, was elected Honorary Life Trustee. The announcement of the election was made by Mr. Heinz, the only other original Trustee actively serving since 1941.

Reorganization for the 1970s

were: Emil Mrak, Chairman, H. E. Carter, J. George Harrar, A. R. Marusi and W. B. Murphy.

At the next meeting of the Trustees on November 5, 1971, the new by-laws were adopted (Appendix B), action taken upon the recommendation of the special committee to double the membership dues of the Foundation, and Dr. Mrak reported the committee's success in arrangements for Dr. W. J. Darby to accept the office of President of The Nutrition Foundation, to become effective January 1, 1972. Clarence Francis, now as a public trustee, had the honor and pleasure of seconding the motion to approve the election—for him, truly a thirty-year anniversary of "The Development of a Good Idea"—his idea, multiplied and expanded since December, 1941, by others of like mind in their concern for the food industry's service to the public.

For Mr. Heinz it was a memorable experience also, since he was the only one of the original company executives who still represented his company on the Board. He had been a very effective leader in numerous respects and especially in persuading executives in other countries to join in organizing nutrition foundations to serve the public in a similar manner and spirit. Acquaintance with Mr. Heinz and members of his staff since early days in Pittsburgh had made clear to me his genuine interest in education and research and the application of science in the public interest. The occasion was a unique experience for me also, since I was the only one of the original public trustees to be present.

Dr. Darby's background and abilities were remarkably suited to the new position. Subsequent to doctorate training in both biochemistry and medicine, he advanced rapidly to become a professor in charge of biochemistry and nutrition in the School of Medicine at Vanderbilt Univer-

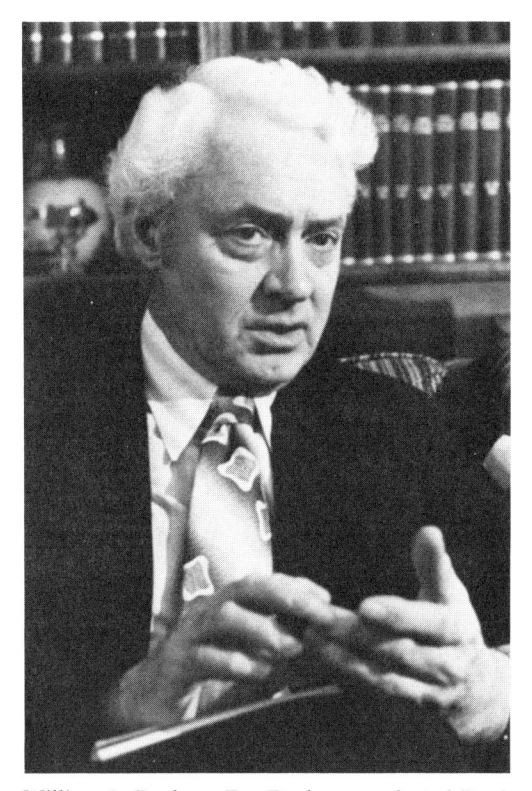

William J. Darby—Dr. Darby was elected President and a Public Trustee of The Nutrition Foundation, effective January 1, 1972.

sity. His research accomplishments in nutrition were closely related to maternal and child health, the identity of a new vitamin (folic acid) and its effectiveness in anemia and sprue, and in the use of clinical methods for identifying nutritional diseases. His contributions were recognized nationally and internationally, including worldwide service with the United Nations agencies WHO, FAO and UNICEF, and the International Union of Nutritional Sciences. He had been the first Chairman of the Protein Advisory Group (WHO/FAO/UNICEF). For many years he had served as a member of the Food and Nutrition Board of the National Academy of Sciences-National Research Council, including the chairmanship of the Committee on

A Good Idea

Food Protection, where he gained familiarity with the problems of industry, their relationship to health, and the role of government agencies. He had served through several years in advisory capacities with the Department of Health, Education and Welfare, the National Institutes of Health, the U.S. Agency for International Development (State Department), the ICNND, and the Food and Drug Administration. He had also served directly with The Nutrition Foundation as an Associate Editor of NUTRITION REVIEWS (1944-1950) and as a member of the Scientific Advisory Committee (1958-1965). Research in which he participated at Vanderbilt University had been supported by the Foundation almost continuously since 1944. He had received the Osborne and Mendel Award of the American Institute of Nutrition and the Joseph Goldberger Award from the American Medical Association, in recognition of basic and medical research, respectively. At the Trustees luncheon on November 5, 1971, Dr. Darby presented his concept of "Nutrition for the 1970s" (Appendix C) which presaged nutrition interests, needs, and opportunities for program development and leadership by The Nutrition Foundation.

The Trustees expressed their confidence in moving ahead vigorously to activate and support the plans essentially as recommended by their committees.

The Nominating Committee recommendations were approved to become effective January 1, 1972, as follows:

Chairman of the Board of Trustees—H. E. Longenecker
Vice Chairman of the Board of Trustees—A. R. Marusi
Chairman of the Executive Committee—H. E. Longenecker
Vice Chairman of the Executive Committee—A. R. Marusi

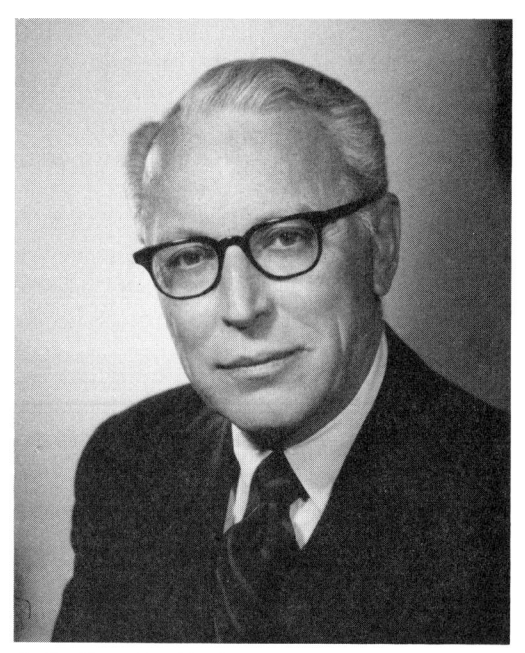

A. R. Marusi—Chief Executive Officer and President of The Borden Company, was Vice President of the Board of Trustees of The Nutrition Foundation, 1972-1975. Mr. Marusi serves as Chairman of the Membership and Finance Committee of The Nutrition Foundation.

Members of the Executive Committee:

Public Trustees:

J. Z. Bowers
Josiah Macy Jr. Foundation

H. E. Carter
University of Arizona

J. G. Harrar
The Rockefeller Foundation

G. W. Irving, Jr.
Federation of American Societies for Experimental Biology

D. R. Lindsay
Duke University

H. E. Longenecker
Tulane University

Reorganization for the 1970s

Emil Mrak
University of California

J. Q. Newton
The Commonwealth Fund

Gretchen Pullen
Swanson Foundation

Frederick Seitz
The Rockefeller University

H. L. Sipple
Naples, Florida

Luther L. Terry
University of Pennsylvania

Industry Trustees:

E. L. Artzt
Procter & Gamble Company

W. O. Beers
Kraftco Corporation

J. W. Evans
American Maize-Products Co.

D. E. Guerrant
Libby, McNeill & Libby

H. C. Harder
CPC International, Inc.

R. S. Hatfield
Continental Can Company, Inc.

V. W. Henningsen, Jr.
Henningsen Foods, Inc.

J. E. Lonning
Kellogg Company

A. R. Marusi
Borden, Inc.

R. W. Reneker
Swift & Company

During 1972 the two positions of vice-president were filled. The Vice Presidents elected were Dr. C. O. Chichester, former Chairman of the Department of Food Science, University of California at Davis, Professor of Food and Resource Chemistry at the University of Rhode Island and Director of the International Food Science programs for Marine Resource Development, and Mr. Richard M. Stalvey for Education and Public Affairs—well known as a gifted writer and interpreter of science for the public. Dr. Chichester had received his doctorate degree in Agricultural Chemistry, followed by a notable career as professor at the University of California. Mr. Stalvey's earlier experience on the staff of the Food and Drug Administration and the American Medical Association's Bureau of Investigation as well as his knowledge of publications and communications admirably fitted him for the responsibilities relative to education and public affairs. In 1973, Kristen W. McNutt, Ph.D., joined with Dr. Sipple in editing the initial Nutrition Foundation Monograph, "Sugars in Nutrition." Subsequently she was appointed to a newly created post as Research Associate of The Nutrition Foundation.

In addition to editing the monograph on sugars, Dr. Horace Sipple helped substantially during the transition in administration beyond 1971. He, together with other members of the staff, agreed to remain in service for a period of several months. Both Dr. Pearson and Dr. Sipple were elected to serve as public trustees of the Foundation. Provision was also made for Mrs. Mary van Sante to continue for at least a year beyond normal retirement age.

Orientation and New Horizons

In advance of the spring meeting of the Board of Trustees on May 5, 1972, tentative budget plans were adjusted to conform with the new organizational structure and expanding program. An opportunity for Dr. Darby to review plans for the future was given at a meeting of the Food and Nutrition Liaison Committee in Naples, Florida, January 26, 1972, when all segments of the Foundation were represented and made aware that a major growth in the Foundation was well underway. His review of the situation is illustrated by the following quotations:

> An aggressive program of communication with current members and recruitment of new members has been organized by the Finance Committee under the Chairmanship of Mr. A. R. Marusi. Regional Chairmen and co-chairmen have been named and . . . meetings with appropriate representatives of member companies and prospective members are scheduled.

Review of Activities

An analysis and review of the activities, commitments and past program has been initiated. You will be interested in a few of the highlights. During the 30 years from 1942 through 1971, the Foundation has awarded research grants totaling $9,461,640. Among the grantees a total of seven have been elected as Nobel Laureates.

The Foundation has provided $141,480 for the support of the distinguished awards made annually by professional societies. These include 20 Joseph Goldberger Awards administered by the American Medical Association, 23 Osborne and Mendel Awards administered by the American Institute of Nutrition, 23 Babcock-Hart Awards administered by the Institute of Food Technologists, and 23 Mary Swartz Rose Awards administered by the American Dietetic Association.

The grant program has included support of the very satisfying group of 43 outstanding young scientists in their first academic positions, who have been designated Future Leaders. That they are in fact Future Leaders may be indicated by the positions to which some of them recently have been appointed. Dr. Myron Winick, as of January 1, 1972, became Professor of Pediatrics and Director of the Institute of Human Nutrition, Columbia University; Dr. Harold H. Sandstead as of July 1, 1971, was named Director of the Human Nutrition Research Laboratory, U.S. Department of Agriculture, Grand Forks, North Dakota. At least four of these young leaders have attained full professorial status and 14 others have been promoted to Associate Professorships since the program's inception in 1967.

The circulation of the monthly scientific review publication, NUTRITION REVIEWS, exceeds 5,200. During the past year approximately 75,000 copies of various educational pamphlets have been sent in response to requests, and some 2,000 inquiries related to nutritional matters have been answered by letter or telephone.

Three other Nutrition Foundations—British, Swedish and Japanese—have been organized in the pattern of this Foundation, the first of its kind in the world.

But, as impressive as this is, it is not enough to meet the needs of the '70s!

Purposes of the Foundation

The purposes of The Nutrition Foundation are:

1. To advance the science of nutrition and to further its use for the health and welfare of mankind;
2. to aid the food and allied industries in serving the public through advances in nutrition and food science; and
3. to pursue these goals as a public non-profit institution dedicated to the improvement of nutrition and health.

To fulfill these purposes the Foundation will:

1. Continue as a non-profit institution to advance the science of nutrition through an expanded and strengthened program of grant support to appropriate research;
2. select certain areas of nutrition research toward which a concentration of funds and efforts can make possible scientific breakthroughs and noteworthy achievements; and
3. provide vigorous leadership in the furtherance of sound nutrition. . . .

Nutrition Information

To bring about improved understanding of nutrition will require a significant expansion of activities in the field of nutrition information. The Foundation alone cannot accomplish these

Reorganization for the 1970s

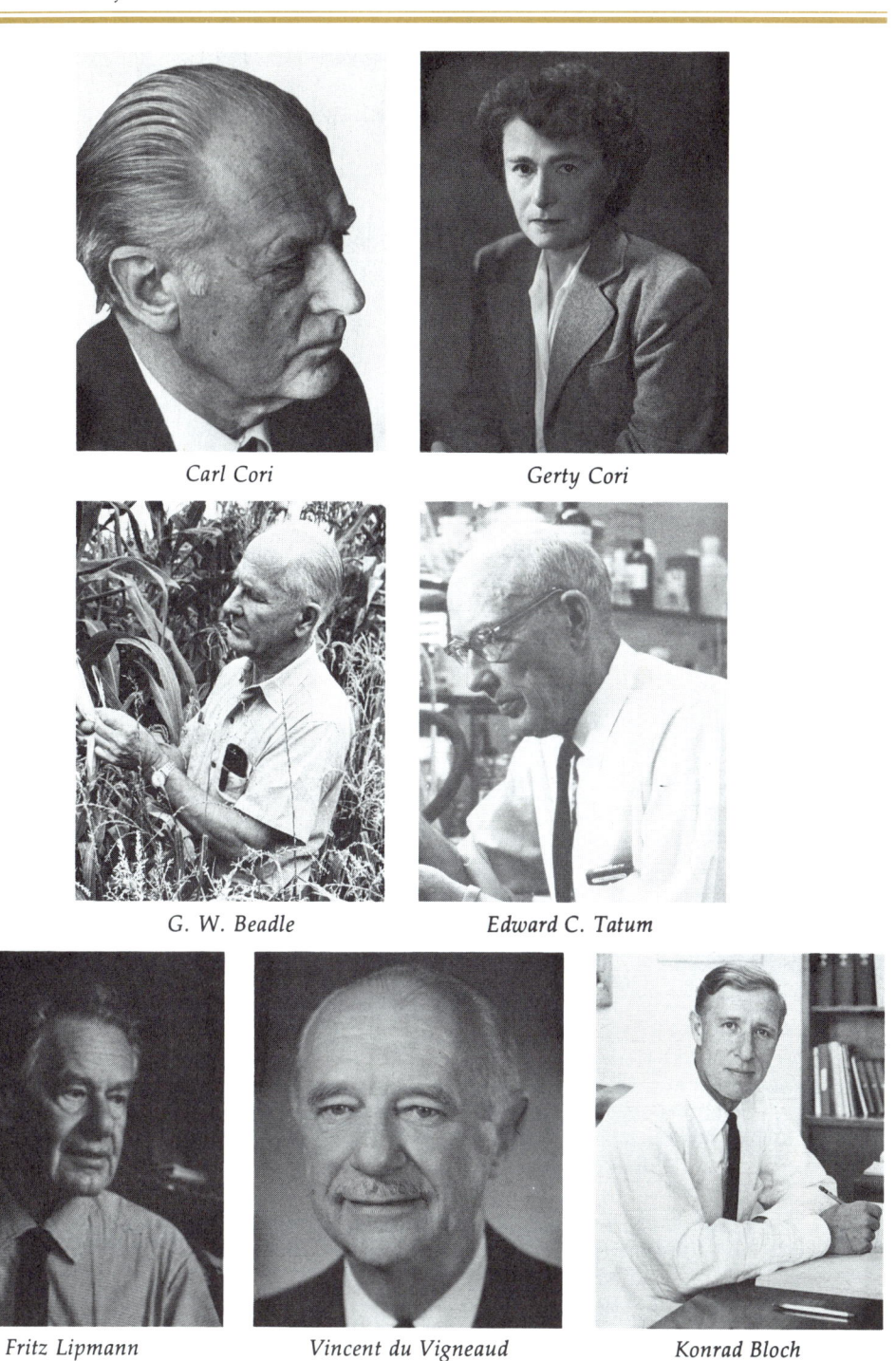

Carl Cori

Gerty Cori

G. W. Beadle

Edward C. Tatum

Fritz Lipmann

Vincent du Vigneaud

Konrad Bloch

Investigators whose early research received support from The Nutrition Foundation and who subsequently were selected as Nobel Laureates.

A Good Idea

tasks. It can coordinate efforts and cooperate with diverse agencies to make more effective use of existing resources. Toward such efforts we have since the first of the year participated in meetings or direct conversations and correspondence with members of the Food and Drug Law Institute, the Food and Drug Administration, the National Academy of Sciences (both the Food Protection Committee and the Food and Nutrition Board), the Council on Foods and Nutrition of the American Medical Association, the National Dairy Council, and committees of the Institute of Food Technologists. Such involvement and coordination of efforts will continue.

These must be long-term efforts, for they cannot be accomplished by a crash program. They must go forward in an orderly, objective manner and must not be diverted by the public crises that recurrently appear. On the other hand, the Foundation can and should act to defuse emotionally charged issues and to provide a scientific voice of reason to reduce misunderstanding and to improve the chances for long-term constructive investigation and action.

The Nutrition Foundation must provide leadership of integrity. It will not become a lobbying agency and must remain scientifically detached in debates affecting any particular segment of the food industry. Its position and public statements cannot possibly satisfy all of the special interests of individual food company members. To be effective as a nutrition authority, it must base its public statements on the latest and soundest findings of nutritional science. These may not always coincide with a member company's interest.

The Foundation should serve as a Center of Nutrition Information. In so doing its service must be coordinated with and supplementary to the services now offered by the National Library of Medicine, the USDA Library at Beltsville, Md., the American Institute of Nutrition, the Council on Foods and Nutrition of the AMA, L.I.F.E., and other agencies. . . .

The Foundation can provide informal assistance to organizations seeking appropriately knowledgeable personnel to work on information and education programs and assist in selecting and obtaining speakers for conferences, public addresses, and forums. It can serve as a medium for identifying centers or groups engaged in research of immediate interest. . . .

The Foundation can also communicate with the public through food editors, teachers and public health professionals by sponsoring meetings of these and similar groups. . . .

Professional Nutrition Education

To build sound programs in nutrition education and information in the professional fields, three simultaneous developments are essential. These are (a) the development of personnel for nutrition, (b) the commitment of significant institutional resources for education and research in the field, and (c) the provision for educational materials and facilitation of communication. The Nutrition Foundation can contribute significantly to professional nutrition education by:

1. Continuing its Future Leaders program, with review of its present form in light of current national resources and needs and past effectiveness, and
2. Establishing a program of support for a limited number of centers of Excellence in Nutrition.

These Centers of Excellence in Nutrition should be in diverse schools and universities and serve as models for similar developments elsewhere. The Foundation should provide substantial long-term support in keeping with the needs and assessed potential and commitment of the institution. Several types of schools or departments are appropriate sites for such centers: schools of medicine, dentistry, agriculture, home economics, food science, nursing, dietetics and the allied medical professions. . . .

A revised and expanded program of educational publications will be given high priority. The principal targets of the information and educational efforts will be the public, students from primary schools through undergraduate colleges, professional and scientific groups (medical, dental, paramedical, agricultural,

Reorganization for the 1970s

educational, food scientists, sociologists, economists, regulatory scientists, writers, and personnel of industry, international agencies and government). To advise on such programs, specially constituted *ad hoc* advisory panels will be convened.

The editor of NUTRITION REVIEWS, Dr. Mark Hegsted, and I agree that we should give high priority to examination by a task force of ways to expand the usefulness and scope of this prestigious journal. Examples of subjects to be considered include the possibility of collaborating with European and Japanese Nutrition Foundations in order to enhance the publication's international coverage, as well as the advisability of publishing informative documented reviews of matters of wide public concern. . . .

Since few scientists read the *Federal Register*, the inclusion of selected brief summaries of regulatory activities might usefully inform the academic nutrition profession on important developments of scientific interest.

A systematic listing of new publications from international agencies and from the National Academy of Sciences-National Research Council, Federal agencies and other sources, could be a unique contribution, as could be a positive listing of recommended publications and teaching aids.

The continuing demand for the publication "Present Knowledge In Nutrition" dictates a need to revise this series.

We propose to publish a series of Nutrition Foundation Monographs similar to the WHO monograph series. Many of these are expected to emerge from symposia sponsored by the Foundation or by other organizations.

A less technical Report Series that deals objectively and informatively with issues of current public nutritional interest will be developed.

I believe the Foundation should stimulate the production of much needed textbooks, certain other teaching aids, and popular books such as paperbacks that can promote understanding and knowledge among the general public.

To improve nutrition teaching in public schools the Foundation will undertake a review of the nutritional content of widely used textbooks and seek means of improving it. This will require close collaboration with selected Federal and state agencies, publishers of textbooks and authors.

Teacher Training, Workshops, Symposia

The Foundation will become informed of the nutritional content of teacher training curricula and by working with appropriate educators will seek to improve this. Further, we propose to stimulate appropriate in-service teacher training efforts in nutrition by working with selected educational agencies at both Federal and state levels. . . .

The Foundation will sponsor and support workshops and symposia on timely subjects of public interest and of research importance. Certain of these may serve, as noted above, as a basis for publication in the Report or Monograph Series. Other workshops may serve primarily to promote informal communication between scientists from academia, industry and government or between scientists and consumers. . . .

Examples of timely topics for workshops or symposia and resulting publications are: (a) the role of fructose, certain other sugars and sugar derivatives in nutrition; (b) modified starches; (c) the economics of food chemical safety; (d) guidelines for good nutritional advertising relative to foods; (e) systems of hospital food service and special convenience foods for therapeutic diets; (f) the responsibility of the scientist in decision-making concerning matters of food safety; (g) identification of industry activities that can be coordinated in the public interest (such as information on food composition, production and evaluation of general nutrition education materials); (h) exchange of information and evaluations of the programs of the several national nutrition foundations—British, Swedish, Japanese and American. The first suggested meeting of the several foundations is tentatively set for September 2, 1972, immediately preceding the International Congress on Nutrition. Such discussions may be helpful to other countries, such as Brazil, where there is interest in establishing a nutrition foundation.

The Nutrition Foundation seems to be an ideal medium for organizing a series of informal conferences on potential future problems that may arise from specific food chemicals of international importance. Discussion by selected scientists from several countries before issues become critical in a single country can help prevent unnecessary, costly, unilateral, and precipitous action by one country that makes similar actions by other countries inescapable.

Research

Through the utilization of *ad hoc* panels and the new Council as provided by the revised by-laws, the program and commitments to research will be reviewed critically and new directions will be considered. The Foundation will then be in position to set priorities for its expanded program. Interests of high priority will be identified in order to provide adequate support for work directed at important questions to produce decisive results.

The time is appropriate to reexamine the basic areas of research recently supported by the Foundation. These are:

a. the relation of nutrition to learning, behavior and the development of the nervous system;
b. appetite, taste and dietary patterns;
c. naturally occurring inhibitors in foods and the availability of nutrients;
d. nutrition education.

The position of the Foundation has been that when adequate support from other sources becomes available for any of these areas, the Foundation may redirect its resources to other aspects of nutrition science judged worthy and in need of support. Recognizing that some nutrition problems can be studied more effectively outside of the United States, the Foundation stands ready to take advantage of such opportunities wherever they occur and are consistent with its priorities and its interests. We shall consider other innovative areas and review our order of priorities in research funding.

Areas that appear to offer innovative opportunities and compete for priorities include concepts basic to methodology for estimating safety or hazard of chemicals and foodstuffs. Although attention will be focused on limited aspects of this problem by others, especially the new National Center for Toxicological Research at Pine Bluff, there are concepts and toxicologic principles that underlie considerations of carcinogenesis, teratogenesis (physical deformities induced during gestation), mutagenesis and other phenomena toward which creative study may best be stimulated by modest support to individual investigators. As illustrations, I would cite the relationship of the phenomenon of anti-thyroid activity to carcinogenesis and the subject of toxicity of excessive intakes of essential nutrients.

Earlier I suggested that the nutritional properties and metabolic effects of various carbohydrates loom as important areas for expansion in the immediate future.

Even a cursory perusal of the subject of food chemistry reveals a host of substances of relatively undefined biologic activity to which we are daily exposed. Is there needed research in relation to natural constituents that deserves stimulatory support from the Foundation?

Do some of the new leads concerning the relationship of host resistance and infection to nutrition offer important, exciting opportunities for discovery?

A number of non-chemical interdisciplinary interests also could provide large returns on research investments by the Foundation. For example, a delineation of the economic impact of some regulatory decisions or predictable effect of alternative decisions in the future. Worthy of attention in this regard are the developments concerning cyclamates, DDT, 2, 4, 5-T, mercury, nitrates and nitrites, Red 2, brominated oils and so on.

Should the Foundation not play a role in stimulating competent interest and more socio-anthropological research on the basis of food attitudes and beliefs, including the origin and appeal of food fads and cults, the public understanding of and attitudes toward additives, pesticides, processed foods, fabricated foods and nutritional improvement of foods? If so, how? Where?

When priorities are determined I do not believe they should be absolute in their limitation on the placement of research funds. A degree of flexibility must exist in order that the wisest and most beneficial use of resources be exploited. Finally, in planning a research grants program

Reorganization for the 1970s

there must be provision for maintaining a vista through which to view promising new concepts.

The first meeting of the newly organized Board of Trustees was held on May 5, 1972. In his opening remarks the Chairman of the Board had a special bit of good news in mentioning that Dr. Darby had been elected to the National Academy of Sciences in recognition of his outstanding accomplishments in research. The same honor has more recently (1973) been extended to D. Mark Hegsted, editor of NUTRITION REVIEWS. Nevin Scrimshaw, a member of the Food and Nutrition Advisory Council, is also a member of the National Academy of Sciences. In earlier years seven of the representatives of the public serving on the Board of Trustees had been elected to the National Academy of Sciences. The Trustee most recently elected a member (1975) is John J. Burns, Vice President of Hoffmann-LaRoche.

With the growth in confidence and enthusiasm among the Trustees and committees, the doubling of the annual contributions of each member company, and anticipated support from non-industry sources, the Trustees projected an early annual budget reaching beyond $2,000,000.

In 1973 Dr. Harrar succeeded Dr. Longenecker as Chairman of the Board of Trustees and of the Executive Committee, and Mr. J. E. Lonning succeeded Mr. Marusi as Vice-Chairman. The leadership of Dr. Harrar gave the Foundation unquestioned national and worldwide assurance of integrity, high standards of program

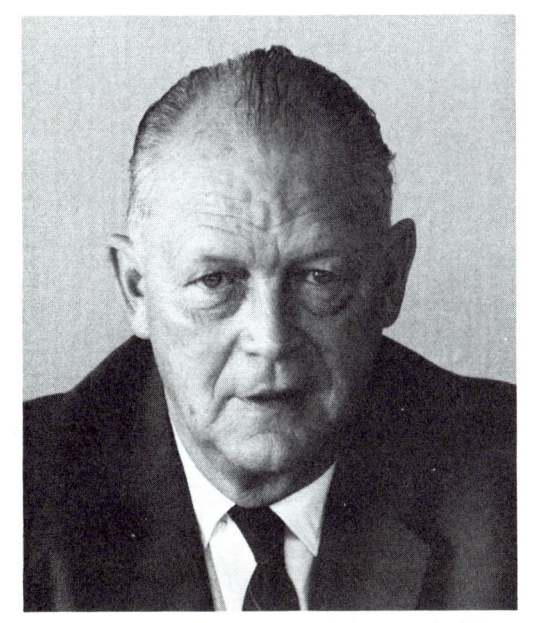

J. George Harrar—Chairman of the Board of Trustees, The Nutrition Foundation 1973-

Dr. Harrar, a distinguished agricultural scientist, served as President of The Rockefeller Foundation 1961-1972. His leadership and vision were major influences in the design and implementation of the Green Revolution.

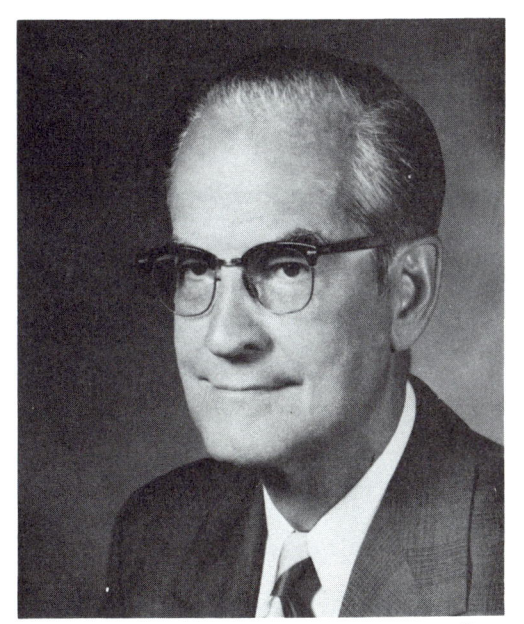

J. E. Lonning—Chief Executive Officer, Kellogg Company. Vice Chairman of the Board of Trustees, 1973-

Mr. Lonning served the U.S. Delegation to the World Food Conference in Rome, November, 1974.

A Good Idea

guidance and efficient administration. Early academic experience at Oberlin College, the University of Puerto Rico, Virginia Polytechnic Institute, the University of Minnesota, Iowa State College and Washington State College had been followed by phenomenal success in building an agricultural research and training program in Mexico, before serving as President of The Rockefeller Foundation (1961-1972).

The transition phase of 1972-73 was one of restaffing, of meetings with the scientific, governmental, industrial and public constituency of the Foundation, and of planning and initiating new activities. As a part of that assessment upon which to project activities, Dr. Darby requested me to prepare a history of the Foundation. The staff undertook a demanding sequence of meetings with nutrition leadership here and abroad, with new advisory groups called for in the reorganizational plan, and with prospective new supporters of the Foundation.

There resulted strengthened conviction concerning three major needs: a unifying communication system between and among the nutrition community; a scholarly examination of the dimensions of risk-benefit embracing the broad aspects of food and nutrition; and development of effective means of promoting nutritional knowledge and understanding. In the final chapter, which summarizes the Foundation's activities from 1972 to 1975, Dr. Darby tells how during that time The Nutrition Foundation has contributed to fulfillment of these needs.

The Fourth Decade: The Program of the 1970s

THE opportunities for leadership inherent in a prestigious, mission-oriented foundation carry heavy responsibilities for effective planning and selection of priorities. The organizational structure of The Nutrition Foundation assures fulfillment of these responsibilities. It provides for use of the widest range of advisory talent drawn from all sections of the scientific and public community.

The Foundation staff represents extensive experience in major academic institutions and in advisory roles to government and industry, and offers recognized competence in education, research, and public and international nutrition considerations. The Food and Nutrition Advisory Council, drawn from academia, government and industry, is composed of outstanding scientists from diverse disciplines. The Food and Nutrition Liaison Committee constitutes a unique pool of talented scientists, educators and science administrators from these same sources. These bodies operate within the framework determined by the Trustees. They have assigned the operative responsibilities of review and recommendations concerning staff, policies, programs and budget to the Executive Committee. This Committee, composed of twenty-one members, with twelve Public Trustees and no more than nine Member Trustees, is chaired by a distinguished Public Trustee. The bylaws require that the Chairman of the Board of Trustees, of the Executive Committee of that Board, and of the Food and Nutrition Liaison Committee be selected from the Public Trustees of the Foundation.

The program and structure of The Nutrition Foundation reflect the wise planning of its founders and the experienced guidance of its Trustees and advisors in constant reassessment of public needs.

In 1970 and 1971, the Trustees—working through two committees, a task force and an outside consulting firm—developed guidelines to meet the responsibilities facing The Nutrition Foundation in the 1970s. These are in line with the purposes set forth in the 1941 Certificate of Incorporation:

A Good Idea

To develop and apply the science of nutrition, in its fundamental conception and practical significance as a basic science of public health;

To aid the food industry in appropriately solving its general and individual problems relating to that science;

To do so by lawful and effective means, as a public institution operated on a non-profit basis and dedicated to improve the food and diet and thus to better the health of the people of the United States of America.

Objectives of activities during the period from January 1, 1972 to the present, in keeping with the guidelines, may be grouped as follows:

I. To provide leadership in the consolidation of objective scientific information basic to understanding nutritional needs and developments, to catalyze communication within the organized scientific community and thereby to reduce duplication of efforts and strengthen the effectiveness of the nation's nutritional scientific resources;
II. To improve public awareness and understanding of nutrition and foods in relation to public health;
III. To encourage acceptance of sound nutrition principles in governmental, academic, industrial and consumer areas;
IV. To improve nutrition education at all levels —professional schools, colleges and universities, high schools, elementary schools— including training and personnel development and an expanded publication program;
V. To continue to advance the science of nutrition through research and education grants as a non-profit organization, and to concentrate grant support in areas within which there may be initiated possible "scientific breakthroughs" and other noteworthy achievements;
VI. To support activities by The Nutrition Foundation that contribute to resolution of the world food and nutrition problems.

The Foundation has established a Nutrition Information Center in its Office of Education in Washington, D.C. The Center is responsible for producing and distributing the Foundation's nutrition education publications and for preparing graphic materials used in Foundation activities. It is the managing editorial office for NUTRITION REVIEWS. Simultaneously, the Executive Offices of the Foundation have been relocated on Fifth Avenue in New York.

Examples of activities supported by the Foundation may be noted under each of the identified program objectives following.

Promotion, Exchange and Assessment of Scientific Information

The Foundation's professional staff serves as members of or liaison representatives to major review and advisory committees, professional, scientific and governmental. The staff maintains continuing communication with other granting agencies and scientific institutions concerning programs and technical matters. The Foundation has encouraged scientific and professional societies to develop organized mechanisms for exchange, communication and coordination of related program interests. Specific examples include:

The National Nutrition Consortium

The Nutrition Foundation assisted the four principal national professional and scientific societies directly concerned with nutrition and food science in establishing the National Nutrition Consortium, Inc. The societies are the American Dietetic Association, American Institute of Nutrition, American Society for Clinical Nutrition and the Institute of Food Technologists. The total membership of the four societies represents over 40,000 professionals. Two additional organizations

The Fourth Decade

have since become affiliated with the National Nutrition Consortium: the Committee on Nutrition of the American Academy of Pediatrics, and the Society for Nutrition Education. (The founding of the latter society and of its publication, *The Journal of Nutrition Education*, was assisted earlier by grants from The Nutrition Foundation.)

The Consortium provides responsible authorities in food science and nutrition with an established forum and common channel of communication, and it serves as a focus for coordinated actions to guide the application of food and nutrition knowledge for the public good. It has developed a statement of guidelines for a national nutrition policy which served as a key document in Congressional hearings on national nutrition policy and in the report of those hearings. It has, at the request of Congressional committees, identified knowledgeable scientists to discuss various nutritional matters under consideration by those committees. These issues include needed support for nutrition education in schools of health sciences, particularly medical schools, and the need for regulation of high dosage nutrient-containing preparations that might lead to excessive toxic intakes of certain nutrients.

In cooperation with the National Committee for Nutrition Labeling Education and with assistance from The Nutrition Foundation, the Consortium has prepared an informative paperback book for consumers entitled, "Nutrition Labeling — How It Can Work For You." This is being promoted directly to the consumer audience and distributed to media personnel (food and science editors, newspapers, trade journals, telecasters and broadcasters), consumer publications, national advertisers, consumer representatives, the National Association of Food Chains, the USDA, the Food and Drug Administration, the Consumer Federation of America, USDA Home Economics Demonstration Agents and Extension Food and Nutrition Program Aides, school nurses, school doctors, dentists, health educators, supervisors of student teacher training in colleges of teacher education, occupational health nurses and others. It is intended as a "primer on nutrition for the layman" and appeals to its readership through the consumer's interest in nutrition labeling. The initial printing is 100,000.

Cooperation Between National Nutrition Foundations

Upon the initiative of The Nutrition Foundation, a meeting was held by staff officers of the British Nutrition Foundation, the Swedish Nutrition Foundation and The Nutrition Foundation during the IX International Congress of Nutrition in Mexico City in 1972. Since that meeting, these three organizations have maintained continuing communication regarding present and future activities and events supported by the respective Foundations. They have agreed regarding interchange of publications, and the republication and translation of material from one Foundation by the others. Representatives of each Foundation are invited to attend symposia and meetings of the other Foundations, to provide consultation relative to planning of programs and evaluation of scientific advances, and to participate in other forms of direct collaboration.

An example of collaboration is the establishment by the three Foundations of The Nutrition Foundations' Award Book selection. The objective of this award is to stimulate and identify authoritative, exceptionally meritorious books dealing with major concepts of food and nutrition so the non-specialized reader may recognize examples of quality books that are well written and scientifically accurate. The author of the selected work receives a prize of £1,000. The initial selection was "The Conquest of Famine" by the distinguished international nutritionist, W. F. Aykroyd. It was published by Chatto and Windus, London, in 1974 and by the Reader's Digest Press, New York, in 1975.

A further collaborative effort was publication of a joint statement by Dr. Leif Hambraeus, Director of the Swedish Nutrition Foundation, and Dr. William J. Darby, President of The Nutrition Foundation, of "Proposed Nutritional Guidelines for Utilization of Industrially Produced Nutrients." This was published in the August, 1975 issue of the Swedish Nutrition Foundation's journal, and was noted in both NUTRITION REVIEWS and the British Nutrition Foundation's Bulletin. Reprints are being widely distributed by the Foundations.

Other foundations interested in joining this international group are being identified and include the Dutch Nutrition Foundation and the Swiss Nutrition Foundation. The international group is encouraging, through continuing discussions with individuals and organizations from other countries, the establishment of similar national Nutrition Foundation programs. Representatives from Chile, Canada, Italy, France and Germany have corresponded with or visited the Foundation's office concerning such developments in their countries. A network of Nutrition Foundations could contribute greatly toward fulfillment of a major international need in education and research, and enhance the effectiveness of both bilateral and international programs of scientific and developmental efforts in food and nutrition.

Saccharin

An example of The Nutrition Foundation's leadership in consolidation of objective scientific information basic to understanding needs and developments was the convening of an international group of scientists with new data pertaining to the safety and toxicology of the artificial sweetener, saccharin. This was accomplished through two workshops held a year apart for the purpose of reviewing experimental design of and data from current studies and the planning of additional needed research. The open exchange of data and discussions among advisors and decision-makers from the U.S. and other nations provided a common base of knowledge relative to all new experimental evidence. At the same time, experimental differences could be identified and resolved by direct scientific exchange rather than debated in the public media by non-scientists.

Hyperkinesis

More recently, The Nutrition Foundation focused upon anxiety created by the publicized hypothesis implicating many widely distributed or highly nutritious foodstuffs and non-designated food additives as influencing the syndrome of "hyperkinesis." The Foundation supported a responsible critical review by a competent group of expert medical and behavioral scientists of all evidence relative to this hypothesis. This was the National Advisory Committee on Hyperkinesis and Food Additives, comprised of fourteen scientists selected and identified by the offices of thirteen major scientific and medical organizations. The Committee sought out and reviewed all relevant published information and conferred with knowledgeable resource personnel and interested investigators. Its report to The Nutrition Foundation, published June 1, 1975, concluded that data from critically designed and executed studies, free of existing deficiencies of design, must be available before firm conclusions can be reached on the Feingold hypothesis. The Committee outlined guidelines for experimental design of future investigations, considered the research opportunities and needs, and recommended needed funding. It concluded that the role of The Nutrition Foundation in clarification of this concern is two-fold:

a. the continuing support of the Advisory Committee for purposes of assessing and coordinating research program activities and evaluating overall developments, and
b. direct support of recommended grants utilizing funds available from a variety of sources. Industry as well as other support for these activities could well be coordinated through administration by The Nutrition Foundation.

The report of the National Advisory Committee has been widely distributed. The Trustees of The Nutrition Foundation are providing a special fund for support of research recommended by the National Advisory Committee and by the Council of the Foundation. Utilization of this support is being coordinated with that which may be available from other sources, including granting and contracting agencies of the Federal government.

Improvement of Public Awareness of Nutrition in Relation to Health

Nutrition Labeling

Dissemination of accurate information concerning questions on nutrition and foods results from activities such as those just described. In addition, the Foundation maintains a continuum of educational activities directed at different target audiences. The subject of nutrition labeling is a case in point. Following publication in the Federal Register of the initial proposal by the Food and Drug Administration concerning nutrition labeling, the Foundation has actively participated in efforts to bring the best and most knowledgeable educational, scientific and consumer resources to bear on this issue. These efforts have included the following activities:

a. The President of the Foundation was the luncheon speaker at the first "Food Industry Briefing on Nutrition Labeling" on April 13, 1972, and the Foundation has co-sponsored and participated in subsequent meetings on February 8, 1973, and May 30-31, 1974.
b. Members of the Foundation staff served on the advisory group assembled by the National Academy of Sciences to review and comment to the Commissioner of Food and Drug on the FDA's initial labeling proposal.
c. A series of special reports on nutrition labeling was published in NUTRITION REVIEWS during 1973. The series was reprinted and widely distributed so the nutrition community and communicators with the public could be kept abreast of developments relative to labeling regulations and, if they so wished, could comment on these to the FDA hearing clerk or Commissioner.
d. The Foundation encouraged and assisted preparation by the Consortium of the educational publication "Nutrition Labeling—How It Can Work For You."
e. The staff of the Foundation has frequently presented scientific and educational aspects of the subject in public talks, on radio and television programs, and in counseling with reporters and other media personnel.

Misinformation and Faddism

Because of the large amount of misinformation and food faddism promul-

A Good Idea

gated by various authors, speakers and the popular press, a seventy-six page supplement to the July, 1974 issue of NUTRITION REVIEWS was published on "Nutrition Misinformation and Food Faddism." "Americans Love Hogwash" was the intriguing title of the lead article by Dr. Edward Rynearson, Emeritus Professor of Medicine at the Mayo Clinic. The guest editor of the supplement, Dr. Philip White, is Director of the Office of Foods and Nutrition of the American Medical Association. This publication was designed to be used as a reference by physicians, teachers, lawyers and others who are called on for advice about nutrition and diet. It includes official statements and reports issued by authoritative scientific societies and advisory boards concerning the dangers of high doses of certain vitamins, critiques of several unsound diets, excerpts from scientific and popular articles on areas of faddism, and a list of recommended books and articles for the layman. While Dr. Rynearson's article deals with many aspects of nutrition misinformation, he focuses much of his attention on the theories put forward in popular books for laymen by writers such as Adelle Davis and Carlton Fredericks.

This supplement has been distributed to practicing physicians, dentists, nurses, food and science editors, writers, television producers, teachers and scientists, and to interested individuals who order it from the Foundation. It serves as a reference text for many college and university courses and has been sold in at least 25 university bookstores. It has been widely referenced in newspaper and magazine articles by writers and columnists. One article alone, a lead story by Max Gunther entitled "The Worst Diet Advice" in *T.V. Guide* for January 11, 1975, reached an estimated 19 million readers. This article was based primarily upon an interview by Gunther with Dr. Philip White of the American Medical Association, and the articles contained in the NUTRITION REVIEWS supplement.

Special Reports to Media

Authoritative scientific summaries and interpretations of the scientific aspect of issues of public interest are the subject of occasional press releases by the Foundation in the form of "SPECIAL REPORTS." These SPECIAL REPORTS are distributed to the print, broadcast and television media, professional organizations, educators, health, nutrition and community leaders and government agencies. Their distribution invariably involves Foundation staff in public dialogue through the media.

An example of such a report was the release on "Food Day" written in response to a growing concern for irresponsible and unscientific attacks on the nation's food supply — attacks through propaganda, much of which is political, being widely disseminated under the guise of nutrition education. Another SPECIAL REPORT was based on the report of the National Committee on Hyperkinesis and Food Additives. These SPECIAL REPORTS provide perspective and authoritative evaluations for the guidance of the nutrition community, media communicators, health and community workers and the public.

Source Materials and Educational Publications

The Foundation publishes and distributes, either free or at minimal cost, educational pamphlets and booklets for the layman on subjects such as obesity, diet for teenagers, and choosing a healthful diet. These are distributed in response to requests from teachers, professionals or the lay public. Requests often originate from viewers of television programs, such as "Feeling Good" produced by the Children's Television Workshop, or read-

The Fourth Decade

ers of national magazines, such as *Family Health,* in which writers refer to or recommend these publications to their readership.

Encourage Broad Acceptance of Sound Nutrition Principles

All educational efforts ultimately may encourage or result in the incorporation of more sound nutrition concepts into spheres of interest of governmental, academic, industrial or consumer groups. However, a number of specific activities of The Nutrition Foundation deserve special mention in this regard. These are:

The Annual Symposia of the Food and Nutrition Liaison Committee

Annually, the Food and Nutrition Liaison Committee holds a two-and-a-half-day symposium that highlights: (a) major important developments and research findings that should be reflected in application; (b) new research interests which may subsequently prove to be of special significance; (c) viewpoints of competent scientists relative to the scientific evidence concerning public issues; and (d) establishment of better international exchange of relevant scientific information concerning questions of food and nutrition. Examples of topics discussed during the years 1972 to 1975 include:

Evidence concerning the state of nutrition of the populations of the United States and Canada as obtained from recent or ongoing surveys.

The changing patterns of food habits and the role of socio-economic influences in these changes.

Infant feeding practices and evidence concerning the nutrient intake of infants.

The special requirements for maintaining the nutrition of the low-birth-weight infant.

The hypothesized role of dietary fiber and the nature of new evidence pertaining to the role of fiber in nutrition.

The role of fiber in reducing availability of certain nutrients, particularly trace elements.

The nutritional effects of chelating substances in foods.

Evaluation of the epidemiologic approach to questions concerning nutrition, food and health.

Influences of diet on oral biology.

Nutrition and aging.

"Hyperkinesis," the minimal brain dysfunction syndrome, and the postulated role of foods and food additives.

The relative role of malnutrition and other environmental factors in determining or influencing intellectual development.

Taste reflexes in infants; the presence of taste preferences in the newborn.

The laboratory evaluation of protein quality and results of a collaborative study sponsored by the American Medical Association and the Food and Drug Administration.

New analytical methods for nutrients and contaminants of importance in maintaining food quality.

The biological availability of nutrients from food, and factors which alter nutrient availability.

New information concerning essential trace elements and the metabolic interaction of trace elements.

A Good Idea

New evidence concerning the possibility of toxic levels of mercury, lead and cadmium in the diet.

Nutrient imbalance.

Mechanisms of appetite control.

The effect of the browning reaction on nutritive value of foods.

Research on high lysine yeast and the nutritional availability of lysine.

The use of fixed enzymes in food processing.

Evidence concerning the role of nitrates and nitrosamines in foods and their implications for health, including results of a cooperative study by the U.S. Department of Agriculture, the Food and Drug Administration and the food industry.

Abstracts of papers presented at the annual Food and Nutrition Liaison Committee meetings are distributed to members of the FNLC, invited attendees and Trustees.

There is an opportunity at these meetings for free exchange and discussion between the invited experts and the audience, consisting of members of the Food and Nutrition Liaison Committee from industry, academia, government and consumer areas. This affords an ideal milieu for developing common understanding by scientists from academia, government and industry of present or potential developments of broad public importance.

Benefit-Risk Decision Making: The Citizens' Commission on Science, Law and the Food Supply

A number of Foundation activities have focused upon an evaluation of benefit-risk considerations, especially private risk versus public benefit and the mechanism of decision making. Staff members of the Foundation have had a long and constant advisory involvement with these matters at every level, including international agencies, departments of the federal government, state agencies, and committees and commissions of national scientific and professional societies. The Nutrition Foundation in concert with the Food and Drug Law Institute, The Rockefeller Foundation, the Josiah Macy, Jr. Foundation and the Commonwealth Fund, encouraged and supported the creation of an independent Citizens' Commission on Science, Law and the Food Supply. This action was partly in response to a call by the Commissioner of the Food and Drug Administration for an independent mechanism to assess the current understanding of the effects of chemicals and "the usefulness of laws that are intended to protect but which ignore the practicality of implementation."

The objectives of the Commission were to develop broad guidelines applicable for:

Identification of considerations involved in the assessment of benefits and risks in applying scientific technology in the production, processing, distribution and use of food for man;

Decision making in matters pertaining to such benefits and risks; and

The design of legal and regulatory processes that will afford maximum public benefits and minimal risks within the varied social, cultural and economic patterns of society which exist world-wide.

The original Board of Directors of the Commission was chaired by Dr. Frederick Seitz, President of Rockefeller University, and was composed of Dr. Allan C. Barnes, Vice President of The Rockefeller Foundation; Dr. John Z. Bowers, President of the Josiah Macy, Jr. Foundation; Dr. H. E. Carter, Coordinator for Interdisciplinary Pro-

The Fourth Decade

grams at the University of Arizona and President of the National Science Board; Dr. William J. Darby, President of The Nutrition Foundation; Dr. J. George Harrar, Life Fellow of The Rockefeller Foundation; Dr. Channing H. Lushbough, Associate Director of Consumer's Union; and Laurence I. Wood, Esq., President of the Food and Drug Law Institute.

An International Planning Board was convened and twelve committees and subcommittees organized. Planning grants from the participating foundations and a contract from the Food and Drug Administration supported staff and office and committee hearings. An *ad hoc* group developed two reports in 1973-74 at the request of the Food and Drug Administration. These were entitled: "Current Ethical Considerations in the Determination of Acceptable Risk with Regard to Food and Food Additives" and "Recent Symposia and Public Conferences Which Considered Some Aspects of the Social and Ethical Implications of Benefit-Risk Decision Making." They served as major sections in a report prepared by the Food and Drug Administration for the Subcommittee on Agriculture-Environmental and Consumer Protection of the Committee on Appropriations, House of Representatives (93rd Congress) at the request of Congressman Whitten, Chairman of the Subcommittee. These were published by the Subcommittee in the report of its hearings, Part 8, Food and Drug Administration "Study of the Delany Clause and other Anti-Cancer Clauses," U.S. Government Printing Office, 1974. The Citizens' Commission's report sets forth broad, useful, widely applicable guiding principles.

These reports and other aspects of the Commission's studies have stimulated and influenced scholarly exchanges in writing and in professional and public symposia and conferences. Examples are the American Association for the Advancement of Science sponsored Gordon Conference on Food and Nutrition in 1974, and the first in the series of Academy Forums sponsored by the National Academy of Sciences, May 1973. Personnel involved in the Commission made decided identifiable contributions to both of these meetings through their presentation of concepts clarified by the deliberation of its committees and related groups. A similar impact of the Commission can be identified in a variety of other conferences and in the writing of many who are concerned with this area of public responsibility.

Nutrition Foundation Senior Scholar

There is an often expressed need for a scholarly approach by non-scientists to humanistic and ethical considerations of issues that relate to research and the application of scientific and technologic knowledge for betterment of the quality of life and health of peoples. Such issues embrace moral and value judgments, human rights and responsibilities, and individual versus societal benefits or risks. These issues have become especially important in relation to meeting food needs and wants under different socio-economic circumstances and within the differing value systems of various cultures.

The scientific community is limited in effectively communicating concepts to thought leaders concerned with moral and ethical judgments that influence utilization of scientific and technologic developments. Scientists, politicians and governmental bodies need the perspective that can be brought to focus by those humanists whose professional backgrounds are in ethics and philosophy and who possess a curiosity concerning science, an appreciation of it and a desire to understand its significance in service to society.

A Good Idea

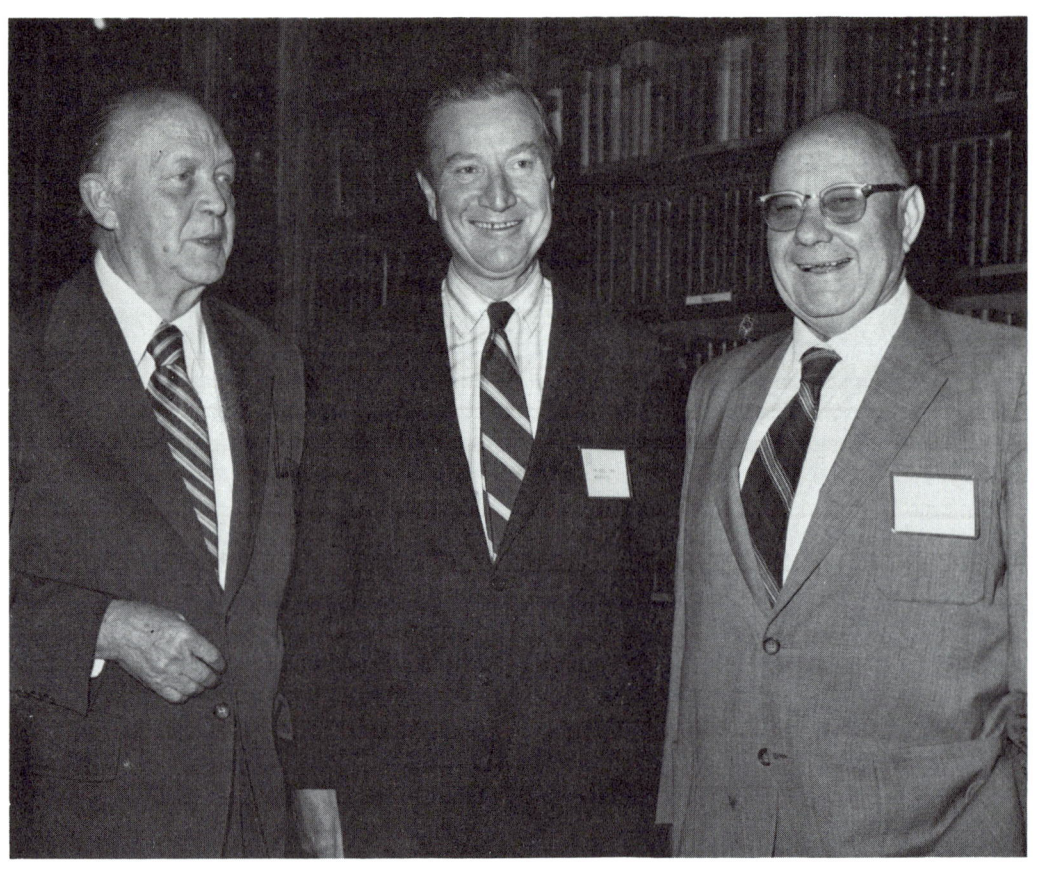

J. George Harrar, Russell E. Train, Emil M. Mrak

Mr. Train, the Administrator of the Environmental Protection Agency (EPA), addressed the Board of Trustees of The Nutrition Foundation at their meeting May, 1975. Dr. Emil Mrak, a Public Trustee of the Foundation, is also Chairman of the Science Advisory Board of EPA.

In recognition of the need to identify leadership in this area, the Trustees of The Nutrition Foundation established support for a Senior Scholar. The Trustees directed that this unique position be filled by a humanist with an interest in the ethical and philosophical questions raised by science and technology. The purpose of the support is to allow a senior humanist the freedom to address himself to such issues relative to food and nutrition.

Professor Samuel E. Stumpf, a distinguished American philosopher, former President of Cornell College, was appointed Senior Scholar of The Nutrition Foundation, effective July 1, 1974.

Dr. Stumpf is Visiting Professor of Medical Ethics in the School of Medicine at Vanderbilt University, was a member of the planning panel of the Citizens' Commission on Science, Law and the Food Supply, and served as Chairman of the subcommittee of that Commission which prepared the report on ethical considerations in the determination of acceptable risk with regard to food and food additives.

During the initial year of his scholar-

The Fourth Decade

ship, he participated in the World Food Conference in Rome; in the Forums of the National Academy of Sciences on "Experiments and Research with Humans: Values in Conflict" and on "Sweeteners"; in the Food and Nutrition Conference of the AAAS Gordon Research Conference; the meeting of the Food and Drug Law Institute; meetings of the American Association for the Advancement of Science; the annual meeting of the Pharmaceutical Manufacturers Association; the annual meeting of the Food and Nutrition Liaison Committee of The Nutrition Foundation and in other scientific symposia dealing broadly with ethical considerations and values. The wide demand for participation of Professor Stumpf in major conferences indicates the recognized need for scholars of his background to become involved with issues raised by science and technology. The understanding which they bring to such issues will contribute to formulation of more rational views and discussions on the part of all segments of society.

Participation in and Support of Scientific Meetings and Symposia

The Foundation has demonstrated cooperation with and support of scientific societies by responding to their requests for assistance in organizing programs and meetings. In response to requests by the American Association for the Advancement of Science (AAAS) and the American Chemical Society, the Foundation's officers have coordinated the planning or chaired programs, particularly symposia at annual meetings of these and other societies.

In numerous instances, officers of the Foundation have responded to requests to give interpretive addresses before broad scientific audiences concerned with problems of nutrition, food quality, safety, benefit-risk decision making, world food needs, the role of food science and technology in the developing regions, new research findings with implications for future planning and decision making, scientific assessment of problems underlying matters of public interest or concern, questions relative to educational research or manpower needs and many similar topics. Examples of these are:

Symposium on Environmental Quality and Food Supply: "Acceptable Risk and Practical Safety, Philosophy in the Decision Making Process," Washington, D.C., October 20, 1972.

Annual Meeting of the National Dairy Council: "Opportunities for the Dairy Industry in Nutritional Research," New Orleans, January 25, 1972.

Kenneth A. Spencer Award for Achievement in Agricultural Chemistry: "Food, Nutrition and Science," Kansas City section of the American Chemical Society, Kansas City, February 24, 1972.

32nd Annual Meeting of the Institute of Food Technologists: "The Scientific Community's Responsibilities for Nutrition and Food Safety," Minneapolis, May 22, 1972.

Annual Joint Convention of the Milk Industry Foundation and the International Association of Ice Cream Manufacturers: "The Scientific Community Looks at Nutrition Labeling," Atlantic City, October 2, 1972.

Food and Nutrition Board: "Food and Nutrition Board — A Perspective," Washington, D.C., December 14, 1972.

BIBRA Lecture: "The Conflict of Nutrition and Toxicology," Royal College of Physicians, London, November 12, 1973.

A Good Idea

American Association for the Advancement of Science (AAAS): "Science and Man in the Americas," Mexico City, June 23, 1973.

Tennessee Governor's Conference on Aging: "Community Health Care and Nutrition Services for Older Adults," Nashville, September 25, 1973.

The World Poultry Conference: "Perspectives on Nutrition," New Orleans, August 12, 1974.

XIV International Biological Symposium: "Balancing the Benefits and Risks of the Application of Science to Agriculture and Food Production," XXV Anniversary of INCAP, Guatemala, December 2-5, 1974.

Kentucky State Medical Association Meeting: "Food Facts and Myths: From Unicorn to Hogwash," Lexington, September 26, 1974.

American Association for the Advancement of Science: "Why Use Food Additives," San Francisco, February 25, 1974.

Marabou Conference on Nutritional Improvement of Foods: "The Concept of Nutrient Density," Sundbyberg, Sweden, August, 31, 1974.

Negus Memorial Lecture: "Technology Assessment and World Food Needs," Virginia Academy of Science, Harrisonburg, May 8, 1975.

Western Regional Conference on Higher Education for Fulbright-Hays Scholars: "Nutrition, Food Needs and Technologic Priorities: The World Food Conference," University of Arizona, Tucson, May 28, 1975.

The Forty-Niners Award Ceremony: "Fads, Fears and Foodways," Chicago, January 25, 1975.

Seventh W. O. Atwater Memorial Lecture: "Nutrition Science—An Overview of American Genius," 58th annual meeting of the American Dietetic Association, San Antonio, October 21, 1975.

The Nutrition Foundation and The Food and Drug Law Institute jointly sponsored the conference "Nutrition: Marketing and the Law." The purpose of the conference was to present important background information on nutrition and on the legal regulation of food products to members of the marketing, advertising, technical, and legal disciplines, who are responsible for product development, marketing, and claims in advertising and labeling.

The Nutrition Foundation also provided financial support to an important symposium on Specifications for Food Chemicals, sponsored by the Food Chemicals CODEX of the Committee on Food Protection, Food and Nutrition Board, National Academy of Sciences-National Research Council. Dr. C. O. Chichester, Vice President of the Foundation, was a member of the organizing committee of the symposium, and Dr. Darby was the opening speaker. This conference critically examined a number of important concepts and developments relative to food chemicals, including quality control procedures, analytical methodology, regulatory matters, manufacturing processes, toxicologic specifications, adequacy of Food Chemicals Codex specifications, the relationship between the Food Chemical Codex and the Codex Alimentarius, specifications and safety evaluation of GRAS substances, and expiration dating for food chemical specifications.

Similarly, The Nutrition Foundation has assisted in review of new evidence concerning the allowances for and intake of folic acid. The eighth edition (1974) of the

The Fourth Decade

Recommended Dietary Allowances pointed out the need for review of this evidence. Accordingly, an International Workshop on the subject was planned by the Food and Nutrition Board and supported in part by a grant from The Nutrition Foundation. The discussions and proceedings of that workshop afford insight into the limitations of the currently published allowance and provide an excellent knowledge base for design of new studies which will permit improved allowances to be estimated.

The Nutrition Foundation, along with other advisory groups, has served to assist the National Academy of Sciences in identifying appropriate subject areas and speakers for its series of public forums on scientific topics, including specifically the first Academy Forum: "How Safe is Safe? —The Design of Policy on Drugs and Food Additives"; the Academy Forum on the ethics of human experimentation, "Experiments and Research with Humans: Values in Conflict"; and the Academy Forum on "Sweeteners—Issues & Uncertainties." Dr. Darby served as a member of the planning committee for the first Forum and, along with Professor Samuel E. Stumpf, Senior Scholar of the Foundation, participated in the other two.

The Nutrition Foundation has participated in similar symposia in collaboration with a wide variety of scientific and educational organizations. Among these are: the AAAS-sponsored Gordon Conferences on Food and Nutrition, the British Nutrition Foundation and the Swedish Nutrition Foundation symposia, the Marabou Conferences, the Western Hemisphere Nutrition Conference, the American Medical Association's Council on Foods and Nutrition, the Food and Drug Law Institute's "Food Up-Date," US AID, WHO, and the American Foundation for the Overseas Blind symposia and conferences on vitamin A deficiency, the Commonwealth Fund's meetings on education, the Institute of Food Technologists and local

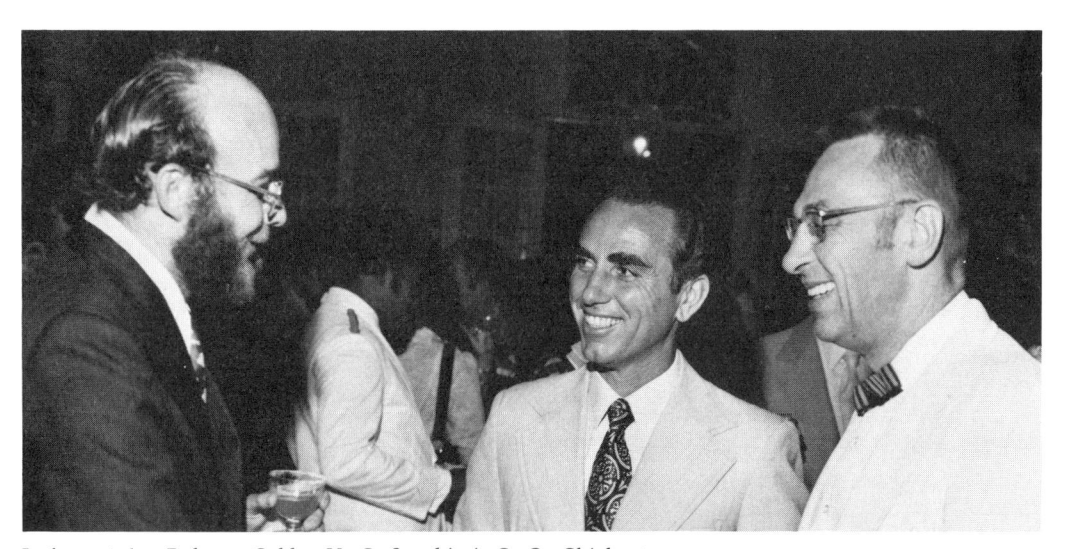

Left to right: *Roberto Cobbe, V. C. Sgarbieri, C. O. Chichester*

Dr. Chichester, Vice President of The Nutrition Foundation, has long been active in assisting the development of food science in Latin America. He received the 1976 International Award of the Institute of Food Technologists for his promotion of education and understanding internationally. Here he confers with fellow participants at the Second Latin American Seminar in Food Science and Technology.

A Good Idea

and regional chapters or sectional meetings of the Institute. Also included are various state organizations, such as the Kentucky Medical Association, the Tennessee Governor's Conference on Aging, the Governor of Georgia's Nutrition Committee, St. Vincent's Medical Center and Jacksonville Hospitals Educational Program symposia, etc. These are in addition to numerous symposia and seminars at the invitation of universities throughout the United States and of others sponsored by leading industrial groups.

Improvement of Nutrition Education at All Levels

Nutrition Education in Medical Centers

Recent efforts of The Nutrition Foundation to stimulate nutrition education throughout the formalized educational system have met with enthusiastic response. The opportunities for immediate effectiveness were especially timely in the field of medical education. This timeliness results from a number of concurrently emerging influences:

> An increasing interest by medical students and young physicians in societal problems and needs, coupled with the general awareness that resulted from post-World War II international activities, of the gravity of malnutrition and hunger in the developing world.
>
> Realization by physicians and surgeons that many therapeutic advances in medicine have attained a new potential that obviously is being limited by a failure to apply nutritional principles.
>
> The increasing availability of sensitive laboratory diagnostic tests for assessing levels of nutriture (state of nutrition).
>
> Increasing recognition of the beneficial influence of a few outstanding academic centers with recognized programs in clinical nutrition established with encouragement and grant support from The Nutrition Foundation.

National Conferences on Nutrition Education in Medicine

In 1963, the Foundation collaborated with the Council on Foods and Nutrition of the American Medical Association in sponsoring a nationwide conference and workshop on nutrition education in medical schools at Chicopee Falls, Massachusetts. Subsequently, grants from the Foundation assisted in the establishment of a nutrition program in the new Mount Sinai Medical School in New York City and at the University of Missouri, Columbia. Only limited interest in such developments had been generated, however, until a second conference was organized and held in 1972 in Williamsburg, Virginia, under the joint auspices of the Council on Foods and Nutrition of the American Medical Association, The Nutrition Foundation, the American Heart Association and the Nutrition Program of the Center for Disease Control (HEW). Several additional foundations, scientific and medical societies, and the Food and Nutrition Board of the National Academy of Sciences-National Research Council cooperated in this second conference which was attended by representatives of a majority of the medical schools in the United States. Some 4,000 copies of the proceedings of the "Conference on Guidelines for Nutrition Education Programs," published by The Nutrition Foundation, have been distributed upon request, not only within the United States, but for use at major educational conferences on medical education in Latin America, the Philippines, the Middle East, Asia and Europe.

The dearth of financial support for special educational programs in nutrition was

The Fourth Decade

highlighted at the Williamsburg Conference. The opportunities and needs, as well as the interests of faculties and students, were documented; essential nutritional concepts which should be understood by students were identified; and the need for continuing education of physicians in nutrition was recognized. The conference pointed to the need for several types of instructional assistance, including development of a useful text (handbook); of effective, coordinated audio-visual instructional materials, and of prototype nutrition laboratory resources. It also strongly reaffirmed the dependence of effective nutrition education in medicine upon associated programs of nutrition research.

The Response of Medical Schools

As a result of recommendations of the conference to stimulate establishment of nutrition centers of excellence and to identify model programs of nutrition education within the medical curriculum, The Nutrition Foundation announced that it would be receptive to applications for grants to establish integrated teaching of nutrition in the curriculum of medical centers. Within three months, seven medical schools communicated to the Foundation their firm plans for such developments and requested grant assistance. So far, 21 institutions have formally requested funds amounting to some $3,300,000.

The Nutrition Foundation also promotes nutrition education in medical centers by helping interested institutions and personnel to formulate program needs and devise organizational structures and curricular alterations that provide a sound basis for seeking financial support. The Foundation assists in communicating needs of programs to other agencies and sources of funding. The Foundation helps to develop teaching materials and catalyze the exchange among interested faculty personnel. These activities have been important influences in establishing a growing number of model programs and initiating communication between and among personnel in medical schools and other organizations interested in medical education in nutrition.

More than one-third of the nation's medical schools have sought advice and counsel from The Nutrition Foundation in seeking to further their capabilities for more adequate nutrition education within their curricula. Almost all of the institutions need additional funds in order to establish or expand their programs. Nevertheless, the experience and guidance of the Foundation, resulting from its wide involvement in medical education, enables it to assist medical schools more effectively to utilize existing resources and interests, as well as to be increasingly effective in obtaining support or assistance.

The Foundation has supported the establishment of new programs of nutrition education within the organizational and teaching structures of the Boston University School of Medicine, the Albany Medical College of Union University, Jefferson Medical College of Thomas Jefferson University, and the Health Center, University of Texas at San Antonio. Simultaneously, it has assisted a number of other medical schools to enrich their nutrition education programs. These include the nutrition unit of the University of California, Davis; the Division of Nutrition of the new Mayo Medical School in Rochester, Minnesota; and, in particular, through the Swanson Center for Nutrition, the nutrition educational programs at Creighton University Medical School and the University of Nebraska in Omaha. Assistance to these and other schools takes a variety of forms, such as support of a Future Leaders Award at the University of California, Davis; consultative service to the Mayo Medical School in

A Good Idea

the areas of curriculum planning and teaching programs; placement of personnel for training; exchange of curricular materials and program concepts. The Foundation's counsel repeatedly is sought for recruitment and placement of personnel. The staff of The Nutrition Foundation and members of its advisory group maintain close communication with the programs assisted in order to identify developments which may be of benefit and interest to others.

The effectiveness and value of these activities are exemplified by contributions to a statewide development in Texas involving six medical schools in that state. Faculty members from these institutions and other professionals meet repeatedly for discussions concerning nutrition education. Papers on this subject presented at one of the Texas meetings were supplemented by additional pertinent information and published by The Nutrition Foundation for distribution to interested educators and other personnel. The report is entitled "The Application of Nutrition in the Health Sciences," and is available from The Nutrition Foundation. This report complements that of the Proceedings of the Williamsburg Conference.

Regional Programs or Centers

Experience increasingly underscores the value of encouraging the establishment of centers or regional programs that coordinate and support nutrition activities in a number of contiguous institutions. The cooperative developments involving the six medical schools in Texas and the Nutrition Committee of the Texas State Medical Association serve as illustrations of effective cooperation. The Swanson Center for Nutrition in Omaha exemplifies another organizational design for an important regional resource. This Center is effective not only within the two medical schools in that City—the University of Nebraska and Creighton University—but is helping to expand the interest in nutrition beyond these schools to other educational institutions, hospitals and community groups in Nebraska.

Another very promising locus for such a development is Pennsylvania, with the concentration of medical schools in Philadelphia, the nutrition teaching program of Thomas Jefferson Medical School and its collaboration with Pennsylvania State University, and the other medical centers in Philadelphia, Hershey and Pittsburgh. The Howard Heinz Nutrition Program in Pennsylvania affords the broadest potential model for this type of program, due to simultaneous developments at the Jefferson University Medical School of Thomas Jefferson University and at Pennsylvania State University. Both institutions receive support from The Nutrition Foundation. Other medical schools in Pennsylvania that have indicated a special interest in nutrition programs are the Hershey Medical School, the Hahnemann Medical School in Philadelphia, and the University of Pittsburgh.

Opportunities for similar coordinated use of resources in regional programs exist elsewhere, especially in the state of Florida and the Chicago area. Discussions have been held with medical and educational leaders in both of these areas about the possibility of effecting a regional type of organization for promoting nutrition education in medicine, and for utilizing maximally the personnel existing in several institutions in the area.

The Nutrition Foundation is encouraging periodic conferences of the staff of participating and interested institutions in order to evolve the most effective type of cooperation suitable to the needs, programs and resources of local clusters of institutions. The Foundation assists these

The Fourth Decade

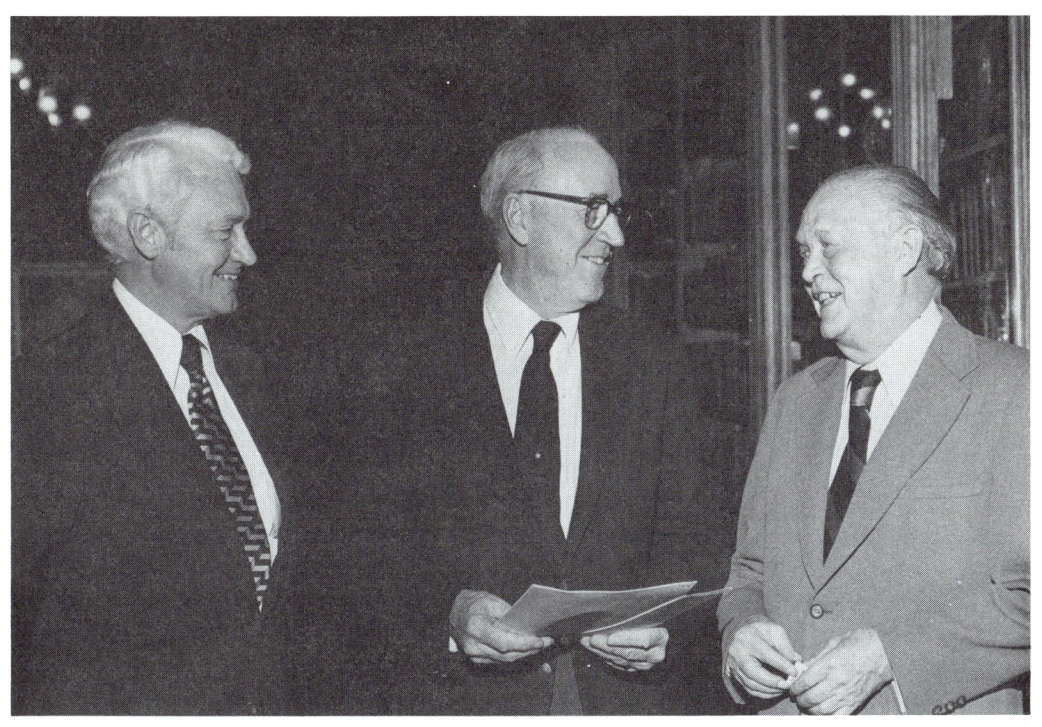

Left to right: *William J. Darby, Edward J. Rosenow, J. George Harrar.*

Dr. Rosenow, Executive Director of the American College of Physicians, receives from Dr. George Harrar, Chairman of the Board of Trustees of The Nutrition Foundation, the commitment of support for the American College of Physicians' Teaching and Research Scholarships in Nutrition.

exchanges by providing input from selected personnel from other schools who have been involved in successful developments within their own institutions.

Support of the American College of Physicians' Teaching and Research Scholars in Nutrition

The prestigious American College of Physicians annually appoints a small number of Teaching and Research Scholars of the College. They are selected by the Fellowships and Scholarships Committee of the Board of Regents of the American College of Physicians from nominees proposed by Chairmen of Departments of Medicine in medical schools. The nominations and selections are made on the basis of the nominee's interest and skills in teaching and research and promise of excellence in future development. Appointments are for a term of three years between the fourth and eighth postgraduate training year.

In recognition of the need to identify nutrition as an important subspecialty of medicine, and to develop a cadre of superior young leaders, the Regents of the American College of Physicians at their meeting of April 1-4, 1974, established two Teaching and Research Scholarships in the field of nutrition. These are being funded by a grant from The Nutritional Foundation.

A Good Idea

The first two scholars in this program began their appointments in July, 1975. They are Lawrence C. Brandt, M.D., who, at Albert Einstein College of Medicine, is studying the production of vitamin B_{12} analogs in a clinical condition associated with blind loops of the gastrointestinal tract; and James V. Miller, M.D., who is continuing studies at the University of New Mexico School of Medicine of the biochemical and nutritional derangements that occur in alcoholic liver disease.

The American College of Physicians with a membership of over 20,000, is the leading organization of internists in the country. It is especially significant that this organization at its annual meeting in 1974, not only established these scholarships in nutrition but awarded three of its Masterships in the College to physicians whose careers have been marked by contributions to nutrition education and research. The recipients were Charles S. Davidson, M.D., William B. Castle Professor of Medicine at Harvard Medical School; Grace A. Goldsmith, M.D., Dean of the School of Public Health and Tropical Medicine at Tulane University; and William J. Darby, M.D., President of The Nutrition Foundation. These activities of the American College of Physicians illustrate the enhanced recognition by leaders in medical practice and education of the important role of nutrition in medicine.

Financial Needs for Nutrition Education in Medical and Health Sciences

There is an urgent need for more support of programs for development of personnel and of effective teaching materials designed to fit within the context of the modern medical school curriculum. In both instances there must be sufficient flexibility to meet the needs of the varying types of teaching programs presently found in medical centers. Today's medical curriculum varies greatly from center to center; the stereotyped highly structured regimen of the past has been modified to permit a freer choice of elective pursuits by the student with increased responsibility for less directed self-study. The integration of nutrition concepts must, therefore, be skillfully designed to compete within this framework with other new and exciting medical advances.

In order to capitalize upon present needs and interests, the timing for encouraging these developments is critical. Accordingly, in November 1973, the Executive Committee and the Board of Trustees of The Nutrition Foundation authorized the creation of a special two million dollar fund to support development of nutrition education in medicine. Special funding for this support is being sought. The initial major contribution toward this goal was a portion of the Howard Heinz Nutrition Program for Pennsylvania. The Howard Heinz Endowment pledged a total of approximately $850,000 over a four year period for supporting a model coordinated nutrition education program within the Commonwealth. A portion of this amount, $205,000, is committed to strengthening and developing nutrition teaching in the Thomas Jefferson Medical School in Philadelphia. Additional initial contributions have come from several member companies of the Foundation, and other funds are being solicited. Even if the total amount sought by The Nutrition Foundation is obtained, it cannot alone adequately meet the needs of this important development nationwide. It is hoped that The Nutrition Foundation's stimulatory efforts and the demonstrated interest and need may result in the allotment of adequate support from larger foundations and from governmental and educational organizations.

The proposed fund from The Nutrition

The Fourth Decade

Foundation would be used to maintain the current upsurge of concern for and interest in the integration of nutrition into clinical medicine; to encourage the establishment of effective teaching units by providing a series of models which exemplify patterns to fit within the diverse teaching programs of medical schools; and, in so doing, to catalyze production and evaluation of effective instructional material for use in programs of undergraduate medical education and postgraduate and continuing education of physicians. Such developments will greatly strengthen and support the efforts of faculty members who seek ongoing continuous support from current sources of funds for medical schools, including federal and state support. Parenthetically, it should be noted that "stimulatory" or "seed" grants from the Foundation have proved to be effective stimuli for procurement of additional funds from other sources accessible to the grantees. These sources include institutional funds assigned by medical schools' administrations, related program or project grants in institutional centers, sources of hospital support (especially Veterans Administration Hospital programs), and reimbursement of charges for diagnostic laboratory procedures and patient consultation. Experience of institutions with well-developed clinical nutrition services, including those for nutritional diagnosis, has been that these services become a significant source of revenue, as do similar services in endocrinology, hematology, or other subspecialties.

At the Williamsburg Conference it was estimated that support of $100,000 annually, committed for a five-year period, would initiate the development within a medical school of a coordinated nutrition program and support the establishment of a staff of two or three members and a nutrition diagnostic laboratory. Such services would be comparable to those of other subspecialties. Costs have increased since that estimate, which represented an approximate average need. Full implementation of a total national program obviously would require a period of five or more years in order to develop personnel and organizational support and programs. One can anticipate that necessary supplementary funds beyond an average allotment of $100,000 to $125,000 per institution could come from other resources available within the medical school and to the involved faculty. The need is immediate, if maximal advantage is to be gained from current therapeutic and preventive medical potential. It is hoped that funding from federal, state and larger foundation sources may be forthcoming promptly to fulfill these needs.

Additional needs exist for similar, although smaller, support to assure incorporation of nutrition into the training and education of other health personnel: in schools of dentistry, public health, osteopathy and allied health professions, including nursing. There is an unfulfilled need for an increased number of more specialized and trained dietitians. The growing educational requirements for this profession were highlighted by the Report of the Study Commission on Dietetics of the American Dietetic Association, "The Profession of Dietetics," The American Dietetic Association, 1972. National planning for nutrition and health services should recognize these resource needs.

Competent ongoing guidance regarding foods and nutrition is a responsibility which rests upon not only the physician, but upon all members of the allied health professions. The latter often maintain a more frequent and leisurely relationship with patients than can the physician. Indeed, members of the allied health professions may have almost daily communication with patients who are under chronic surveillance during periods of adjustment to new life styles. It is at these times that the provision of detailed nutritional guidance is most essential. For example, considerable nutrition education is involved in readjusting the dietary habits of patients maintained in renal dialysis, the ambulatory patient dependent in part upon total parenteral nutrition ("hyper-alimentation"), patients with inborn errors of metabolism, subjects with chronic malabsorption resulting from conditions such as gluten enteropathy, and patients who receive continuous therapy with the increased number of drugs known to have nutritional impacts, such as diuretics, anti-metabolites in cancer therapy, and oral contraceptives. The long-term therapy of the "terminal" cancer patient to prevent cachexia, or the continuing dietary management of cardiovascular disease, are as demanding as dietary surveillance of the insulin-treated diabetic. In management of the latter, there is a long established pattern of nutritional re-education by the medical care team with much teaching of the patient by the dietitian. The same need for nutritional counseling must be fulfilled for the many other types of patients who require it today.

Nutrition Education in Colleges and Universities

Since its origin, the Foundation has had a significantly beneficial impact upon the graduate education of the student who majors in nutrition. This has been provided through: (a) grant support to university faculties for research, and the opportunity these funds have given for support of students; (b) the instructional quality and usefulness of NUTRITION REVIEWS and other publications; (c) the inspirational stimulation of the Foundation's awards program; and (d) its continual effort to identify and encourage particularly able young faculty members through the Future Leaders Award program. These activities are continuing, and career opportunities for this level of personnel remain excellent.

The Land Grant Institutions

Leadership in nutrition education at undergraduate as well as graduate levels traditionally has resided in land grant institutions. This leadership stems from the initial appropriation by the Congress in 1874 of a $10,000 special fund for studies in human nutrition under the direction of Wilbur Olin Atwater, who often is called "Father of American Nutrition." Atwater served as the first director of a state (Connecticut) agricultural experiment station, then first director of the federal office of experiment stations. After retirement from the latter post in 1891, he continued as the first director of the federal program in human nutrition and worked incessantly to secure funds for use, as he wrote to his friend, Rev. Emory J. Haynes, D.D., of Boston, April 20, 1873: "to have the men and the investigations that will prove stimulating to the undergraduates and to the intellectual life of the college."

Greensboro Workshop on the Role of the Land Grant Universities in Nutrition Education

The 1890 colleges (Black land grant colleges) generally have not shared in the nutrition leadership that resides primarily in the 1862 land grant institutions. In 1972, in recognition of the need for greater support for work in nutrition and health within the 1890 schools, Congress appropriated supplementary funds specifically for these institutions, to be dispersed in the form of grants. A shortage of personnel and other resources limited the effectiveness of utilization of these funds. Accordingly, the U.S. Department of Agriculture

The Fourth Decade

and The Nutrition Foundation, in conjunction with representatives of the Black land grant institutions, developed plans and support for a workshop to consider how more effective programs of education, research, personnel development and leadership for applied nutrition may be promoted through land grant colleges, with particular emphasis on the 1890 institutions. Planning was assisted by representatives of the American Institute of Nutrition and the Society for Nutrition Education.

The workshop was held in Greensboro, North Carolina, October 1-4, 1973, and the proceedings were published and distributed by The Nutrition Foundation. The workshop was attended by 180 teachers and scientists from land grant universities, from 1890 schools, the U.S. Department of Agriculture, HEW, industry, and from a wide variety of other universities, colleges and medical centers. The workshop afforded a first opportunity for establishing communication and, in many instances, subsequent collaboration between the spectrum of personnel and organizations which can provide support to the 1890 schools. Effective cooperation has been established in several programs since the workshop and a subsequent follow-up assessment is projected.

Nutrition in the General Education Programs in Colleges

The Nutrition Foundation also fosters general courses in food and nutrition for the non-science major and nutrition education for teachers and teachers-in-training in colleges, undergraduate schools and universities. Most college graduates, including teachers, have not been exposed to any basic formal background in foods and nutrition. Consequently, when they seek information they often turn to non-authorities, authors of popular selling books or to television show personalities. In a few universities, effective instructors have successfully attracted a relatively large enrollment in general courses designed to examine scientifically issues of public concern regarding food. Similar properly planned learning experiences are highly desirable for all teachers or teachers-in-training, especially those who may not have other exposure to biology or health and nutrition education. The teacher who will specialize in home economics, health or biology also can profit from and should experience a more intensive background in nutrition and foods.

Another current problem is presented by graduate scientists. Seldom directed toward a career in general education, they usually do not become familiar with or competent in the most effective use of educational theory and practice or with communication techniques and media that are readily available and adaptable to instructional purposes.

The Nutrition Foundation, therefore, is supporting and promoting multidisciplinary teaching aimed at filling these needs.

Nutrition Instruction for the General College Student

At Pennsylvania State University, a course for the general college student combining lecture and guided self-instruction has been accredited for the University's general degree requirements. This course has been offered during four successive quarters. Enrollment has been greatly oversubscribed at each offering, and it is projected that the course will reach 1,200 students annually. Self-instructional material used has been repeatedly assessed and appropriately revised to provide a background of general principles. Issues of con-

A Good Idea

cern to the student are dealt with in a seminar atmosphere, affording an opportunity to illustrate the use of the principles presented in self-study packets. Again, assessments accompany each stage of the development.

At Florida Atlantic University, Dr. Daniel Melnick has developed a course aimed at a similar student level. A teaching manual built primarily around issues has been prepared for this course. It has been revised after each course offering in keeping with the assessment of student reaction, and now has been printed for wider distribution in other institutions, including Pennsylvania State University, for assessment and further development. The Nutrition Foundation is assisting through grant support and other means in this development.

Nutrition Education for Teachers

The Heinz Nutrition Education Program in Pennsylvania

In order to penetrate the educational systems at both university and elementary and secondary school levels, there must be active and enthusiastic involvement by the knowledgeable professional educator. Identification of the nutrition principles to be taught and their application should be a responsibility jointly shared by professionals in education, foods, nutrition and health. The nutrition program at Pennsylvania State University, supported by the Foundation with funds provided by the Howard Heinz Endowment, has been outstanding in blending the competences and interests of these groups.

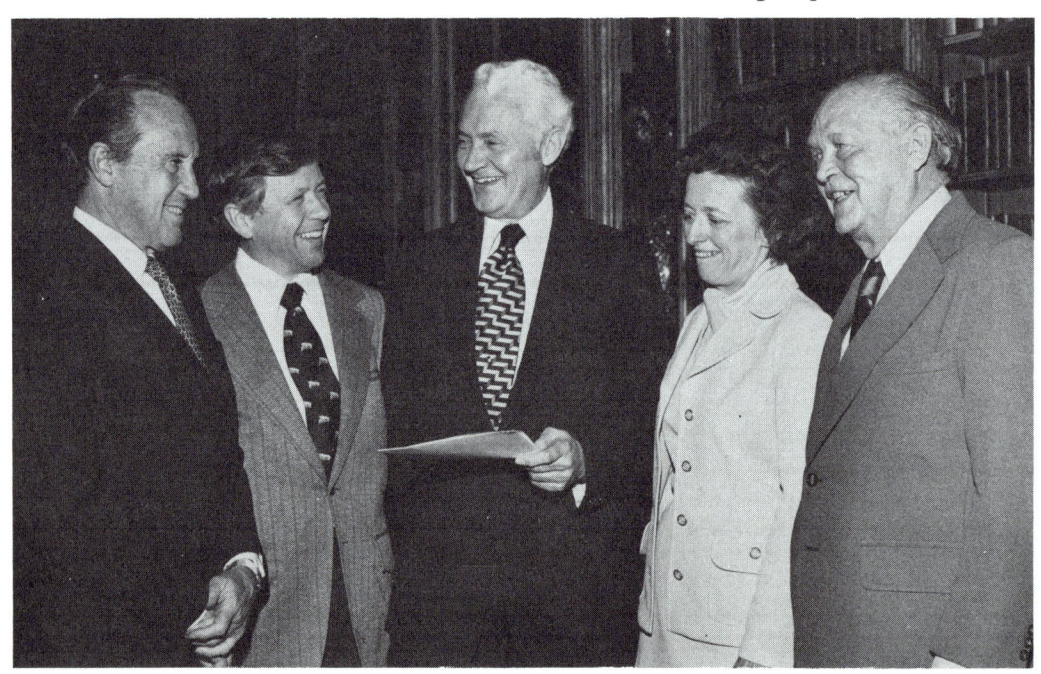

Left to right: H. J. Heinz, II, Donald Ford, William J. Darby, Helen Guthrie, J. George Harrar

Mr. H. J. Heinz announces a grant from the Howard Heinz Endowment through The Nutrition Foundation to support the development of a model program of nutrition education in Pennsylvania. Drs. Ford and Guthrie represent Pennsylvania State University, a recipient institution along with Jefferson Medical School of Thomas Jefferson University.

The Fourth Decade

Following an evaluation of past efforts in nutrition education in school systems in Pennsylvania and elsewhere in the United States, the faculty of the nutrition program and the College of Education at Pennsylvania State University are jointly developing and implementing throughout elementary and secondary schools a program for teaching designed within a framework of nutrition concepts. Incorporated at all phases are thoughtfully planned and informative assessments. Simultaneously, in-service training or renewal courses in nutrition are given for the teachers who are involved.

Curricular material in nutrition has been integrated in grades four through six in two school regions one urban, and one rural. A team of educators and nutritionists from the Pennsylvania State University has developed curriculum plans that incorporate nutrition information into the health, language, arts, science and mathematics components of the school curriculum. They also are determining the necessary preparatory work to facilitate school and community support. An evaluation of goals and effectiveness has been incorporated throughout this program and is supervised by the Center for Cooperative Research with Schools, the faculty of which has extensive experience in curriculum evaluation. This evaluation will provide the basis for subsequent refining, remodeling and planning of the curriculum and supporting materials to be developed and used in the initial grade levels. A similar plan subsequently will be followed for extension of such teaching both upward and downward throughout schools, from kindergarten through the twelfth grade.

Wide interest in this program has been stimulated through conferences with key educators and personnel, including participants at the annual meeting of the Council of Organizations for Education (COE) in Pennsylvania. The first teacher-training course offered in the summer of 1975 was oversubscribed.

A Pennsylvania State University Committee, the PENN (Pennsylvania Educators and Nutritionists for Nutrition) has been organized as a planning group for the design and implementation of the School of Nutrition Education program. Members of the faculty are working with the Penn State Educational Television Studio in preparing and producing a one hour program dealing with consumer issues in nutrition. They also are seeking to develop a series of half-hour programs and accompanying learning materials which can be utilized for credit for continuing education for teachers and for other viewers.

The potential for cooperative development of audio-visual materials with other institutions is being explored, including the utilization of a similar series in preparation at Michigan State University. The Nutrition Foundation encourages such cooperation which can lead to improved effectiveness and wider utilization of educational resources.

The nutrition education program at Pennsylvania State was initiated by assembling a well planned nutrition education conference in July 1974—a conference participated in by members of the faculty at that university, as well as other experts in the fields of education, nutrition, communication, medicine, public health, sociology and marketing. This workshop addressed itself to nutrition developments relative to educational needs of health professionals, lay and adult audiences, general college students, teachers in training and in-service—all within the broad framework of nutrition and human development as interpreted at the opening session by Dean Donald H. Ford of the College of Human Development at

Pennsylvania State University. This conference and the proceedings, published by Pennsylvania State University, serve as an admirable background against which this program is developing.

Conferences on Nutrition Education

Preceding the exciting developments in Pennsylvania, The Nutrition Foundation participated in planning and support of two symposia on the subject of nutrition education at Columbia University's Teachers College. These symposia included a valuable perspective of the earlier vigorous program of nutrition within that college and a description of material especially useful to those concerned with the integration of nutrition into school curricula within the framework of the modern educational system. The proceedings are available from Columbia University Teachers College.

Among other educational symposia assisted by the Foundation was an international conference on nutrition education sponsored jointly by the American Institute of Nutrition and the International Union of Nutritional Sciences in Guadalajara, Mexico, 1972. This conference addressed itself to the problems of transmitting nutritional information to different ethnic groups. Major areas of discussion concerned food habits research and nutrition education; the methodology of information transfer by use of mass media, particularly in developing countries; the role of commercial firms; personnel needs and training; evaluation of programs; and nutrition in formal education. The papers from this meeting are distributed by UNICEF.

Nutrition Foundation Educational Materials and Guides

The obvious need for identifying and preparing appropriate educational material for use at differing levels was a major factor in the establishment of The Nutrition Foundation's Information Center. Because of the vast number of inquiries received, particularly from teachers and teachers-in-training, the Foundation's Office of Education compiled an INDEX OF NUTRITION EDUCATION MATERIALS—booklets, pamphlets, audio-visual aids—available from federal agencies, professional societies and health and educational organizations and foundations. This INDEX, with more than 4,000 copies already distributed, is being widely used not only by teachers but by community workers, health workers and communicators of all types. A supplement is in preparation.

Other educational publications sponsored or prepared by the Foundation range from those for the lay public to the fourth edition of "Present Knowledge in Nutrition." These various publications are of supportive value in diverse teaching programs.

Nutrition Foundation Monographs

Educational materials sponsored by the Foundation include authoritative monographs that summarize scientific knowledge within a broad area and consolidate relevant advances in that area from diverse disciplines. Nutrition Foundation monographs include:

"Sugars in Nutrition," edited by Horace L. Sipple and Kristen W. McNutt, 768 pages, Academic Press, Inc., New York, 1974

"Protein-Calorie Malnutrition," edited by Robert E. Olsen, 467 pages, Academic Press, Inc., New York, 1975

"Trace Elements in Human Health and Disease," in 2 volumes, edited by

The Fourth Decade

Ananda S. Prasad, Academic Press, Inc., New York, 1976.

Nutrition Reviews

The critical review journal, NUTRITION REVIEWS, contains authoritative review articles by distinguished international scientists; authoritative, critical and informative reviews and interpretive summaries of important original clinical and experimental research; selected excerpts from classic publications that marked milestones in nutrition research; and informative special reports of governmental and organization actions. NUTRITION REVIEWS is widely used by the professional nutrition community—university professors, food scientists, graduate students, physicians, home economists and dietitians. Science writers and news media personnel also find it useful. A special student rate encourages its use by students. Over 2,000 of some 8,000 subscribers are from outside the United States.

Present Knowledge in Nutrition

This succinct summary of scientific advances in nutrition, "Present Knowledge in Nutrition," is widely employed as a text or supplementary reading in universities, colleges, graduate schools and medical schools and other schools of the health sciences, and it serves as a reference for pro-

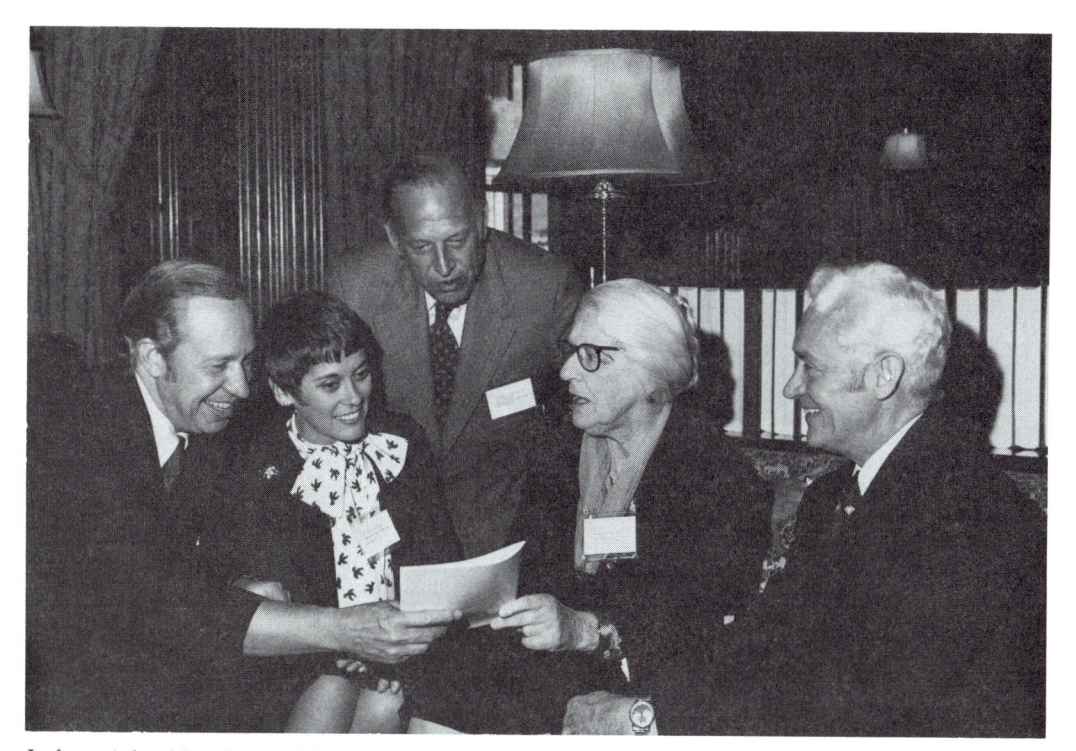

Left to right: *Marvin Cornblath, Kristen W. McNutt, Richard M. Stalvey, Cicely D. Williams, William J. Darby.*

Dr. Cornblath and the Department of Pediatrics, University of Maryland sponsored a symposium on nutrition in young children and The Nutrition Foundation published a special issue of NUTRITION REVIEWS to mark the 80th year of the distinguished international physician, Dr. Cicely D. Williams. Dr. Williams introduced the term kwashiorkor into the medical literature.

A Good Idea

fessional scientists in the field of nutrition and for teachers. Initially consisting of lead articles reprinted from NUTRITION REVIEWS, the fourth edition, 1976, systematically covers scientific developments and present state of knowledge concerning human nutrition. It includes the biochemistry, physiology, and the state of scientific understanding of all nutrients known to be required by man. This edition, like the earlier one, no doubt will be widely accepted in colleges and graduate teaching programs.

Supplements and Special Issues of NUTRITION REVIEWS

A Special Supplement to the July, 1974 issue of NUTRITION REVIEWS, entitled "Nutrition Misinformation and Food Faddism," has proved to be of exceptional interest to a very broad spectrum of readers, including the general public, physicians, students, teachers, newspaper and magazine writers, government officials, dentists, and college and university students.

A special issue of NUTRITION REVIEWS to mark the eightieth year of Cicely D. Williams, the distinguished international physician who described and named the syndrome of kwashiorkor (protein-calorie malnutrition), was published in November, 1973. This issue makes available to the student of nutrition the almost inaccessible earlier works of Dr. Williams, many of which initially were published in reports that are not available in collections in the United States. This publication and

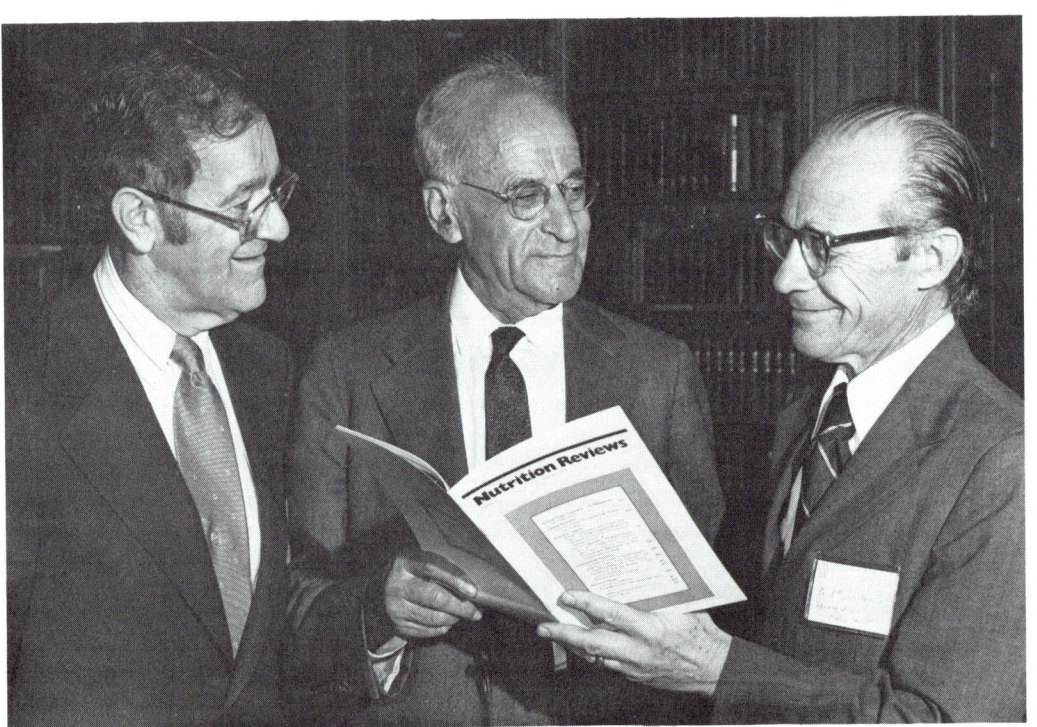

Left to right: *Samuel Goldblith, Samuel Lepkovsky, D. Mark Hegsted*

Dr. Mark Hegsted, Editor of NUTRITION REVIEWS, shows Drs. Goldblith and Lepkovsky a reprint of a "Nutrition Classic," two of Dr. Lepkovsky's papers on pyridoxine. Photographed at a meeting of the Board of Trustees of The Nutrition Foundation and marking Dr. Lepkovsky's 75th birthday.

The Fourth Decade

The Nutrition Foundation monograph on protein-calorie malnutrition illustrate the overall planned effort of the Foundation to make available to scholars needed informative basic scientific material relating to major nutritional problems or issues.

Reprint Series of Source Books and Classics

A reprint series of highly valuable classical works in the field of nutrition, jointly selected and sponsored by The Nutrition Foundation, the British Nutrition Foundation and the Swedish Nutrition Foundation is being initiated with the re-publication of Graham Lusk's "The Science of Nutrition," fourth edition (1928). This reference work originally was published by W. B. Saunders Company, Philadelphia, and is reprinted by permission. A second source book in this series will be Alfred Hess's "Scurvy, Past and Present" (1920), originally published by J. B. Lippincott Company.

Each issue of NUTRITION REVIEWS reprints the critical portions of a classic, original contribution to the science of nutrition, which probably would not have been read in the original by today's student. Such educational perspective develops in students an understanding important for their interpretation of the modern-day wide swings of fashionable interests in science and public affairs.

Current Publications of The Nutrition Foundation

(Published by the Foundation or with Foundation support)

Books and Education Aids

"Sugars in Nutrition," a Nutrition Foundation Monograph, edited by Horace L. Sipple and Kristen W. McNutt, 768 pages, Academic Press, Inc., New York, 1974.

"Protein-Calorie Malnutrition," a Nutrition Foundation Monograph, edited by Robert E. Olsen, 467 pages, Academic Press, Inc., New York, 1975.

"Trace Elements in Human Health and Disease," a Nutrition Foundation Monograph, in 2 volumes, edited by Ananda S. Prasad, Academic Press, Inc., New York, 1976.

"Nutrition Education Materials," published by The Nutrition Foundation, Office of Education and Public Affairs, 170 pages, Washington, D.C., 1975.
—Lists 1,000 pamphlets, booklets and audio-visual materials. Assists teachers and general public in acquiring useful teaching aids and educational materials.

"A Teaching Manual on Food and Nutrition for Non-Science Majors," Daniel Melnick, Ph.D., The Nutrition Foundation, Washington, D.C., 1975.

"Teenage Nutrition and Physique," Dr. Ruth L. Hueneman, Charles C. Thomas, Springfield, Illinois, 1974.

"Saving a Child from Xerophthalmia—A Disease of Darkness," produced by The Nutrition Foundation and the American Foundation for Overseas Blind, New York, 1975.
—Educational aid for professionals and para-professionals, including color slides and diagrams.

Nutrition Foundations' Award Book

W. R. Aykroyd, "The Conquest of Famine," Chatto & Windus, London, 1974, and Reader's Digest Press, New York, 1975, 216 pages.

Proceeedings of Symposia Developed with Support by the Foundation

"Conference on Guidelines for Nutrition Education Programs," Williamsburg,

A Good Idea

Virginia, June 25-27, 1972, 105 pages.
—Proceedings of a national conference on nutrition education in medical schools.

"The Application of Nutrition in the Health Sciences," Houston, Texas, February 9, 1974, 51 pages.
—Proceedings of a meeting on nutrition education in medical and dental schools.

"Workshop on the Role of Land Grant Institutions in Applied Human Nutrition," Greensboro, North Carolina, October 1-4, 1973, 118 pages.
—Proceedings of a workshop on development of education programs, research and training of personnel in nutrition.

"Conference on Education in Nutrition—Looking Forward from the Past," Teachers College, Columbia University, New York, February 26-27, 1975, 59 pages.
—Proceedings of a conference on nutrition education for school teachers.

"Proceeedings of Nutrition Education Conference," Pennsylvania State University, July 21-24, 1974, 102 pages.
—Proceedings of a broad conference on nutrition understanding and educational needs.

"Vitamin A Deficiency and Blindness Prevention," American Federation for the Blind and American Foundation for the Overseas Blind, Inc., New York, 1974, 74 pages.
—Proceedings of two workshops on vitamin A deficiency.

NUTRITION REVIEWS: Volume 1, 1941-Volume 34, 1976

Published monthly by The Nutrition Foundation's Office of Education and Public Affairs, Washington, D.C. Editorial Office, School of Public Health, Harvard University, Boston, Massachusetts. Includes authoritative, interpretative summaries of clinical and experimental nutrition research, special reports of government and organization activities, and selected excerpts from publications marking milestones in nutrition research.

Special Reprints from NUTRITION REVIEWS

R. Guarth Hansen, Ph.D., "An Index of Food Quality," NUTRITION REVIEWS, Vol. 31, No. 1, 1973.

"Nutrition Labeling and Standards of Identity," reprinted from NUTRITION REVIEWS, Vol. 31, Nos. 1, 4 and 8, 1973 and Vol. 32, No. 1, 1974.

J. George Harrar, Ph.D., "Nutrition and Numbers in the Third World," W. O. Atwater Memorial Lecture, NUTRITION REVIEWS, Vol. 32, No. 4, April, 1974.

"Guidelines for a National Nutrition Policy," proposed by the National Nutrition Consortium, Inc., NUTRITION REVIEWS, Vol. 32, No. 5, May, 1974.

H.A.P.C. Oomen, M.D., "Vitamin A Deficiency, Xerophthalmia and Blindness," NUTRITION REVIEWS, Vol. 32, No. 6, 1974.
—Available with 12 full color slides, mounted on slide strips, with individual magnifying viewer.

William J. Darby, M.D., "Nutrition, Food Needs and Technologic Priorities: The World Food Conference," NUTRITION REVIEWS, Vol. 33, No. 8, August, 1975.

Pamphlets and Booklets

Published by The Nutrition Foundation, Office of Education and Public Affairs, Washington, D.C.

Your Diet: Health Is in the Balance

The Fourth Decade

—valuable, non-technical booklet discussing the need for nutrients and the variety of foods in which they are found

Choosing Foods to Fit Your Life
—a brochure explaining how a variety of food patterns can provide sound nutrition

Food Choices—The Teenage Girl
—a non-technical booklet discussing diets which meet the nutritional needs of the teenage girl

Nutrition for Athletes
—a primer on nutrition designed for use of coaches and high school and junior high school teachers

Obesity
—a basic discussion of obesity and its prevention and a medically sound program for weight control

Food—A Key to Better Health
—an elementary presentation of fundamentals of a good diet, prepared for use of Nutrition Aides in conjunction with the USDA

Special Reports

"FOOD DAY," analysis and critique of "Food Day" activities. Produced and distributed by The Nutrition Foundation, Office of Education and Public Affairs, Washington, D.C., March 28, 1975, 5 pages.

"Report of the National Advisory Committee on Hyperkinesis and Food Additives to The Nutrition Foundation," published and distributed by The Nutrition Foundation, Office of Education and Public Affairs, Washington, D.C., June 1, 1975, 19 pages.

"Proposed Nutritional Guidelines for Utilization of Industrially Produced Nutrients," prepared jointly by The Nutrition Foundation, and the Swedish Nutrition Foundation, Naringsforskning, no. 2, 1975, pp. 113-120.

Grants for Research and Education

Challenging Opportunities

Research is the germ plasm of science, without which our modern species would become extinct. Decline of interest in or challenge of research within any area of knowledge promptly results in decreased appeal of the subject for the brightest young minds when competition from other opportunities for creative scholarship arises. Those who remain devotees of a subject which undergoes such loss become intellectually sterile and usually impotent.

These facts and the challenging opportunities for research in nutrition in the 1970's and their promising rewards are strong motivating reasons for greater support to research.

The upsurge of enthusiastic interest in nutrition reflects the expanded horizons of research which followed the realization that nutrition has extraordinarily broad significance in health and disease and is not merely a matter of preventing classical deficiency diseases. The application of new methods and concepts in the study of human needs in health and disease, coupled with the demand to know more about the composition of foods and the significance of non-essential nutrients and other substances present in foodstuffs have further expanded and heightened interest. These influences, coupled with the deceleration of federal grant support, led to an enormous increase in requests for research grant funds from The Nutrition Foundation. The increase in requests has continued and the demands of promising proposals far exceed those which can be funded.

A Good Idea

Simultaneously, the expressed interest of the Foundation in publication, development of education materials, symposia and stimulation of new organizations have provoked additional requests for grant support for these activities. A moderate increment in the funds dispersed for use by grantees has been sustained. Grants for 1972-75 have totaled as follows: 1972-$450,000; 1973-$490,000; 1974-$670,000. The increment in 1974 is due in large measure to increased funding that became available through funds from the Howard Heinz Endowment and from special contributions for nutrition education.

Support given in the educational field, in addition to the programs at Pennsylvania State University and Thomas Jefferson Medical School has included sizeable funding for initiating nutrition education programs in the medical schools at Albany, Boston University School of Medicine, and the Health Center, University of Texas at San Antonio, plus final payments on commitments at Mt. Sinai, Columbia University, and the University of Missouri.

Other support important in education is assistance in developing teaching materials like the teaching manual on nutrition issues by Dr. Melnick. Grants for support of major international symposia planned to produce monographs in needed areas are especially effective in focusing research as well as educational interests on important new knowledge and research needs. Similarly, support for examining specific questions through symposia or workshops can represent excellent investments in needed research.

As examples of the latter, the Foundation has assisted the National Academy of Sciences in developing two symposia, one dealing with new evidence concerning folic acid metabolism and requirements of man and the other with aspects of the background materials for the Food Chemicals Codex. While it is impossible to quantitate the impact of such investments in research and education, indications are that the exchange at symposia and workshops frequently constitutes benchmarks or consolidation of evidence that leads to subsequent major discoveries, application and educational activities.

Major Interests

The major interests supported by research grants during the period 1972-1975 are categorized in the following pages.

Malnutrition, Intellectual Development and Behavior

Final observations in the major study of Dr. Joaquin Cravioto in Mexico of the influence of malnutrition on intellectual development and behavior are completed and numerous scientific papers describing the findings have been published. Dr. Cravioto is preparing a series of book-length reports. A major contribution of this study has been the identification of the relative role of malnutrition *per se* and of the absence or paucity of stimulatory experiences in conditioning retardation of the underpriviledged, malnourished child. His critical approach and careful attention to observational details have resulted in improvements in methods of study and observational standards. Indeed, Dr. Cravioto served as Chairman of an international workshop on methodology and a participant in the associated symposium on malnutrition in learning sponsored by the Swedish Nutrition Foundation, the World Health Organization and the National Institute of Child Health and Human Development in Sweden in 1973. The resulting monograph of the Swedish Nutrition Foundation contains contributions by the following in-

The Fourth Decade

vestigators whose research has been supported by The Nutrition Foundation: Dr. Joaquin Cravioto, Dr. Robert R. Zimmermann, Dr. Myron Winick, and Dr. Joseph M. Brozek.

The increasing evidence from studies in experimental animals of the influence of malnutrition upon emotional derangements and aggressiveness also has been of great interest.

Chemical Senses

Another research area of considerable importance, particularly in recent efforts to evaluate the role of sugars in the diet, is that of the taste and taste preferences of the newborn. Studies supported by the Foundation have demonstrated that the newborn infant possesses taste preferences and readily distinguishes between preparations of differing degrees of sweetness. The newborn exhibits a preference for the sweeter sugars, sucrose and fructose, rather than the less sweet sugars, glucose and lactose, and for moderate concentration of sugar over a very low or high concentration. Taste preference of an infant or adult, however, does not assure advantage or disadvantage in health. Techniques for these studies were evolved with support by Nutrition Foundation grants.

Appetite and Amino Acid Nutriture

The role of nutrient composition *per se* in determining appetite or food preferences is a subject of investigation supported by The Nutrition Foundation. Work at the University of California, Davis, has extended considerably the appreciation of the appetite-depressing effect of certain amino acid imbalances, an effect reminiscent of the rapid loss of appetite noted in some of Professor William C. Rose's early investigations of amino acid deficiencies in young men.

Nutrient Requirements and Biological Availability of Nutrients

In attempting to estimate human nutrient requirements, it is increasingly recognized that chemical methods to measure total quantity alone are insufficient to determine the nutritional availability of particular nutrients as they are present in different foodstuffs. Nutrients may be present in forms that are more or less available, or unavailable. Materials accompanying the nutrient in the diet may alter, and frequently impair, the absorption of the nutrient from the gastrointestinal tract. Hence, studies of biological availability of nutrients in man become increasingly important in estimating the nutritional value of foods. The Foundation supports research in this area being conducted at the University of Illinois, the University of Rhode Island and the University of Chicago.

Grants from The Nutrition Foundation to the University of California, Vanderbilt University, Massachusetts Institute of Technology, and the National Academy of Sciences bear on these considerations in relation to folic acid. Dr. E. L. R. Stokstad of the University of California, Berkeley, has devised a method for quantitatively estimating the availability to man of this vitamin from foodstuffs. He has ascertained that there exists in certain foods, notably orange juice, an influence that reduces the availability of the vitamin.

Trace Elements and Fiber

Dr. John Reinhold, working at Pahlavi University, Shiraz, has pursued the question of interference with availability of dietary zinc. Earlier it has been hypothesized that phytate was the major factor present in whole cereals, particularly corn, which reduced the availability of dietary zinc. In recent investigations, he has found

A Good Idea

that dietary fiber is more active in reducing the availability of zinc than is phytate. This observation is especially timely in view of the emphasis currently placed upon the desirability of increased fiber in the diet. It opens for further study a new aspect of the question of dietary fiber.

The question of biological availability of micronutrients is especially important in the instance of trace elements. Growing recognition of the importance of trace elements and the necessity for monitoring intake levels has led policy-making groups, governmental regulatory agencies and public health agencies to seek information on dietary intake and man's need for these elements. Trace elements, in one manner or another, may be related to several human disease conditions: diabetes, hypertension, hyperlipidemias, endocrinologic disturbances, growth defects, dental caries, goiter, anemia, osteoporosis, and even genetic defects. Dr. Harold H. Sandstead, Director of the USDA Nutrition Laboratory on Trace Elements at Grand Forks, North Dakota, and an alumnus of The Nutrition Foundation's Future Leaders Award program, and Dr. William J. Darby were members of two expert groups convened by the World Health Organization in Geneva, to review the world-wide situation in this area of information. These committees dealt with human requirements of trace elements and the evidence pertaining to hypothesized relationships between trace elements and cardiovascular disease. Dr. Darby served as chairman of the WHO Expert Committee on Trace Elements in Man. The discussions and resultant report highlight evidence for man's requirement of iodine, fluoride, copper, iron, zinc, chromium and magnesium, as well as the potential chronic toxic effects of cadmium, mercury and lead. Evidence is emerging from animal studies of a dietary need for nickel, tin, selenium, silicon, molybdenum and vanadium. The Nutrition Foundation currently supports investigations on the possible role of silicon in bone healing in man, epidemiologic studies of the possible relationship between the level of chromium intake and human diabetes, and the relationship of lead toxicity to calcium intake.

World Food and Nutrition Problems

Although the program of The Nutrition Foundation is oriented mainly toward the improvement of nutritional health and support of research in institutions within the United States, the Foundation also has had major impacts throughout the world. This is true particularly with regard to activities and responsibilities of the international agencies and organizations concerned with the developing world. That the Foundation should maintain an awareness of and responsiveness to current world nutrition needs not only is logical from a humanitarian standpoint, but important because of the contribution which science and technology developed in the United States may make, by adaptation and transfer, to meeting needs elsewhere.

The dominant position of the United States as a producer and exporter of food in quantities essential to meet pressing needs abroad casts the U.S. in a uniquely responsible role in matters of world food production and utilization. There is no national limit on the application and significance of scientific knowledge. A discovery in a developing country may soon find important application in the United States or other highly industrialized societies, as is clearly illustrated by our present knowledge of zinc in nutrition. Human zinc deficiency was highlighted in studies in the Middle East and the above noted observa-

The Fourth Decade

tion on zinc and fiber was also made there. These findings have obvious significance to the U.S. at present.

Repeatedly during 1974, world leadership expressed concern for matters of food supply, under-nutrition and population numbers—a concern eloquently voiced by Dr. J. George Harrar, Chairman of the Board of Trustees of The Nutrition Foundation, in the W. O. Atwater Lecture, "Nutrition and Numbers in the Third World," on February 28, 1974. This lecture was published in NUTRITION REVIEWS and received even wider circulation by being reprinted in *BioScience*. At the May 1974 meeting of the Trustees, Dr. Harrar highlighted the importance of international events planned for that year in a pointedly frank analysis of the gravity of the world food and population problem. He emphasized a responsibility for appropriate involvement of The Nutrition Foundation in activities that can help to broaden understanding and that may contribute to alleviation of the problem.

The widespread concern for these problems has been increased by the changing world economic situation. The seriousness of the situation was underscored by action of the Executive Board of UNICEF at its 1974 session in adopting its declaration that a worldwide emergency for children in developing countries is resulting from the current economic crisis; by the convening in November 1974 of the World Food Conference, and by numerous subsequent international actions.

In anticipation of such events, The Nutrition Foundation initiated efforts to promote understanding of the nature of the world food and nutrition problems, and of the role of industrial technology and science in meeting these needs. These efforts included repeated emphasis during public and international forums of the risks of world food shortages due to restrictions on

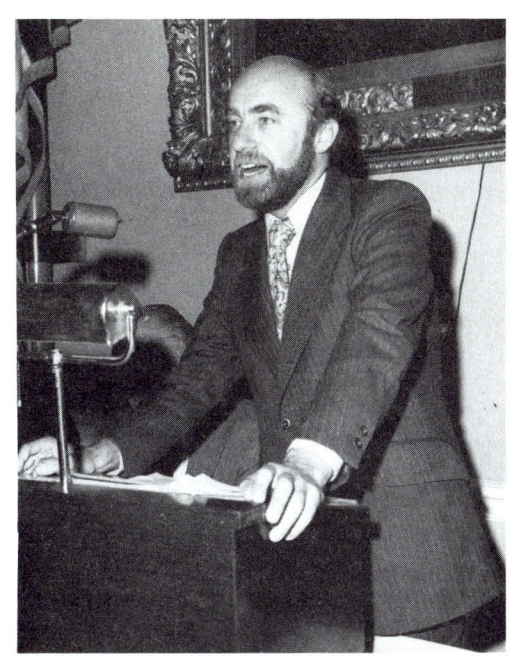

Alan Berg—Dr. Berg addressed the Trustees of The Nutrition Foundation on food and nutrition in international development at a semi-annual luncheon meeting. He is Senior Nutrition Advisor in the Agriculture and Rural Department at the World Bank and long has contributed to more appropriate recognition of key roles of food and nutrition in international programs of development.

or prohibition of useful technologic aids. Indeed, the activities of the Citizens' Commission on Science, Law and the Food Supply were planned to provide a sound analysis of benefit-risk decision making which bears so directly upon these problems. Well publicized considerations of these questions have been published and distributed.

The selection of W. R. Aykroyd's book *The Conquest of Famine* as the first Nutrition Foundations' Award Book was a further action to promote understanding of this problem. Similarly, publication of the second Nutrition Foundation monograph, "Protein-Calorie Malnutrition" and collaboration with the Worldmark Press in compiling the Protein Advisory Group

A Good Idea

(PAG) Compendium address other important aspects of the world problem.

The Nutrition Foundation was invited as one of the non-government organizations to participate in the World Food Conference in Rome, November 5-15, 1974.

A status review of these and related activities was published in NUTRITION REVIEWS, August 1975, summarizing the response of The Nutrition Foundation and indicating the role envisioned for this and similar organizations. It is based in large part upon the assessments made by several colleagues associated with The Nutrition Foundation who participated in the World Food Conference. They included trustees of the Foundation: Dr. J. George Harrar; Mr. Henry J. Heinz II; Mr. J. E. Lonning; Rev. Theodore M. Hesburgh; The Nutrition Foundation's Senior Scholar, Dr. Samuel E. Stumpf; and a member of the Food and Nutrition Liaison Committee, Dr. John Luck. The President of the Foundation attended as a representative of the Non-Government Organizations (NGO).

Despite the surprising and frustrating involvement of international politics in such a basic humanitarian endeavor, the Conference, according to Mr. J. E. Lonning, Vice Chairman of The Nutrition Foundation's Board of Trustees and a member of the U.S. Delegation,

> ... must be viewed as a success in that it represented an opening dialogue. Without such collective action future solutions to the problem of world hunger would not be possible.

Important recommendations concerning policies to improve nutrition contained in the provisional report of the World Food Conference emphasize:

Nutrition education for the public and in formal curricula;

The desirability and feasibility of meeting nutrient requirements through fortification;

The responsibility of governments for taking action strengthening and modernizing consumer education services, food legislation, food control programs and marketing practices aimed at protection of the consumer;

The importance of governments associating non-governmental organizations whose programs include nutrition-related activities with their nutritional efforts, particularly in the areas of food and nutrition programs, nutrition education and feeding programs for the most vulnerable groups.

These and other recommendations of the Conference predictably cast the framework within which science, government and industry must function together in the future in order to meet their responsibilities.

The Nutrition Foundation obviously has given high priority to education, as well as to other activities emphasized by the Rome Conference. Prior to the Conference, the Foundation had provided outstanding leadership for sound nutritional planning of foods and their use. Toward such an objective, The Nutrition Foundation, in consort with colleagues in Sweden and Britain, has prepared and published "Proposed Nutritional Guidelines for the Use of Industrially Produced Nutrients." Guidelines, internationally applicable, will aid in the proper development and adoption of technologic innovations as called for by the recommendation of the Congress.

The Nutrition Foundation is cooperating with WHO, USAID, and the American Foundation for the Overseas Blind (AFOB) in finalizing a document on control of avitaminosis A and xerophthalmia, a re-

The Fourth Decade

port that stems from a meeting held at Djakarta in December, 1974. The Foundation, with the cooperation of UNICEF, AFOB and USAID, is also preparing and distributing appropriate educational materials on this subject adapted for a wide range of health workers. Such collaborative associations of governmental and non-governmental organizations can facilitate attainment of the goal of the World Food Conference.

It is toward meeting "the trust of the future"—the growing development and application of knowledge concerning nutrition to satisfy the needs of man and to "make imperfect man comfortable, happy and healthy"—that The Nutrition Foundation is dedicated.

Appendix

A. Excerpts from the Organizational Meeting of the Board of Trustees March 12, 1942.

B. By-Laws of The Nutrition Foundation, Revised and Adopted November, 1971.

C. "Nutrition in the 1970's" Address to the Board of Trustees of The Nutrition Foundation November 5, 1971.

D. Selected References Illustrative of Research Supported by The Nutrition Foundation, 1942-1975.

E. Future Leader Awardees, The Nutrition Foundation 1964-1975.

F. Recipients of Awards Supported by The Nutrition Foundation

G. The Food and Nutrition Board, Twenty-Five Years in Retrospect, 1940-1965.

Appendix A

Excerpts from the Organizational Meeting of the Board of Trustees
March 12, 1942

Minutes of the organizational meeting of the Board of Trustees of *The Nutrition Foundation, Inc.*, held at the Waldorf-Astoria Hotel in the City and State of New York, on March 12, 1942, at 3:00 p.m.

Present:

Mr. James S. Adams, President, Standard Brands Incorporated
Mr. Frederick Beers, Vice President, National Biscuit Company
Mr. Carlyle H. Black, Vice President, American Can Company
Mr. Cason J. Callaway, Hamilton, Ga.
Dr. W. C. Coffey, President, University of Minnesota
Mr. Carle C. Conway, Chairman, Continental Can Company
Dr. Karl T. Compton, President, Massachusetts Institute of Technology
Mr. Daniel W. Creeden, President, Libby, McNeill & Libby
Mr. Charles Wesley Dunn, General Counsel, Associated Grocery Manufacturers of America, Inc.
Mr. J. Stafford Ellithorp, Jr., Vice President, Beech-Nut Packing Company
Mr. Clarence Francis, President, General Foods Corporation
Mr. Henry J. Heinz, II, President, H. J. Heinz Company
Mr. John Holmes, President, Swift & Company
Dr. Charles G. King, University of Pittsburgh
Mr. J. Preston Levis, President, Owens-Illinois Glass Company
Mr. James McGowan, Jr., Vice President, Campbell Soup Company
Reverend Hugh O'Donnell, President, Notre Dame University
Dr. Thomas Parran, Surgeon General, United States Public Health Service
Mr. Russell G. Partridge, Vice President, United Fruit Company
Mr. George V. Robbins, Vice President, California Packing Corporation
Mr. Ole Salthe, New York City
Mr. Morris Sayre, Vice President, Corn Products Refining Company
Mr. George A. Sloan, New York City
Mr. R. Douglas Stuart, First Vice President, Quaker Oats Company
Dr. Stephen S. Wise, Rabbi, Free Synagogue, New York City

Proceedings:

1. Mr. John Holmes, Chairman of the Organization Committee of Founder Manufacturers, called the meeting to order. On motion by Mr. Holmes, duly carried, Dr. Karl T. Compton was elected as Temporary Chairman. The Temporary Chairman appointed Mr. Ole Salthe as Temporary Secretary.

2. The Temporary Chairman stated that *The Nutrition Foundation, Inc.*, was incorporated on December 24, 1941, pursuant to the Membership Corporations Law of the State of New York; and he submitted a certified copy of its certificate of incorporation. On motion duly made and carried, it was

Resolved, that the certified copy of the certificate of incorporation of *The Nutrition Foundation, Inc.*, submitted by Dr. Compton, be added to the permanent records of this corporation.

The Temporary Chairman read the list of incorporators of this corporation. They are:

Appendix

Mr. Frederick Beers
Mr. Carlyle H. Black
Mr. Carle C. Conway
Mr. Daniel W. Creeden
Mr. Alfred W. Eames
Mr. J. Stafford Ellithorp, Jr.
Mr. Clarence Francis
Mr. H. J. Heinz, II
Mr. John Holmes
Mr. J. P. Levis
Mr. James McGowan, Jr.
Mr. Morris Sayre
Mr. Thomas L. Smith
Mr. R. Douglas Stuart
Mr. Russell G. Partridge

The Temporary Chairman read the statement of the purposes of this corporation, prescribed in its certificate of incorporation. This statement provides:

The purposes for which the corporation is formed are:

(1) To develop and apply the science of nutrition, in its fundamental conception and practical significance as a basic science of public health;

(2) To aid the food industry in appropriately solving its general and individual problems relating to that science; and

(3) To do so by lawful and effective means, as a public institution operated on a non-profit basis and dedicated to improve the food and diet and thus to better the health of the people of the United States of America.

3. The Temporary Chairman submitted a draft of By-Laws of *The Nutrition Foundation, Inc.*, prepared by Mr. Charles Wesley Dunn and approved by the original founder manufacturers; and he recommended their adoption by the Board, as authorized by law. In making this recommendation the Temporary Chairman noted that the incorporators of this corporation are the original members of its Board of Trustees; and that all such members, except two, namely, Mr. Thomas L. Smith and Mr. Alfred W. Eames, were present. . . . On motion duly made and carried, it was

Resolved, that the Board approves and adopts the By-Laws of *The Nutrition Foundation, Inc.*, submitted by Dr. Compton and as so amended; and hereby makes them the By-Laws of this corporation.

4. The Temporary Chairman called for the election of additional members of the Board. In doing so he stated that the By-Laws provide, in Article II: the Board of Trustees of this corporation shall consist of members appointed by its founder members, on the basis of one representative for each, and of additional members, representing sustaining members of this corporation and the general public, elected by the Board; and its membership shall be not less than 5 nor more than 50. The Temporary Chairman noted that the members of the Board appointed by the founder members of this corporation are:

Mr. James S. Adams
  Standard Brands Incorporated
Mr. Frederick Beers
  National Biscuit Company
Mr. Carlyle H. Black
  American Can Company
Mr. Carle C. Conway
  Continental Can Company
Mr. Daniel W. Creeden
  Libby, McNeill & Libby
Mr. J. Stafford Ellithorp, Jr.
  Beech-Nut Packing Company
Mr. Clarence Francis
  General Foods Corporation
Mr. Henry J. Heinz, II
  H. J. Heinz Company
Mr. John Holmes
  Swift & Company
Mr. J. Preston Levis
  Owens-Illinois Glass Company
Mr. James McGowan, Jr.
  Campbell Soup Company
Mr. Russell G. Partridge
  United Fruit Company
Mr. George V. Robbins
  California Packing Corporation
Mr. Morris Sayre
  Corn Products Refining Company
Mr. R. Douglas Stuart
  Quaker Oats Company.

The Temporary Chairman further noted that there are no sustaining members of this corporation, as yet. On motion duly made and carried, the following were elected as additional members of the Board representing the general public:

Mr. Cason J. Callaway, Hamilton, Georgia,
Dr. W. C. Coffey, President, University of Minnesota,
Dr. Karl T. Compton, President, Massachusetts Institute of Technology
Mr. Charles Wesley Dunn, Attorney, New York, N.Y.
Rev. Hugh O'Donnell, President, Notre Dame University,

Appendix

Dr. Thomas Parran, Surgeon General, United States Public Health Service,
Dr. Ray Lyman Wilbur, Chancellor, Stanford University,
Mr. M. L. Wilson, Assistant Director in charge of Nutrition, Office of Defense Health and Welfare Services, Federal Security Agency,
Dr. Stephen S. Wise, Rabbi, Free Synagogue, New York, N.Y.

5. The Temporary Chairman announced that the Board was now organized to do business; and that a quorum was present. He noted that the By-Laws provide, in Article II: The Board of Trustees of this corporation shall control it, determine its administration, establish its policies, govern its conduct, expend its funds, and in all ways manage its affairs; and it shall have all the lawful powers necessary to do so.

The Temporary Chairman then explained the membership of *The Nutrition Foundation, Inc.* He stated that the By-Laws provide, in Article I: The membership of this corporation shall consist of three classes, namely, founder members, who shall be the food and related manufacturers named in the Schedule annexed to the By-Laws; sustaining members, who shall be other representatives of the food and related industries, elected by the Board; and public members, who shall be representative of the general public, elected by the Board. He read the names of the original founder members and noted that the By-Laws authorize the Board to elect additional founder members, in its discretion. The founder members are:

American Can Company
Beech-Nut Packing Company
California Packing Corporation
Campbell Soup Co.
Continental Can Co.
Corn Products Refining Co.
General Foods Corporation
H. J. Heinz Company
Libby, McNeill & Libby
National Biscuit Company
Owens-Illinois Glass Company
Quaker Oats Company
Standard Brands Incorporated
Swift & Company
United Fruit Company

Mr. John Holmes stated that the original founder members have invited the Coca-Cola Company to become an additional founder member; and that said Company has accepted this invitation. On motion duly made and carried, the Coca Cola Company was elected an additional founder member.

The Temporary Chairman noted that the Coca Cola Company has appointed Mr. Ralph Hayes, a Vice President of said Company, as its representative on the Board of this corporation.

Mr. John Holmes read a letter dated February 27, 1942, which he received from Mr. Henry A. White, President of the Hawaiian Pineapple Company, Limited. Said letter provides:

"This will acknowledge receipt of your letter of February 2nd, in which you cordially extend an invitation to the Hawaiian Pineapple Company, Limited, to become a Founder Member of the Nutrition Foundation, Incorporated.

"I am satisfied that under the guidance of executives representing the firms enumerated in your letter sound and conservative policies will be pursued by the Foundation, and consequently valuable contributions will be made by it to the general cause of better nutrition.

"But for the war I would be prepared to recommend to our Board of Directors that this company avail itself of the privilege extended of becoming a founder member. Our operations are confined to a war area, and as a result we face grave uncertainties. Until conditions become clarified I do not feel that the company would be justified in incurring such a substantial commitment and I should therefore like to ask whether it would be possible to grant us additional time to reach a decision. We would greatly appreciate being permitted until the end of the current year to indicate our desire of becoming a founder member, the same date as other members.

"Would you be kind enough to submit this request to the other founder members and let me know whether the granting of such a concession meets with their approval?"

On motion duly made and carried, it was agreed that the invitation for founder membership extended to the Hawaiian Pineapple Company, Limited, be continued, as requested by it; with the hope that conditions will permit said Company later to accept this invitation.

Following the discussion of membership in this corporation, on motion duly made and carried, it was

Resolved, that no founder or sustaining member of *The Nutrition Foundation, Inc.*, shall refer to his membership in this corporation in his advertisement of his products; or make any other commercial reference to said membership.

Appendix

6. The Temporary Chairman called for the election of the Chairman of this Board. He stated that the By-Laws provide, in Article III: The Board of this corporation shall include a Chairman of the Board, who shall be the principal officer of this corporation; and the Board shall prescribe his term, powers and duties, and compensation (if any). On motion duly made and carried, Dr. Karl T. Compton, President of Massachusetts Institute of Technology was elected Chairman of the Board of Trustees of *The Nutrition Foundation, Inc.*, for a term of one year, without compensation, but with an expense allowance, and he was vested with the powers and duties of the principal officer of this corporation. Thereupon Dr. Compton assumed office accordingly.

7. The Chairman called for the election of additional officers of The Nutrition Foundation, Inc. He stated that the By-Laws provide, in Article III: The officers of this corporation shall also include a President of the corporation, who shall be its executive officer; and a Scientific Director, who shall be a nutrition scientist. He further stated that the By-Laws, in said Article, authorize the Board to elect other officers of this corporation; and provide that the Board shall prescribe the term, powers and duties, and compensation (if any) of each officer of this corporation, additional to the Chairman of its Board. On motion duly made and carried, the following additional officers of *The Nutrition Foundation, Inc.*, were elected:

President
  Mr. George A. Sloan, for a term of one year beginning on February 1, 1942. Mr. Sloan was elected on the condition and agreement that he serves this corporation on a part-time basis.

Scientific Director
  Dr. Charles Glen King, for a term of five years beginning on February 1, 1942, and vested with the powers and duties of the scientific officer of this corporation.

Treasurer
  Mr. Morris Sayre, for a term of one year beginning on January 1, 1942, without compensation, and vested with the powers and duties of the financial officer of this corporation.

Assistant Treasurer
  Mr. Holly Callender, for a term of one year beginning on January 1, 1942, vested with authority to assist the Treasurer under whose direction he shall act at all times.

Executive Secretary
  Mr. Ole Salthe, for a term of one year beginning on March 1, 1942, and vested with the powers and duties of the administrative officer of this corporation acting under the direction of its president. Mr. Salthe is also to serve as Secretary of the Board of Trustees.

The Chairman stated that Mr. Charles Wesley Dunn has offered to execute the legal business of this corporation, without compensation. On motion duly made and carried, the Board accepted this offer.

On motion duly made and carried, Mr. George A. Sloan, President of this corporation, and Dr. Charles Glen King, Scientific Director of this corporation, were elected additional members of the Board representing the general public, each for the term of his office.

8. The Chairman called for the appointment of committees of *The Nutrition Foundation, Inc.* He stated that the By-Laws provide, in Article IV: The Board of this Corporation shall appoint or approve its committees; they shall include an executive committee, appointed from the Board, and expert advisory committees; and the Board shall prescribe the term, powers and duties, and compensation (if any) of each such committee. On motion duly made and carried, the following committees were appointed:

Executive Committee
  Dr. Karl T. Compton, Mr. George A. Sloan, Dr. Charles Glen King, Mr. Morris Sayre, Mr. John Holmes, Mr. Clarence Francis, Dr. W. C. Coffey—all members of the Board of Trustees. The term of this Committee is the calendar year of 1942; it serves without compensation; and it has the powers and duties involved by its representation of the Board during the period between its meetings.

Scientific Advisory Committee
  Dr. F. G. Boudreau, Director, Milbank Memorial Fund, New York, N.Y.; Dr. C. A. Elvehjem, University of Wisconsin, Madison, Wis.; Dr. Icie M. Hoobler, Children's Fund of Michigan, Detroit, Mich.; Col. P. E. Howe, Surgeon General's Office, United States Army, Washington, D.C.; Dr. E. V. McCollum, Johns Hopkins University, Baltimore, Md.; Dr. L. A. Maynard, Cornell University, Ithaca, N.Y.; Dr. J. R. Murlin, University of Rochester, Rochester, N.Y.; Dr. Roy C. Newton, Swift & Company, Chicago, Ill.; Dr. Lydia J. Roberts, Department of Home Economics, University of Chicago, Chicago, Ill.; Dr. W. C. Rose, University of Illinois, Urbana, Ill.; Dr. W. H. Sebrell, National Institutes of Health, Bethesda, Md.; Dr. H. C. Sherman, Columbia University, New York, N.Y.; Dr. F. F. Tisdall, University of Toronto, Toronto, Canada; Dr. R. R. Williams, Chemical Director, Bell Telephone Laboratories, New York, N.Y. The term of this Committee is the

Appendix

calendar year of 1942; it serves without compensation; and it has the advisory powers and duties implied by the name.

Food Industry Advisory Committee

Dr. Roger Adams, Professor of Chemistry, University of Illinois, representing the Coca-Cola Company, Wilmington, Del.; Mr. H. A. Barnby, Director, Packaging Research Division, Owens-Illinois Glass Company, Toledo, Ohio; Dr. Frederick C. Blanck, Chief Research Chemist, H. J. Heinz Company, Pittsburgh, Pa.; Dr. Lawrence V. Burton, Editor, Food Industries, New York, N.Y.; Dr. Charles N. Frey, Research Director, Standard Brands Incorporated, New York, N.Y.; Dr. Frank L. Gunderson, Director of Nutrition, Quaker Oats Company, Chicago, Ill.; Dr. W. H. Harrison, Technical Adviser, Continental Can Company, Washington, D.C.; Mr. Norman F. Kennedy, Director of Research, Corn Industries Research Foundation, New York, N.Y.; Dr. Edward F. Kohman, Chemical Research Department, Campbell Soup Company, Camden, N.J.; Mr. Donald Maveety, Director of Research, National Biscuit Company, New York, N.Y.; Dr. Robert W. Pilcher, Assistant Manager, Research Department, American Can Company, Maywood, Ill.; Dr. G. L. Poland, Director of Research, United Fruit Company, New York, N.Y.; Mr. Alan C. Richardson and Mr. James McConkie, Research Laboratory, California Packing Corporation, San Francisco, Cal.; Dr. H. E. Robinson, Assistant Chief Chemist and Nutritionist, Swift and Company, Chicago, Ill.; Dr. James A. Tobey, Director of Nutrition, American Institute of Baking, New York, N.Y.; Mr. Lewis W. Waters, Vice President in charge of Research and Development, General Foods Corporation, New York, N.Y. The term of this committee is the calendar year of 1942; it serves without compensation; and it has the advisory powers and duties implied by its name.

9. The Chairman suggested that *The Nutrition Foundation, Inc.*, might beneficially engage a public relations representative, during its formative period; and there was general concurrence. On recommendation by the President it was duly moved and carried, that this corporation appoint the John Price Jones Corporation, acting through its Vice President, Mr. David Church, as the public relations representative of this corporation, under the direction of its President, for a period of six months beginning on March 1, 1942, at a fee of $900 for said period.

10. The Chairman called for a financial report by the Treasurer. The Chairman stated that the By-Laws provide, in Article VI, that the funds of this corporation shall consist of voluntary contributions to it. The Treasurer reported that: each founder member has agreed to contribute $50,000 to this corporation, payable in total amount or at the rate of $10,000 per year for a 5-year period; and therefore the sixteen founder members have agreed to contribute an aggregate amount of $800,000. Of that amount this corporation has already received $350,000, deposited to its credit with the Chemical Bank & Trust Company in New York City. The Chairman noted that, on the basis of the Treasurer's report, the funds of this corporation now available for expenditure in 1942 amount to $160,000.

11. The Chairman called for a budget recommendation by the President. The Chairman stated that the By-Laws provide, in Article VI, that the funds of this corporation shall be expended on the basis of a budget adopted or approved by its Board.

The President recommended the following budget of this Corporation for the calendar year of 1942:

Grants for research	$ 75,000.00
Office Expense (including travel, etc., itemized statement attached)	52,879.21
Additional grants, etc., to be approved by the Board or its Executive Committee	22,120.79
	$150,000.00

In recommending the budget the President noted that: it was prepared on the basis of 1942 contributions by fifteen founder members aggregating $150,000, which amount has since been increased to $160,000 by the election of the Coca-Cola Company as an additional founder member; the general policy of this budget was to divide the 1942 funds of this corporation on the basis of alloting half for research and half for other expenses. On motion duly made and carried, it was

Resolved, that the Board approves the 1942 budget of this corporation recommended by its President, subject to any revision thereof later made by the Board or the Executive Committee.

On motion duly made and carried, it was

Resolved, that the Board approves the lease of the Foundation offices in the Chrysler Building, New York City, negotiated by the President of this corporation, and authorizes him to execute said lease.

13. The Chairman stated that the Board should take action with respect to scientific discoveries made as a result of support by this corporation, from the standpoint of the public interest. On suggestion by him and after discussion and on motion duly made and carried, it was

Appendix

Resolved, that in handling or disposing of all scientific discoveries made in the course of work supported by this Foundation, the best interests of the public shall be the sole determining consideration; and that any and all such scientific discoveries shall be public property.

Further resolved, that the subject of such scientific discoveries is referred to the Executive Committee for study and a report to this Board of policy in further detail, with respect thereto.

14. The Chairman called for a statement by the Scientific Director of this corporation. A copy of said statement is attached to these Minutes. In this statement the Scientific Director recommended the following general program of scientific action by the Foundation: (1) scientific research, on a long-range basis, to discover new fundamental knowledge in the field embraced by the science of nutrition, for better public health; (2) scientific research, on a current basis, to solve immediate public health problems in that field; (3) scientific research, on a war basis, to aid our Government in dealing with emergency problems in that field; and (4) dissemination of scientific knowledge developed in that field, for educational purposes, in order that the science of nutrition may be more effectively applied for better public health.

This statement invoked favorable comment. On motion duly made and carried, it was

Resolved, that the Board approves, in principle, the scientific program for this Foundation thus recommended by its Scientific Committee for action.

15. The Chairman then suggested that the Board adopt a broad resolution directing the Executive Committee to develop and execute the 1942 program of general action by this corporation. On motion duly made and carried, it was

Resolved, that the Executive Committee is hereby directed and authorized to develop and execute the 1942 program of general action by this Foundation, consistent with its 1942 budget and pursuant to the policies established by its Board of Trustees, on the basis of the recommendations by its officers and advisory committees.

The discussion of this resolution indicated a Board opinion that said initial program of the Foundation requires very careful study from a policy standpoint. Therefore the Chairman announced that he will call a special meeting of this Board to receive a report by the Executive Committee with respect to that program, and to act on such report.

16. The Chairman explained details of the inaugural dinner of the Foundation. The Reverend Hugh O'Donnell, speaking for the public members of the Board, congratulated the founder members of this corporation on establishing it in the public interest.

The meeting adjourned at 5:30 p.m.

Original By-Laws of The Nutrition Foundation, Inc. (adopted March 12, 1942)

Introduction

The Nutrition Foundation, Inc., is a corporation organized pursuant to the membership Corporations Law of the State of New York. Its purposes, prescribed by the certificate of incorporation, are:

(1) To develop and apply the science of nutrition, in its fundamental conception and practical significance as a basic science of public health;

(2) To aid the food industry in appropriately solving its general and individual problems relating to that science; and

(3) To do so by lawful and effective means, as a public institution operated on a non-profit basis and dedicated to improve the food and diet and thus to better the health of the people of the United States of America.

Article I

Members

Section 1. The membership of the corporation shall consist of three (3) classes, namely, founder members, sustaining members, and public members.

Section 2. The founder members shall be the food and related manufacturers named in the Schedule annexed to these by-laws. The sustaining members shall be other representatives of the food and related industries, elected by the board of trustees. The public members shall be representatives of the general public, elected by the board.

Section 3. Members shall each have all the rights in the corporation, prescribed by the board of trustees. Members shall each have only the financial obligation to the corporation, voluntarily contracted by them in writing.

Appendix

Section 4. Any member may resign from the corporation on written notice to it and subject to the payment of his financial obligation to it. Any member may be suspended or expelled from the corporation, by a two-thirds vote of the board of trustees, for cause.

Article II
Board of Trustees

Section 1. The board of trustees of the corporation shall consist of members appointed by its founder members on the basis of one representative for each; and of additional members, representing sustaining members and the general public, elected by the board. The board shall at all times include representatives of the general public, to assure its public character; and it shall be organized to secure its public conduct. The membership of the board shall be not less than five (5) nor more than fifty (50); and non-voting alternate representatives on it shall be permitted.

Section 2. The board of trustees shall control the corporation, determine its administration, establish its policies, govern its conduct, expend its funds, and in all ways manage its affairs; and it shall have all the lawful powers necessary to do so.

Article III
Officers

Section 1. The board of trustees shall determine and elect the officers of the corporation; and it shall prescribe the term, powers and duties, and compensation (if any) of each.

Section 2. The officers shall include a chairman of the board of trustees, who shall be the principal officer of the corporation and a representative of the general public; a president of the corporation, who shall be its executive officer; and a scientific director, who shall be a nutrition scientist. Any two offices may be held by the same person.

Article IV
Committees

Section 1. The board of trustees shall determine and appoint or approve the committees of the corporation; and it shall prescribe the term, powers and duties, and compensation (if any) of each.

Section 2. The committees shall include an executive committee, appointed from the board of trustees, and expert advisory committees.

Article V
Meetings

Section 1. There shall be an annual meeting of the corporation, each calendar year; and the board of trustees is empowered to call special meetings of the corporation in its discretion. Each annual or special meeting shall be held at the time and place and for the purposes prescribed by the board.

Section 2. The meetings of the board of trustees shall be held, in its discretion, at the time and place and for the purposes prescribed by it.

Section 3. Any meeting of the corporation or the board of trustees may be held without the State of New York. One third of its members shall constitute a quorum at any meeting of the corporation or the board.

Article VI
Funds

Section 1. The funds of the corporation shall consist of voluntary financial contributions to it; and they shall be expended on the basis of a budget adopted or approved by the board of trustees.

Section 2. The board of trustees shall prescribe the fiscal year of the corporation.

Article VII
Seal

Section 1. The seal of the corporation shall be circular in form and shall be inscribed with the name of the corporation and with the state and year of its incorporation.

Section 2. The board of trustees may change the form or inscription of the seal, in its discretion.

Article VIII
Amendments

Section 1. The board of trustees shall have power to amend these by-laws.

Section 2. The board of trustees shall have general power to make, alter, amend, and repeal by-laws of the corporation.

RESUME OF STATEMENT PRESENTED BY
DR. CHARLES G. KING
TO THE BOARD OF TRUSTEES
CONCERNING THE PROGRAM OF
THE NUTRITION FOUNDATION, INC.

March 12, 1942

The Board of Trustees and Officers seem to be in full agreement that the major emphasis in the program to be undertaken by The Nutrition Foundation should be upon four types of activity:

(1) Research work with a long time value to provide basic information and guidance in the science of nutrition.

Appendix

(2) Research studies with a more immediate bearing upon public health problems.

(3) Research projects that have immediate bearing upon the war emergency, both for the armed forces and for the civilian population.

(4) Promotion of educational work to help bridge the gaps between scientific information and the channels in which such information may become effective.

1. Examples of the more theoretical types of investigation that appear to be of outstanding importance at the present time may be indicated as follows:

(a) Continued studies should be directed toward the isolation and identification of the remaining vitamins, particularly those in the B-Complex.

(b) Much work remains to be done to establish whether or not such elements as fluorine, bromine, silicon, nickel, aluminum, and boron are essential, either for animal nutrition or for human nutrition.

(c) Physiological and biochemical studies are needed to supply a much better picture of the reconstruction of foodstuffs inside the body. For example, we know something of the interconversion of sugars, proteins, and fats, but we know relatively little about the specific chemical reactions that are involved and we do not understand very clearly how far a body can adjust itself in making such interconversions from one foodstuff to another. Problems of this nature are not only fundamental in physiology and biochemistry but they establish basic principles and, in the long run, enable the physician to reach a higher level of medical practice. Diabetes and fatty livers may be cited as pathological conditions that bear a close relationship to such studies.

(d) Each of the vitamin and mineral elements (and to some extent the fragments from proteins and fats) has specific functions within the animal and human body. These functions need to be clarified to give meaning and understanding to the whole field of nutritional requirements.

(e) Each type of experimental animal, when studied in detail, shows individual variations in its nutritional requirements; hence, a new principle in the science of nutrition that can be supplied by the study of one animal becomes of greater value in terms of human nutrition if supplementary studies are made with many different types of experimental animals. Such studies would also, in the long run, make an outstanding contribution to agriculture.

2. Studies of a more practical nature:

(a) Among the most striking reports in the whole literature of nutrition pertaining to human health, has been the series of papers published from the University of Toronto's School of Medicine (Dr. F. F. Tisdall, et al.). These studies provide a convincing "proof of the pudding." In brief, within a group of about 400 mothers and their infants, the occurrence of various types of illness—such as colds, diarrhea, and pneumonia—was about four times greater among those receiving a typical low-income diet than among those on a similar diet that had been supplemented with enough of the common protective foods to bring the nutritional level to a "good diet" status. It would be of tremendous significance if more studies of that kind could demonstrate that in typical American areas improved food intake could contribute so much to better health.

(b) Intensive surveys are needed to provide more information concerning the extent of malnutrition in the United States and Canada. Such surveys should be carried out with the best techniques that have been devised, including chemical tests as a part of the medical examinations. Of critical importance to this kind of study is the development of better chemical methods of diagnosis so that the physician will have objective evidence in terms of specific chemical analyses to supplement or to guide general impressions gained by physical examinations. The development of better methods of analysis also makes a valuable contribution to the food industry.

(c) At both ends of the human life span the normal intake of foodstuffs tends to be severely restricted. Old people tend to develop finicky food habits, and infants are to a very large degree restricted to cow's milk as a basic or sole food. From a chemical point of view, we know that cow's milk differs in many respects from mother's milk. We know too that the common modifications of cow's milk do not provide formulas for infant feeding that are adequate for the nutrition of infants. Some of the food manufacturing firms are making progress in this direction, but there is need for much more study of the problem jointly by biochemists and nutritionists.

Appendix

(d) The present high incidence of defective and decayed teeth in our American population, representing all age groups and all economic levels, presents a problem of very great importance in terms of public health. Most of us have been shocked to find that approximately 20 to 25% of the rejections of men called for selective service, on medical grounds, have been because of defective teeth. There is much evidence to indicate that nutrition is one of the most important factors in the development of good teeth and in the prevention of dental caries. Perhaps the science of nutrition cannot solve the problem completely, but there is good reason to believe that it could make a great contribution toward a practical solution of the problem.

3. The members of both Advisory Committees and the members of the Board of Trustees are apparently all in agreement that the Foundation program should include a substantial contribution to problems of immediate importance to the national war emergency. Activities in this area will need to be guided carefully to avoid unnecessary encroachment upon work that can be done to better advantage by the food industries directly, or by the national government. However, from discussions with Colonel Paul E. Howe of the Surgeon General's Office, and with others who are very close to the problems of the armed forces, it is apparent that there will be activities in which the Foundation should participate. Work of this nature might consume a generous portion of our immediate budget, but it seems clear also that we should not lose sight of the long time contribution that the science of nutrition can make both during war time and during peace time.

4. There are at least two kinds of service in the field of nutritional education in which The Nutrition Foundation should be able to participate very helpfully:

(a) At present there are, and will no doubt continue to be, areas in the science of nutrition where there is a critical need for comprehensive reviews (covering all of the work that has been done to date) by authorities who are outstanding scholars in those special fields, so that those working in other fields of nutritional science will have more effective guidance. For example, Dr. Rose might prepare a review of the field of protein metabolism and protein requirements that would be of value to nearly everyone working or actively interested in the field of nutrition.

(b) Another area where there is a continuous need for careful supplementation of existing scientific literature is in providing summaries of scientific findings in such a form that they will be available within a short time to those who are especially interested in health, food technology, or in education in the field of nutrition.

In other words, there should be a provision for more effectively bridging the gaps between research laboratories and the various channels of putting the science of nutrition into practical effect. Preliminary contacts have been made with The Institute of Nutrition through the editor, Dr. George Cowgill, and it is very likely that the scientific, educational, and trade journals will welcome collaboration of the type indicated.

Appendix B

By-Laws of
The Nutrition Foundation, Inc.
(adopted November 1, 1971)

Introduction

The Nutrition Foundation, Inc. was incorporated in 1941 pursuant to the Membership Corporation Law of the State of New York. Its purposes are:

(1) To advance the sciences and knowledge of food and nutrition and to further their use for the health and welfare of mankind.

(2) To aid the food and allied industries in serving the public through advances in nutrition and food science.

(3) To pursue these goals as a public, non-profit institution dedicated to the improvement of nutrition and health.

Article I

Members

Section 1. Members shall include food producers, processors, purveyors, related industries and such additional organizations, or individuals engaged in food and allied fields, or interested in furthering food and nutritional research, information and education. Members shall be required to make a membership commitment of three years, which commitment shall be maintained on a three-year forward basis. Members shall follow the schedule of dues established by the Board of Trustees.

Section 2. Members shall each have all the rights in the Foundation prescribed by the Board of Trustees. Members shall each have only the financial obligation to the Foundation voluntarily contracted by them in writing.

Section 3. Any member may resign from the Foundation by written notice and subject to payment of its financial obligations to the Foundation. Any member may be suspended or expelled from the Foundation for cause by a two-thirds vote of the Trustees.

Article II

Board of Trustees

Section 1. The Board of Trustees of the Foundation shall consist of (a) Member Trustees, one designated representative from each Member shall serve as such; and (b) Public Trustees, who shall be non-industry representatives of the general public, and shall be elected by the Trustees. The Board of Trustees may not, however, exceed the maximum number of Trustees authorized by the Foundation's Certificate of Incorporation, as amended.

Section 2. The Board of Trustees shall control the Foundation, determine its administration, establish its policies, govern its conduct, expend its funds and manage its affairs. The Board of Trustees may delegate to the Executive Committee or to the appropriate officers such responsibilities as it sees fit.

Article III

Executive Committee

Section 1. The Executive Committee shall be elected by the Board of Trustees from among its members by a majority vote thereof. The Executive Committee shall include the Chairman of the Board of Trustees, and the President of the Foundation as ex officio members, and up to twenty-one additional members. Twelve of the members of the Executive Committee shall be elected from among the Public Trustees, one of whom shall be the Chairman of the Executive Committee, and nine of the members shall

Appendix

be elected from among the Member Trustees, one of whom shall be the Vice Chairman of the Executive Committee. The members of the Executive Committee shall be elected for three-year terms and shall be divided into three classes as determined by the Board of Trustees, each made up of one-third of the total members or seven members, three of whom shall be Member Trustees and four of whom shall be Public Trustees, so that the term of each class shall expire every three years with one of said classes being elected at each annual meeting. No member of the Executive Committee may be elected for successive three-year terms. One-third of the members of the Executive Committee shall constitute a quorum.

Section 2. The Executive Committee shall be responsible for operating the Foundation within the policies established by the Board of Trustees. Accordingly, the Executive Committee shall approve senior staff positions, prescribe the compensation, including fringe benefits, of the President and all the staff, and make recommendations to the Board of Trustees regarding policies, program and budgets of the Foundation. It shall report is actions to the Board of Trustees.

Article IV

Officers

Section 1. The Board of Trustees shall determine and elect the officers of the Foundation; and prescribe the term, powers and duties of each.

Section 2. The officers shall include a Chairman of the Board of Trustees who shall be a public Trustee, who shall serve on a voluntary basis; a Vice Chairman of the Board of Trustees who shall be a Member Trustee serving on a voluntary basis; a Chairman of the Executive Committee who shall be a Public Trustee serving on a voluntary basis; a Vice Chairman of the Executive Committee who shall be a Member Trustee serving on a voluntary basis; the President of the Foundation who shall be a full time employee and the Chief Executive Officer of the Foundation; and two Vice Presidents who shall be full time employees, one of whom shall also serve as Treasurer and be responsible for staff operations. One Vice President shall be responsible for the implementation of research programs, the other shall be responsible for nutrition education and public affairs.

Section 3. The Chairman and Vice Chairman of the Executive Committee shall be elected for a two-year period effective January 1.

Section 4. The paid staff of the Foundation, in addition to the full time officers named in Section 2, shall include such other full time staff as may be approved by the Executive Committee. The compensation of full time officers other than the President shall be recommended by the President and approved by the Chairman of the Board of Trustees and the Chairman of the Executive Committee, subject to the policies established by the Board of Trustees.

Section 5. The Chairman of the Board of Trustees shall preside at all meetings of the Board of Trustees, except that in his absence the Vice Chairman of the Board of Trustees shall preside, and in the absence of both, the President shall preside. The Chairman of the Executive Committee shall preside at meetings of that Committee, and in his absence the Vice Chairman of the Executive Committee shall preside, and in the absence of both, the President shall preside.

Article V

Committees other than Executive Committee

Section 1. The Board of Trustees shall determine and appoint or approve the standing committees of the Foundation; and it shall prescribe the term, powers and duties of each. Task forces may be appointed by the President.

Committees shall include: (1) A Nominating Committee, to be appointed annually from among the Board of Trustees by the Chairman of the Board of Trustees with the approval of the Executive Committee. The Nominating Committee shall present at each annual meeting of the Board of Trustees names for nomination of Public Trustees, officers of the Foundation, and members of the Executive Committee and other committees.

(2) The Food and Nutrition Liaison Committee shall consist of representatives designated by Members, each Member being entitled to designate one representative, preferably with scientific training, and such representatives from the general public as may be designated by the President with the approval of the Executive Committee. The Chairman shall be a Public Trustee and the Vice Chairman a Member Trustee. The responsibilities of the Food and Nutrition Liaison Committee shall include a periodic review of scientific areas of interest to the Foundation, with a view to identifying broad new research and educational interests which the Foundation should consider, as well as other activities appropriate to the Foundation. In addition, the Food and Nutrition Liaison Committee shall serve as a pool from which the President may appoint ad hoc task forces to consider various developments, including evaluation of specific research and educational proposals and assistance in locating and evaluating various institutions and individuals with the capabilities to conduct the research projects recommended by the Food and Nutrition Liaison Committee.

(3) The Food and Nutrition Advisory Council shall

Appendix

consist of twelve representatives from public institutions, government and industry (at least four of whom shall be from industry), designated by the President with the approval of the Executive Committee. The responsibilities of the Council shall include making recommendations concerning research grants and advising on research training and educational policy matters. The responsibilties of the Council shall also include public affairs subjects concerning information, press releases, and publications. Where specialized technical competence for assessment of specific research, educational or public affairs matters is needed, ad hoc forces may be appointed by the President and the findings and recommendations of such task forces shall be made available to the Food and Nutrition Advisory Council.

(4) The Finance Committee shall consist of at least seven Member Trustees appointed by the Executive Committee. these appointments shall be for varying terms. The Finance Committee will be responsible for financial and membership matters, including the solicitation of funds from industry and of new members of the Foundation.

Article VI

Meetings

Section 1. There shall be an annual meeting of the Board of Trustees of the Foundation each calendar year. The Chairman of the Board of Trustees or the President may call special meetings, with the approval of a majority of the Executive Committee.

Section 2. Meetings of the Board of Trustees shall be held at its discretion, at the time and place and for the purposes prescribed by them. One-fourth of the members shall constitute a quorum.

Section 3. The Executive Committee shall meet twice annually and at other times at the discretion of the Chairman of the Board of Trustees, the Chairman of the Executive Committee or the President.

Article VII

Funds

The amount of membership payments shall be established by the Board of Trustees.

The Funds of the Foundation will consist of membership payments and such other funds as may become available and accepted by the Trustees. The funds shall be expended on the basis of a budget adopted or approved by the Board of Trustees.

Article VIII

The Board of Trustees shall have the power to make, alter, amend and repeal the Bylaws of the Foundation.

Appendix C

"Nutrition in The 1970's"
Address to The Board of Trustees
November 5, 1971

William J. Darby, M.D., Ph.D.
President-elect

Those of us concerned with foods and nutrition are from time to time easily lulled into false judgment of the dimensions of the field (and perhaps of our responsibilities). I recall a few years ago the lament of one of our distinguished nutrition scientists that nutrition was a dead field now that all of the vitamins had been discovered.

The science of nutrition has moved through periods of emphasis on energy, protein, the vitamins, essential amino acids, the major minerals (especially calcium, phosphorus, and iron) and some trace elements. More recently we are in an era of the lipids; one can now recognize the beginning of an era of the carbohydrates (sugars).

There is a tendency to regard the essential nutrients as a somewhat fixed list catalogued by the Food and Nutrition Board in its Recommended Dietary Allowances. Indeed, nutrition education has been based traditionally on such a list of nutrient requirements, drily presented in a dogmatic style that characterizes a Sunday School lesson. Either one eats "right" or "wrong," with all the connotations of "righteousness" and "sinfulness" attached to the proper or improper use of foods.

At the same time, the public has been subjected to palpably exaggerated claims of health benefits, to promotion through all communication media of overt misuse of foods and beverages, concentrates and nutrient preparations from many sources, from some producers, manufacturers, marketers, scientists, even governmental agencies and from outright charlatans. There is small wonder that a questioning "now" generation turns to anti-establishment sources as creditable authorities in nutrition.

One can dismiss this creditability gap as part of today's rebellion against authority and the established order, which it does in fact in part represent. But merely to dismiss it without understanding its genesis and to assume that it will go away like Fletcherism, the Charleston, or other cults or vogues would prove disastrously naive—naive because this questioning generation is in the main serious, intelligent and determined to set things right in a troubled world, disastrous because in accomplishing their objectives they press often for restrictive measures that can seriously impair the potential for food production, processing, and distribution and compromise our ability to meet the increasing food needs of the world population. It is urgent, therefore, that we reexamine the understanding of nutrition in the 1970's.

For a simple start let us inquire as to the state of knowledge concerning requirements or standards of intake of essential nutrients. The original Recommended Dietary Allowances of the then Committee on Food and Nutrition, National Research Council, was distributed in May 1941, and the table contained proposed quantitative standards for calories, protein, calcium, iron, vitamins A and D, and thiamine, riboflavin, niacin, and ascorbic acid (ten nutrients). It recognized the need to give consideration to other members of the B-complex group, "such as vitamin B_6 and pantothenic acid," but realized that no specific values could be given for an amount of these required

---

Adapted from a talk presented at the meeting of the Trustees of The Nutrition Foundation, Inc., New York City, November 5, 1971. Reprinted from NUTRITION REVIEWS 30:27-31, 1972.

Appendix

in the human diet. The report did not even mention vitamin E, folacin, vitamin B$_{12}$, phosphorus, iodine, or magnesium, for which quantitative estimates of allowances (for a total of 16 nutrients) are tabulated in the most recent 1968, seventh edition, of the Recommended Dietary Allowances. The text of the latter edition discusses the need for 17 other factors: vitamin K, biotin, choline, copper, fluorine, chromium, cobalt, magnesium, molybdenum, selenium, and zinc, sodium, potassium, chloride, water, carbohydrates, and fats—and, indeed, recognizes the role of ethyl alcohol in the diet. We can anticipate that future editions may tabulate quantitative estimates for a number of the other nutrients. Recently presented evidence for a requirement of certain species for nickel and perhaps vanadium likely will be added, as will newer information concerning interrelationships or interactions of a variety of trace elements (molybdenum and copper; cadmium and zinc).*

Perusal of the RDA tables reveals rather marked differences in the quantitative estimates for most nutrients over the period of these revisions. Estimates have decreased for needs of calories, thiamine, niacin, ascorbic acid, and calcium.

Too little attention has been given to the varying biological availability of nutrients in different foods or combinations and the influence of processing, of patterns of diet and of certain additives (for example, chelating agents on inorganic nutrients). This has become painfully clear as a result of our experience with iron enrichment of cereals and bread. Biological availability must be reckoned with in future setting of allowances and the 1970's will see more research directed to this problem.

Our questioning generation is not unaware of some of these developments. Indeed, they are in part too concerned about them because they are not sufficiently informed and they fail to understand that the general usefulness of science is based on *existing* knowledge. The fact that we will know more in ten years is not a reason to deny us the benefits of existing scientific knowledge. Indeed, science is properly likened to that spiral staircase from each level of which one increases his horizon, and the application, the relevance if you will, of science depends upon the horizon of the moment. Such is the understanding of nutrition that must be reached. Only with such understanding will the fallacies of organic gardening, the Zen macrobiotic diet, of "natural" food cults, the whole of over-zealous nutritional consumerism be recognized and the effects of such movements minimized.

A major dimension, therefore, of nutrition in the 70's should be promotion of *understanding* of nutrition—I hesitate to call this nutrition education, for it is a broader need than the teaching by rote of the nutritional alphabet.

A knowledge of the scientific aspects of food—its composition, nutritive value, safety—is not enough to influence food use. Indeed, one is struck with the ignorance that exists relative to the origin of food habits. There is a "science" of food acceptability, systems for appraising the organoleptic qualities, the mouth feel, the acceptability of a food to a more or less receptive population. But so little is known as to the historical, socio-cultural, or religious forces that determine food beliefs and attitudes, that these usually are recognized subconsciously, if at all. The social implications of food vary from one period of time to another. In our own country understanding these variations from one culture to another and the reasons for them is especially important if we are to educate nutritionally the many subcultural groups that make up America.

It is true that the major market for foods is that 90 or so percent of the population that is sufficiently homogeneous so that their acceptance of a product can be tested. But the other 10 per cent or so who constitute the food subcultures are of concern as nutritional risks—they constitute groups whose taboos and attitudes render them refractory to the educational approach that is successful with the majority. They include the ones who disbelieve, who fear, who distrust the scientist, the industrial force, the government. Their attitude may pertain in fact only during particular times, such as pregnancy, or shortly after delivery. A cultural anthropologic approach to understanding food habits is essential if we are to succeed educationally.

It is of interest that many groups, motivated in one way or another, are attempting to get on a nutritional education bandwagon. This signals the receptivity of the public, but makes it even more urgent that there be knowledgeable, understanding, sound leadership with adequate prestige to make the best possible use of the resources and energies available for these pur-

---

*The Eighth Edition (1974) of Recommended Dietary Allowances tabulates quantitative recommendations for 18 nutrients, zinc and magnesium being added to those tabulated in 1968. Meaningful alterations in the level of allowances, based upon new research information, were made in 3 nutrients (protein, vitamins C and E). The text of the Eighth Edition discusses 17 additional nutrients for which evidence of essentiality exists but the information is insufficient to establish a quantitative estimate of recommended dietary allowance. It is recognized, also, that the allowance set forth for some nutrients is based upon tenuous or indirect evidence, and hence subject to repeated reexamination. This further endorses the need for continuing support for research on nutrient requirements and availability. (Wm. J. Darby, August, 1975)

Appendix

poses, and with the vision to understand the scope needed.

In this connection it is of much interest that the "Health Professions Educational Assistance Amendments of 1971" requires each institution to submit a plan to the Secretary of HEW that sets forth the manner in which it would develop educational programs in areas of recognized national needs. This act calls for submission of a plan in the school's application relating to specific programs or projects in at least three of nine categories. The categories include curriculum improvement; interdisciplinary training; increased emphasis at schools of medicine, osteopathy, and dentistry on clinical pharmacology; use and abuse of drugs and alcohol; assessment of efficiency of various therapeutic regimens; *and in schools of medicine and osteopathy, programs on nutrition*. This action will accelerate interest in improving nutrition teaching in schools of health professions, especially in medical schools.

Will students in these schools respond to the subject of nutrition? In schools with strong leadership in nutrition they do. More precise methods for assessing nutritional status in man are a broad and challenging opportunity for nutrition in the 1970's. They will make possible a more objective assessment of the nutritional level of the population and will provide sensitive diagnostic tools for the physician to use in caring for his patients. Lack of methods for the physician's use has kept nutrition at an empirical level in most medical practices. With more laboratory procedures being developed, and the educational recognition of nutrition in medicine, we can anticipate a ground-swell of utilization of the science of nutrition in practice of many branches of medicine. This is beginning, with the thrilling results of complete parenteral nutrition in surgical, medical, and pediatric cases; the application of nutritional concepts in the management of the hyperlipemias; the long-term maintenance of the growing population of patients on the artificial kidney; etc. I believe that the 1970's will see the return of the emphasis on nutrition in medicine given by Hippocrates:

"For the art of medicine would not have been invented at first, nor would it have been made a subject of investigation (for there would have been no need of it), if when men were indisposed, the same food and other articles of regimen which they eat and drink when in good health were proper for them . . . But now necessity itself made medicine to be sought out and discovered by men, since the same things when administered to the sick, which agreed with them in good health, neither did nor do agree with them . . . ."

The past decade has seen an outburst of interest in trace elements. The earliest clinical interests concerned not their beneficial nutritional effects but the toxic effects of excesses. We are now examining the range of safety between the optimal beneficial level of trace nutrients and the minimal toxic levels. In rats, for instance, 1 p.p.m. of dietary selenium as selenite produces maximal growth, but 3 p.p.m. and above cause growth depression and symptoms of selenium toxicity, giving a 1:3 ratio of optimum to toxic level. Studies of this sort may ultimately have some bearing on the interpretation of so-called margins of safety in the toxicologic evaluation of chemicals, now arbitrarily set at 1:100.

Concern for occurrence of detectable levels of mercury, cadmium, lead, arsenic, and other trace and heavy metals in foodstuffs well might be tempered by reflecting on lessons learned in relation to selenium, zinc, and fluorine. It is not unreasonable to inquire whether these substances, or any element in the periodic table, may not, in fact, be essential nutrients. The decade ahead will see attention to this question.

Detection and interpretation of significance to inorganic substances in the environment, their origin, metabolism, and conversion in the ecosystem, are matters germane to and inseparable from nutrition. The New York Academy of Sciences recently hosted a conference on "Geochemical Environment in Relation to Health and Disease." The topics included distribution and availability of trace elements to plants (emphasizing areas of excess and deficiency); availability of trace elements to animals; sampling of trace elements in rocks, soils, waters, and plants; methodology and problems of analysis; animal and human health in relation to geochemical environment. Specific attention was given to cardiovascular diseases, cancer, and infectious diseases.

This newer dimension of nutrition, nutritional toxicology, is not limited to inorganic substances or trace elements in excess, but embraces a multitude of previously unsuspected or undetected chemicals, some of which are not purposefully or consciously introduced directly into the food production system. For example, all of us recently have become uncomfortably conscious of the polychlorobiphenyls (PCB's). More recently the presence in certain samples of foods of hexachlorobenzene and hexachlorobutyldiane has been recognized.

The multitude of compounds currently of interest from the standpoint of nutritional toxicology include chemical additives, food colors, substances on the GRAS list, an evergrowing list of mycotoxins, and an astounding array of naturally occurring toxicants in foods (the content of some of which may be altered by genetic or cultural factors).

To cope with the demands, new methodology ur-

Appendix

gently is needed to permit dependable screening of materials for their potential effects in man, especially for any evidence of carcinogenesis, mutagenesis, and teratogenesis. Current protocols are relatively crude and costly. The basis for extrapolation of findings to conditions of low dose exposure in man must be improved. To address itself to these needs there now is being established at the site of the biological section of the U.S. Army's Arsenal at Pine Bluff, Arkansas, the new National Center for Toxicological Research. The Center's program is initially responsive to the needs of the FDA and EPA, later to other signatory agencies with program needs for research and development suitable to the Center. It is anticipated that there will be participation by other federal agencies, universities, and industry.

The initial focus of the program will be on the effects of low dose, long-term administration of potentially hazardous chemicals with regard to development and evaluation of methodology for animal studies and projection to the human. The creation of this Center and its projected incremental support indicate clearly another large dimension for nutrition in the decade of the 70's.

Safety is not the only attribute of our foods that one predictably can expect to be studied intensively during this decade. Matters of nutritional quality are also under examination. We have moved a long way since the 1940-1941 deliberations over flour and bread enrichment! Predictably we shall move much farther in the 1970's.

But the successful application of science so often calls for revision of information or inventory. So it is with food science as a result of the success of scientific agriculture. We have experienced the "green revolution"; we have experienced the application of genetics to design varieties adaptable to mechanical harvesting, shipping, and other technologic needs. Some data on the nutrient content of most of these new varieties exist, but our tables of food composition do not reflect these values. Furthermore, present tables are limited because newer reliable methods of assay for a number of nutrients now recognized as essential have not been systematically applied to our foods. A new major effort to modernize a table of food composition for the United States is needed. This should take into account the effects of improved processing procedures and technology as well.

A related new dimension for the future is production of nutrient-enriched unconventional foodstuffs, such as unicellular protein, through application of knowledge of the biosynthetic chemistry. Wide vistas for nutrient production exist in the application of such basic nutritional biochemical information.

Formerly we spoke of the marriage of Agriculture and Medicine, performed by Nutritional Science. Today and tomorrow perhaps we should think of a polygamous wedding involving Agriculture, Medicine, Industry, Biochemistry, Communications, and the Environmental Sciences, again performed by Nutritional Science.

Appendix D

Selected References Illustrative of Research Supported by The Nutrition Foundation 1942-1975

The role of the amino acids in human nutrition.
W. C. Rose, W. J. Haines and J. E. Johnson (University of Illinois).
J. Biol. Chem. 146:683 (1942).

Transmethylation as a metabolic process in man.
V. du Vigneaud and S. Simmonds (Cornell University).
J. Biol. Chem. 146:685 (1942).

The increase of B vitamins in germinating seeds.
P. R. Burkholder and I. McVeigh (Yale University).
Proc. Nat. Acad. Sci. 28:440 (1942).

Provitamin A and vitamin C in the genus lycopersicon.
R. E. Lincoln, F. P. Ascheile, J. W. Porter, G. W. Kohler and R. M. Caldwell (Purdue University).
Botanical Gazette 105:113 (1943).

Further experiments on the role of the amino acids in human nutrition.
W. C. Rose, W. J. Haines and J. E. Johnson (University of Illinois).
J. Biol. Chem. 148:457 (1943).

The utilization of the methyl groups of choline in the biological synthesis of methionine.
S. Simmonds, M. Cohn, J. P. Chandler and V. du Vigneaud (Cornell University).
J. Biol. Chem. 149:519 (1943).

Cardiovascular adjustments of man in rest and work during exposure to dry heat.
H. L. Taylor, A. E. Henschel and A. Keys (University of Minnesota).
Am. J. Physiol. 139:583 (1943).

Unsaturated synthetic glycerides, VIII.
B. F. Daubert and A. B. Baldwin (University of Pittsburgh).
J. Am. Chem. Soc. 66:1507 (1944).

Further studies on the relationship between xanthopterin, folic acid and vitamin M.
J. R. Totter, V. Mims and P. L. Day (University of Arkansas).
Science 100:223 (1944).

Component fatty acids of early and mature human milk fat.
A. R. Baldwin and H. E. Longenecker (University of Pittsburgh).
J. Biol. Chem. 154:255 (1944).

Sources of acetic acid in the animal body.
K. Bloch and D. Rittenberg (Columbia University).
J. Biol. Chem. 155:243 (1944).

An inositolless mutant strain of neurospora and its use in bioassays.
G. W. Beadle (Stanford University).
J. Biol. Chem. 156:683 (1944).

Investigations of amino acids, peptides and proteins, Part XVIII.
M. S. Dunn, S. Shankman, M. N. Camien, W. Frankl and L. B. Rockland (University of California).
J. Biol. Chem. 156:703 (1944).

The minimum ascorbic acid need of adults.
E. D. Kyhos, E. S. Gordon, M. S. Kimble and E. L. Severinghaus (University of Wisconsin).
J. Nutrition 27:271 (1944).

Congenital malformations induced in rats by maternal nutritional deficiency. VI. The preventive factor.
J. Warkany and E. Schraffenberger (University of Cincinnati).
J. Nutrition 27:477 (1944).

Appendix

The amino acid requirements of the chick.
H. J. Almquist and C. R. Grau (University of California).
J. Nutrition 28:325 (1944).

Cooking losses at Army and Navy training camps at land grant institutions.
R. Reder, et al. (Oklahoma Agricultural Experiment Station).
South. Coop. Report No. 10 (1945).

Aviation nutrition studies, Part I. Effects of pre-flight and in-flight meals of varying composition with respect to carbohydrate, protein and fat.
C. G. King, H. A. Bickerman, W. Bouvet, C. J. Harrer, J. R. Oyler and C. P. Seitz (Columbia University).
J. Aviation Med. 6:69 (1945).

Vitamin A in relation to aging and to length of life.
H. C. Sherman, H. L. Campbell, M. Udiljak and H. Yarmolinsky (Columbia University).
Proc. Nat. Acad. Sciences 31:107 (1945).

A survey of the incidence of dental caries in the Rhesus monkey.
J. H. Shaw, C. A. Elvejhem and P. H. Phillips (University of Wisconsin).
J. Dental Research 24:129 (1945).

Human milk studies, Part XXVII. Comparative values of bovine and human milks in infant feeding.
J. M. Lawrence, B. L. Herrington and L. A. Maynard (Cornell University).
Am. J. Dis. Child. 70:193 (1945).

Human milk studies, Part XIX. Implications of breast feeding and their investigation.
I. G. Macy, H. H. Williams, J. P. Pratt and B. M. Hamil (Children's Fund of Michigan).
Am. J. Dis. Child. 70:148 (1945).

The effect of anterior pituitary extract and of insulin on the hexokinase reaction.
W. H. Price, C. E. Cori and S. P. Colowick (Washington University).
J. Biol. Chem. 160:663 (1945).

The relationship between vitamin M and the Lactobacillus casei factor.
P. L. Day, V. Mims and J. R. Totter (University of Arkansas).
J. Biol. Chem. 161:45 (1945).

The relative absorption and utilization of ferrous and ferric iron in anemia as determined with the radioactive isotope.
D. F. Hahn, E. Jones, R. C. Lowe, G. R. Meneely and W. Peacock (Vanderbilt University).
Am. J. Physiol. 143:191 (1945).

Enzyme studies on a temperature sensitive mutant of neurospora.
W. D. McElroy and H. K. Mitchell (Stanford University).
Fed. Proc. 3:376 (1946).

Absorption of radioactive iron by school children.
W. J. Darby, P. F. Hahn, R. C. Steinkamp and M. M. Kaser (Vanderbilt University).
Fed. Proc. 5:231 (1946).

Biological value of proteins in relation to the essential amino acids which they contain. Part III. Comparison of proteins with mixtures of the amino acids.
J. R. Murlin, L. E. Edwards, S. Fried and T. A. Syzmanski (University of Rochester).
J. Nutrition 31:715 (1946).

Thiamine, riboflavin, nicotinic acid, pantothenic acid and ascorbic acid content of restaurant foods.
H. P. Sarett, M. J. Bennett, T. R. Riggs and V. H. Cheldelin (Oregon State College).
J. Nutrition 31:755 (1946).

Adenosine deaminase from *Aspergillus oryzae*.
H. K. Mitchell and W. D. McElroy (Stanford University).
Arch. Biochem. 10:351 (1946).

Composition of the human placenta. III. Lipid content.
J. P. Pratt, C. Roderick, M. Coryell and I. G. Macy (Children's Fund of Michigan).
Am. J. Obst. Gynec. 52:783 (1946).

The Use of Synthetic *L. casei* Factor in the Treatment of Sprue.
W. J. Darby, E. Jones, and H. C. Johnson.
Science 103:108 (1946).

Effect of Synthetic *Lactobacillus casei* Factor in Treatment of Sprue.
W. J. Darby, E. Jones, and H. C. Johnson.
J. Am. Med. Assoc. 130:78 (1946).

The effect of the dietary level of methionine on the rate of transmethylation reactions in vivo.
M. Cohn, S. Simmonds, J. P. Chandler and V. du Vigneaud (Cornell University).
J. Biol. Chem. 162:343 (1946).

Synthesis of cholesterol in surviving liver.
K. Bloch, E. Borek and D. Rittenburg (Columbia University).
J. Biol. Chem. 162:441 (1946).

The effect of tryptophane on the synthesis of nicotinic acid in the rat.
F. Rosen, J. W. Huff and W. A. Perlzweig (Duke University).
J. Biol. Chem. 163:343 (1946).

Appendix

The activity of pyridoxal phosphate in tryptophane formation by cell-free enzyme preparations.
W. W. Umbreit, W. A. Wood and I. C. Gunsalus (Cornell University).
J. Biol. Chem. 165:731 (1946).

Relation of amino acid imbalance to niacin-tryptophane deficiency in growing rats.
W. A. Krehl, L. M. Henderson, J. de la Huerga and C. A. Elvehjem (University of Wisconsin).
J. Biol. Chem. 166:531 (1946).

The amino acid requirements of twenty-three lactic acid bacteria.
M. S. Dunn, S. Shankman, M. N. Camien and H. Block (University of California).
J. Biol. Chem. 168:1 (1947).

Self selection of diet, Part VI. The nature of appetites for B vitamins.
E. M. Scott and E. L. Verney (University of Pittsburgh).
J. Nutrition 34:471 (1947).

The effects of caloric restriction on skeletal growth.
P. Handler, G. J. Baylin and R. H. Follis, Jr. (Duke University).
J. Nutrition 34:677 (1947).

Interrelationships of dietary fat and tocopherols.
K. E. Mason and L. J. Filer (University of Rochester).
J. Am. Oil Chem. Soc. XXIV:240 (1947).

Studies on carotenoid metabolism. VII. The site of conversion of carotene to vitamin A in the rat.
F. A. Mattson, J. W. Mehl and H. J. Deuel (University of Southern California).
Arch. Biochem. 15:65 (1947).

Serum iron levels in adolescent girls.
F. A. Johnston (University of Chicago).
Am. J. Dis. Child. 74:716 (1947).

The effect of wartime starvation in Holland upon pregnancy and its product.
C. A. Smith (Harvard University).
Am. J. Obst. Gyn. 53:599 (1947).

Goals for nutrition education for elementary and secondary schools.
Dept. of Nutrition, Harvard School of Public Health (1947).

Commercially dehydrated vegetables—further observations on oxidative enzymes and other factors.
M. F. Mallette, C. R. Dawson (Columbia University), W. L. Nelson and W. A. Gortner (Cornell University).
Indus. Eng. Chem. 39:1345 (1947).

Work at high altitude. III. The production of lactic and pyruvic acids during work at ground level and at increasing altitudes to 15,000 feet.
T. E. Friedemann, A. C. Ivy, S. C. Harris, B. B. Sheft and V. M. Kinney (Northwestern University).
Quart. Bull. Med. School 21:228 (1947).

A survey of the ascorbic acid content of fruits, vegetables and some native plants grown in Ontario, Canada.
J. H. L. Truscott, W. M. Johnstone, T. G. H. Drake, J. R. Van Haarlem and C. L. Thomson (Ontario Agricultural College).
Dept. of National Health & Welfare, Ottawa, Canada, January, 1947.

Chronic moderate hypervitaminosis D in young dogs.
J. B. Hendricks, A. F. Morgan and R. M. Freytag (University of California).
Am. J. Physiol. 149:319 (1947).

The Physiological Effects of the Pteroylglutamates in Man—With Particular Reference to Pteroylglutamic Acid (PGA).
W. J. Darby.
Vitamins and Hormones V:119 (1947).

The Influence of Pteroylglutamic Acid (A Member of the Vitamin M Group), on Gastrointestinal Defects in Sprue. A Study of Interrelationships of Dietary Essentials.
W. J. Darby, E. Jones, H. F. Warden and M. M. Kaser.
J. Nutrition 34:645 (1947).

A micromethod for the microbiological determination of amino acids.
L. M. Henderson, W. L. Brickson and E. E. Snell (University of Wisconsin).
J. Biol. Chem. 172:31 (1948).

An *in vivo* effect of pteroylglutamic acid upon tyrosine metabolism in the scorbutic guinea pig.
C. W. Woodruff and W. J. Darby (Vanderbilt University).
J. Biol. Chem. 172:851 (1948).

Crystalline d-glyceraldehyde-3-phosphate dehydrogenase from rabbit muscle.
G. T. Cori, M. W. Stein and C. F. Cori (Washington University).
J. Biol. Chem. 173:605 (1948).

The pantothenic acid content of coenzyme A by chick assay.
D. M. Hegsted and F. A. Lipmann (Harvard University & Massachusetts General Hospital).
J. Biol. Chem. 174:89 (1948).

Appendix

The determination of diketo-1-gulonic acid, dehydro-1-ascorbic acid, and 1-ascorbic acid in the same tissue extract by the 2.4-dinitrophenylhydrazine method.
J. H. Roe, M. B. Mills, M. J. Oesterling and C. M. Damron (George Washington University).
J. Biol. Chem. 174:201 (1948).

The determination of iron in small volumes of blood serum.
H. B. Burch, O. H. Lowry, O. A. Bessey and B. Z. Berson (Public Health Research Institute of the City of New York).
J. Biol. Chem. 174:791 (1948).

Effect of amino acids on the growth of rats on niacin-tryptophan-deficient rations.
L. V. Hankes, L. M. Henderson, W. L. Brickson and C. A. Elvehjem (University of Wisconsin).
J. Biol. Chem. 174:873 (1948).

Fluorometric measurements of riboflavin and its natural derivatives in small quantities of blood serum and cells.
H. B. Burch, O. A. Bessey and O. H. Lowry (Public Health Institute of the City of New York).
J. Biol. Chem. 175:457 (1948).

The effect of vitamin deficiencies upon the metabolism of cardiac muscle *in vitro*. II. The effect of biotin deficiency in ducks with observations on the metabolism of radioactive carbon-labeled succinate.
R. E. Olson, O. N. Miller, Y. J. Topper and F. J. Stare (Harvard University).
J. Biol. Chem. 175:503 (1948).

Comparative growth on diets containing ten and nineteen amino acids, with further observations upon the role of glutamic and aspartic acids.
W. C. Rose, M. J. Oesterling and M. Womack (University of Illinois).
J. Biol. Chem. 176:753 (1948).

The site of conversion of carotene to vitamin A.
F. H. Mattson (University of Southern California).
J. Biol. Chem. 176:1467 (1948).

Congenital malformations induced in rats by maternal vitamin A deficiency. II. Effect of varying the preparatory diet upon the yield of abnormal young.
J. Warkany and C. B. Roth (University of Cincinnati).
J. Nutrition 35:1 (1948).

Dental caries in the cotton rat. Part X. The effect of fluidity of the ration.
E. P. Anderson, J. K. Smith, C. A. Elvehjem and P. H. Phillips (University of Wisconsin).
J. Nutrition 35:371 (1948).

The determination of minimum vitamin requirements for growth.
D. M. Hegsted and R. L. Perry (Harvard University).
J. Nutrition 35:399 (1948).

The need for and interrelationship of folic acid, antipernicious anemia liver extract, and biotin in the pig.
T. J. Cunha, R. W. Colby, L. K. Bustad and J. F. Bone (State College of Washington).
J. Nutrition 36:215 (1948).

Anemia and edema of chronic choline deficiency in the rat.
R. W. Engle (Alabama Polytechnic Institute).
J. Nutrition 36:739 (1948).

Self selection of diet.
E. M. Scott (University of Pittsburgh).
Trans. Am. Assn. Cereal Chem. VI:126 (1948).

Metabolism of women during the reproductive cycle. Part XVI. The effect of multi-vitamin supplements on the secretion of vitamin A in human milk.
M. Lesher, A. Robinson, J. K. Brody, H. H. Williams and I. G. Macy (Children's Fund of Michigan).
J. Am. Diet. Assn. 24:12 (1948).

Microorganisms associated with dental caries in the cotton rat.
E. J. Wakeman, J. K. Smith, M. Zepplin, W. B. Sarles and P. H. Phillips (University of Wisconsin).
J. Dental Research 27:489 (1948).

The biochemical assessment of nutritional status during pregnancy.
W. J. Darby, R. O. Cannon and M. M. Kaser (Vanderbilt University).
Obst. Gyn. Survey 3:704 (1948).

Vitamin A acetate as a vitamin A standard.
N. B. Guerrant, M. E. Chilcote, H. A. Ellenberger and R. A. Dutcher (The Pennsylvania State College).
Anal. Chem. 20:465 (1948).

The nutrition of the mouse. V. Long-term maintenance of two strains on synthetic and on stock diets.
P. F. Fenton, G. R. Cowgill and M. A. Stone (Yale University).
Proc. Soc. Exp. Biol. Med. 67:27 (1948).

The evaluation of vitamin M (folic acid).
P. L. Day (University of Arkansas).
J. Ark. Med. Soc. XLIV:253 (1948).

Parenteral nutrition. VI. Fat emulsions for intravenous nutrition: the turbidimetric determination of

Appendix

infused fat in blood after intravenous administration of fat emulsions.
R. P. Geyer, G. V. Mann and F. J. Stare (Harvard University).
J. Lab. Clin. Med. 33:175 (1948).

Parenteral nutrition. IV. Improved techniques for the preparation of fat emulsions for intravenous nutrition.
R. P. Geyer, G. V. Mann and F. J. Stare (Harvard University).
J. Lab. Clin. Med. 33:153 (1948).

Appraising the nutritional status of mothers and infants.
C. A. Smith and H. C. Stuart (Harvard University).
Am. J. Publ. Health 38:369 (1948).

Microbiological determination of cytosine, uracil and thymine.
R. B. Merrifield and M. S. Dunn (University of California).
Arch. Biochem. 16:339 (1948).

The new vitamin A reference standard and its use in evaluating the vitamin A potency of fish oils.
H. A. Ellenberger, N. B. Guerrant and M. E. Chilcote (Pennsylvania State College).
J. Nutrition 37:185 (1949).

The wrist stiffness syndrome in guinea pigs.
S. E. Smith, M. A. Williams, A. C. Bauer and L. A. Maynard (Cornell University).
J. Nutrition 38:87 (1949).

Purified amino acids as a source of nitrogen for growing rat.
G. B. Ramasarma, L. M. Henderson and C. A. Elvehjem (University of Wisconsin).
J. Nutrition 38:177 (1949).

Nutrition studies during pregnancy. V. Relation of maternal nutrition to condition of infant at birth: study of siblings.
B. S. Burke, S. S. Stevenson, J. Worcester and H. C. Stuart (Harvard University).
J. Nutrition 38:453 (1949).

Experimental rat caries. II. Location, sequence and extent of carious lesions produced in the Norway rat when raised on a generally adequate, finely powdered, purified ration.
R. F. Sognnaes (Harvard University).
J. Nutrition 39:139 (1949).

Tryptophan and nicotinic acid studies in man.
H. P. Sarett and G. A. Goldsmith (Tulane University).
J. Biol. Chem. 177:461 (1949).

Unidentified factors required by *Lactobacillus casei*. IV. Evidence for two growth factors in purified liver extracts.
L. J. Daniel, H. T. Peeler, L. C. Norris and M. L. Scott (Cornell University).
J. Biol. Chem. 177:917 (1949).

The purification and properties of a triacetic acid-hydrolyzing enzyme.
W. M. Connors and E. Stotz (University of Rochester).
J. Biol. Chem. 178:881 (1949).

A fluormetric method for the determination of pteroylglutamic acid.
V. Allfrey, L. J. Teply, C. Geffen and C. G. King (Columbia University).
J. Biol. Chem. 178:465 (1949).

The effect of pteroylglutamic acid and related compounds upon tyrosine metabolism in the scorbutic guinea pig.
C. W. Woodruff, M. E. Cherrington, A. K. Stockell and W. J. Darby (Vanderbilt University).
J. Biol. Chem. 178:861 (1949).

The utilization of acetate for the synthesis of fatty acids, cholesterol, and protoporphyrin.
L. Ponticorvo, D. Rittenberg and K. Bloch (Columbia University).
J. Biol. Chem. 179:839 (1949).

Oxidation of fatty acids and tricarboxylic acid cycle intermediates by isolated rat liver mitochondria.
E. P. Kennedy and A. L. Lehninger (University of Chicago).
J. Biol. Chem. 179:957 (1949).

Molybdenum metabolism and interrelationships with copper and phosphorus.
C. L. Comar, L. Singer and C. K. Davis (University of Florida).
J. Biol. Chem. 180:913 (1949).

The metabolism of uric acid in the normal and gouty human studied with the aid of isotopic uric acid.
J. D. Benedict, P. H. Forsham and D. Stetten, Jr. (Harvard University).
J. Biol. Chem. 181:183 (1949).

Chemical and biological studies related to the metabolic function of vitamin E.
P. D. Boyer, M. Rabinovitz and F. Liebe (University of Minnesota.)
Ann. N. Y. Acad. Science 52:188 (1949).

Studies on vitamin E deficiency in the monkey.
L. J. Filer, Jr., R. E. Rumery, P. N. G. Yu and K. E. Mason (University of Rochester).
Ann. N. Y. Acad. Sci. 52:284 (1949).

Appendix

Vitamin E deficiency, dietary fat, and spinal cord lesions in the rat.
C. N. Luttrell and K. E. Mason (University of Rochester).
Ann. N. Y. Acad. Sci. 52:284 (1949).

Work at high altitude. IV. Utilization of thiamine and riboflavin at low and high dietary intake; effect of work and rest.
T. E. Friedemann, A. C. Ivy, F. T. Jung, B. B. Sheft and V. M. Kinney (Northwestern University).
Quart. Bull. Med. School 23:177 (1949).

Work at high altitude. VI. The effect of diet on other factors on the rise of lactic and pyruvic acids, and the lactate-pyruvate ratio in human subjects at simulated high altitudes.
T. E. Friedemann, A. C. Ivy, V. M. Kinney, B. B. Sheft and S. C. Harris (Northwestern University).
Quart. Bull. Med. School 23:438 (1949).

Nutrition and dental caries.
J. H. Shaw (Harvard University).
Fed. Proc. 8:536 (1949).

Amino acid requirements of man.
W. C. Rose (University of Illinois).
Fed. Proc. 8:546 (1949).

Nutrition, renal lesions and hypertension.
C. H. Best and W. S. Hartroft (University of Toronto).
Fed. Proc. 8:610 (1949).

Spectrophotometric studies of the oxidation of fats. VIII. Coupled oxidation of carotene.
R. T. Holman (University of Minnesota and A. & M. College of Texas).
Arch. Biochem. 21:51 (1949).

New York State Nutrition Survey. I. A nutrition survey of public school children.
M. Trulson, D. M. Hegsted and F. J. Stare (Harvard University).
J. Am. Diet. Assn. 25:595 (1949).
II. A one-day study of food intake of adults.
J. Am. Diet. Assn. 25:669 (1949).

Determination of amino acids by microbiological assay.
M. S. Dunn (University of California).
Physiological Reviews 29:219 (1949).

Further experiments with vitamin A in relation to aging and to length of life.
H. C. Sherman and H. Y. Trupp (Columbia University).
Proc. Nat. Acad. Sci. 35:90 (1949).

Caloric intakes in relation to the quantity and quality of protein in the diet.
D. M. Hegsted and V. K. Haffenreffer (Harvard University).
Am. J. Physiol. 157:141 (1949).

Pernicious anemia and related anemias treated with vitamin B_{12}.
E. Jones, W. J. Darby and J. R. Totter (Vanderbilt University).
J. Hematology IV:827 (1949).

Diabetes mellitus in early infancy treated without dietary restrictions.
George M. Guest (University of Cincinnati).
Acta Paediatrica 38:196 (1949).

The influence of diet on iron absorption. I. The pathology of iron excess.
T. D. Kinney, D. M. Hegsted and C. A. Finch (Harvard University).
J. Exp. Med. 90:137 (1949).

Hypervitaminosis A in the dog.
Charlotte L. Maddock, S. Burt Wolbach and Stephen Maddock (Harvard University).
J. Nutrition 39:117 (1949).

Variable Response to Vitamin B_{12} of Megaloblastic Anemia of Infancy.
C. W. Woodruff, H. W. Ripy, J. C. Peterson and W. J. Darby.
Pediatrics 4:723 (1949).

Pernicious Anemia of Pregnancy; Failure of Vitamin B_{12} Therapy; Successful Treatment with Folic Acid; Report of a Case.
R. H. Furman, W. B. Daniels, Jr., L. L. Hefner, E. Jones and W. J. Darby.
Am. Practitioner 1:146 (1950).

Isolation of porphyrins from biological materials by partition chromatography.
J. Lucas and J. M. Orten (Wayne University).
J. Biol. Chem. 191:287 (1951).

The metabolism of 1-^{14}C-L-ascorbic acid in guinea pigs.
J. J. Burns, H. B. Burch and C. G. King (Columbia University).
J. Biol. Chem. 191:501 (1951).

Liver and intestinal xanthine oxidases in relation to diet.
W. W. Westerfeld and D. A. Richert (State University of New York).
J. Biol. Chem. 192:35 (1951).

The calcium balance of adult human subjects on high- and low-fat (butter) diets.

Appendix

F. R. Steggerda and H. H. Mitchell (University of Illinois).
J. Nutrition 45:201 (1951).

Vitamin B6 phosphates, growth factors for leuconostoc mesenteroides.
V. H. Cheldelin, A. P. Nygaard, H. A. Kornberg and R. J. Williams (Oregon State College).
J. Bacteriology 62:134 (1951).

The metabolism of desoxyribose nucleosides in *E. coli*.
L. A. Manson and J. O. Lampen (Washington University).
J. Biol. Chem. 193:539 (1951).

The nature of phosphorylations accompanying the oxidation of pyruvate.
S. S. Barkulis and A. L. Lehninger (University of Chicago).
J. Biol. Chem. 193:597 (1951).

A study of test dose excretion of five B-complex vitamins in man.
F. T. Lossy, G. A. Goldsmith and H. P. Sarett (Tulane University).
J. Nutrition 45:213 (1951).

"Steatitis" or "yellow fat" in the mink, and its relation to dietary fats and inadequacy of vitamin E.
K. E. Mason and G. R. Hartsough (University of Rochester).
J. Am. Vet. Med. Assn. 119:72 (1951).

Iron Metabolism in Human Pregnancy as Studied with the Radioactive Isotope, FE^{55}.
P. F. Hahn, E. L. Carothers, W. J. Darby, M. Martin, C. W. Sheppard, R. O. Cannon, A. S. Beam, P. M. Densen, J. C. Peterson and G. S. McClellan.
Am. J. Ob. and Gyn. 61:477 (1951).

Citrovorum Factor and Folic Acid in Treatment of Megaloblastic Anemia in Infancy.
C. W. Woodruff, J. C. Peterson and W. J. Darby.
Proc. Soc. Exp. Biol. Med. 77:16 (1951).

Serum vitamin A in normal and A-deficient monkeys.
B. L. Truscott and G. van Wagenen (Yale University).
Yale Journal Biol. & Med. 25:139 (1952).

The influence of diet on iron absorption. III. Comparative studies with rats, mice, guinea pigs and chickens.
D. M. Hegsted, C. A. Finch and T. D. Kinney (Harvard University).
J. Exp. Med. 96:115 (1952).

The determination of thiamine and thiamine phosphates in small quantities of blood and blood cells.
H. B. Burch, O. A. Bessey, R. H. Love and O. H. Lowry (Public Health Research Institute of New York).
J. Biol. Chem. 198:477 (1952).

Food for your heart. A manual for patient and physician.
Prepared for the American Heart Association, Inc. by the Dept. of Nutrition (Harvard School of Public Health, Harvard University).
Published 1952. American Heart Association, 48 pp.

Metabolism of L-ascorbic acid, dehydro-1-ascorbic acid and diketo-1-gulonic acid in the guinea pig.
C. M. Damron, M. M. Monier and J. H. Roe (George Washington University).
J. Biol. Chem. 195:599 (1952).

The utilization of purine nucleosides for nucleic acid synthesis in the rat.
B. A. Lowry, J. Davoll and G. B. Brown (Sloan-Kettering Institute for Cancer Research, N.Y.).
J. Biol. Chem. 197:591 (1952).

The origin of L-ascorbic acid in the albino rat.
H. H. Horowitz, A. P. Doerschuk and C. G. King (Columbia University).
J. Biol. Chem. 199:193 (1952).

Metabolism of cardiac muscle. VI. Competition between L(+)-lactate uniformly labeled with ^{14}C and ^{14}C-carbonyl-labeled pyruvate.
M. Brin and R. E. Olson (Harvard University).
J. Biol. Chem. 199:475 (1952).

Structure of glycogens and amylopectins. III. Normal and abnormal human glycogen.
B. Illingsworth and G. T. Cori (Washington University).
J. Biol. Chem. 199:653 (1952).

Utilization of glucose-1-^{14}C for the synthesis of phenylalanine and tyrosine.
C. Gilvarg and K. Bloch (University of Chicago).
J. Biol. Chem. 199:689 (1952).

Nutrition resurvey in Bataan, Philippines, 1950.
H. B. Burch, J. Salcedo, Jr., E. O. Carrasco and C. L. Intengan (Columbia University).
J. Nutrition 46:239 (1952).

Dental caries in the cotton rat. XIII. Effect of whole grain and processed cereals on dental caries production.
M. A. Constant, P. H. Phillips and C. A. Elvehjem (University of Wisconsin).
J. Nutrition 46:271 (1952).

Appendix

The occurrence of calcinosis syndrome in the cotton rat. II. Pathology.
M. A. Constant, P. H. Phillips and D. M. Angevine (University of Wisconsin).
J. Nutrition 47:327 (1952).

A trail of research in sulfur chemistry and metabolism.
Vincent du Vigneaud (Cornell University).
Cornell University Press, 1952, pp. 191.

Influence of food intake on ketosis, mineral balance and survival of alloxan-diabetic rats.
W. A. Brodsky, N. Nelson and G. M. Guest (Children's Hospital, Cincinnati).
Metabolism 1:68 (1952).

Effect of diet upon body growth and organ size in the rat after partial nephrectomy.
T. Addis, R. W. Lipmann, W. Lew, L. J. Poo and W. Wong (Stanford University).
Am. J. Physiol. 168:114 (1952).

Conversion of glucose to galactose in the mammary gland.
J. M. Barry (University of California).
Nature 169:878 (1952).

Cortisone and matrix formation in experimental scorbutus and repair therefrom.
S. B. Wolbach and C. L. Maddock (Children's Hospital, Boston).
AMA Arch. Pathology 53:54 (1952).

A theory concerning the mechanism of fatty acid oxidation and synthesis and of carbon dioxide fixation.
H. A. Lardy (University of Wisconsin).
Proc. Nat. Acad. Sci. 38:1003 (1952).

Hypervitaminosis A and the skeleton of growing chicks.
S. B. Wolbach and D. M. Hegsted (Children's Hospital, Boston).
AMA Arch. Pathology 54:30 (1952).

Serum lipoproteins and cholesterol levels in normal subjects and in young patients with diabetes in relation to vascular complications.
N. R. Keiding, G. V. Mann, H. F. Root, E. Y. Lawry and A. Marble (Harvard University).
J. Am. Diabetes Assn. 1:434 (1952).

Studies in nutrition education.
F. E. Whitehead (Harvard University).
J. Am. Diet. Assn. 28:622 (1952).

Effects of acidosis on insulin action and on carbohydrate and mineral metabolism.
G. M. Guest, B. Mackler and H. C. Knowles, Jr. (University of Cincinnati).
Diabetes I:276 (1952).

A balanced diet.
Prepared for the Nutrition Foundation, by L. J. Bowser, M. F. Trulson and F. J. Stare (The Dept. of Nutrition, Harvard University).
Published 1952. The Nutrition Foundation, 24 pp.

Protective action of stock diets against the cancer inducing action of 2-acetyl-aminofluorene.
R. W. Engel and D. H. Copeland (Alabama Polytechnic Institute).
Cancer Research 12:211 (1952).

The influence of dietary casein level on tumor induction with 2-acetyl-aminofluorene.
R. W. Engel and D. H. Copeland (Alabama Polytechnic Institute).
Cancer Research 12:905 (1952).

An improved procedure for the synthesis of enantiomeric α-lecithins.
E. Baer and J. Maurukas (University of Toronto).
J. Am. Chem. Soc. 74:158 (1952).

Acyl migrations in partially acylated, polyhydroxylic systems.
A. P. Doerschuk (Columbia University).
J. Am. Chem. Soc. 74:4202 (1952).

Synthesis of L-Ascorbic-1-^{14}C acid from D-sorbitol.
L. L. Salomon, J. J. Burns and C. G. King (Columbia University).
J. Am. Chem. Soc. 74:5161 (1952).

Vitamin D and citrate metabolism: studies on rachitic infants.
H. E. Harrison and H. C. Harrison (The Johns Hopkins University).
Yale J. of Biol. & Med. 24:273 (1952).

Physiological changes in plasma proteins characteristic of human reproduction.
I. G. Macy (Children's Fund of Michigan) and H. C. Mack (Harper Hospital).
Published 1952. Children's Fund of Michigan, 170 pp.

Sterochemical configuration and provitamin A activity.
L. Zechmeister, H. J. Deuel, Jr., H. H. Inhoffen, J. Leeman, S. Greenberg and J. Ganguly (University of Southern California).
Arch. Biochem. Biophys. 36:80 (1952).

Studies of the distribution of vitamin A as ester and alcohol and of carotenoids in plasma proteins of several species.

Appendix

J. Ganguly, N. I. Krinsky, J. W. Mehl and H. J. Deuel, Jr. (University of Southern California).
Arch. Biochem. Biophys. 38:275 (1952).

Microbiological synthesis of ^{14}C-uniformly labeled L(+)-and D (-)-lactate.
M. Brin, R. E. Olson and F. J. Stare (Harvard University).
Arch. Biochem. & Biophys. 39:214 (1952).

The conversion of glucose-6-^{14}C to ascorbic acid by the albino rat.
H. H. Horowitz and C. G. King (Columbia University).
J. Biol. Chem. 200:125 (1953).

Lactose synthesis in the mammary gland perfused with 1-^{14}C-glucose.
E. Dimant, V. R. Smith and H. A. Lardy (University of Wisconsin).
J. Biol. Chem. 201:85 (1953).

Synthesis of phosphatides in isolated mitochondria.
E. P. Kennedy (University of Chicago).
J. Biol. Chem. 201:399 (1953).

The non-enzymatic oxidation of α-keto-glutarate. I. The effects of manganous ions and amino acids.
G. Kalnitsky (State University of Iowa).
J. Biol. Chem. 201:817 (1953).

An elevated xanthine oxidase in livers of vitamin-E deficient rabbits.
J. S. Dinning (University of Pittsburgh).
J. Biol. Chem. 202:213 (1953).

The conversion of ^{14}C-labeled glucose to glucuronic acid in the guinea pig.
J. F. Douglas and C. G. King (Columbia University).
J. Biol. Chem. 202:865 (1953).

A survey of the literature on dental caries.
National Research Council.
Publication No. 225.

Nutritional intake of children. I. Calories, carbohydrate, fat and protein.
V. A. Beal (University of Colorado School of Medicine).
J. Nutrition 50:223 (1953).

Studies on renal juxtaglomerular cells. I. Variations produced by sodium chloride and desoxycorticosterone acetate.
P. M. Hartroft and W. S. Hartroft (University of Toronto).
J. Exp. Med. 97:415 (1953).

Gene expression in neurospora mutants requiring nicotinic acid or tryptophan.
D. Newmeyer and E. L. Tatum (Stanford University).
Am. J. Botany 40:393 (1953).

Effect of weight reduction and caloric balance on serum lipo-protein and cholesterol levels.
W. J. Walker, E. Y. Lawry, D. E. Love, G. V. Mann, S. A. Levine and F. J. Stare. (Peter Bent Brigham Hospital & Harvard University).
Am. J. Med. 14:654 (1953).

Arteriovenous glucose differences, metabolic hypoglycemia and food intake in man.
T. B. Van Itallie, R. Beaudoin and J. Mayer (Harvard University).
J. Clin. Nutrition I:208 (1953).

An analysis of the syndrome of malformations induced by maternal vitamin A deficiency.
J. G. Wilson, C. B. Roth and J. Warkany (University of Cincinnati).
Am. J. Anatomy 92:189 (1953).

Maternal-fetal nutritional relationships—effect of maternal diet on size and content of the fetal liver.
C. A. Smith, J. Worcester and B. S. Burke (Harvard University).
Obstetrics and Gynecology 1:46 (1953).

Nutritional factors in hemodynamics, III. Importance of vitamin C in maintaining renal VEM mechanisms.
R. P. Akers and R. E. Lee (Cornell University Medical College).
Proc. Soc. Exp. Biol. Med. 82:195 (1953).

Exercise and weight control. Frequent misconceptions.
J. Mayer and F. J. Stare (Harvard University).
J. Am. Diet. Assn. 29:340 (1953).

Effects of acidosis on utilization of glucose in erythrocytes and leucocytes.
H. Graubarth, B. Mackler and G. M. Guest (University of Cincinnati).
Am. J. Physiol. 172:301 (1953).

Studies on the structure of sphingomyelin. II. Performic and periodic acid oxidation studies.
G. Marinetti, J. F. Berry, G. Rouser and E. Stotz (University of Rochester).
J. Am. Chem. Soc. 75:313 (1953).

On the crystallization, structure and infrared spectra of saturated L-α-lecithins.
E. Baer (University of Toronto).
J. Am. Chem. Soc. 75:621 (1953).

The enzymatic oxidation of d- and 1-B-hydroxybutyrate.

Appendix

A. L. Lehninger and C. D. Greville (The Johns Hopkins University).
J. Am. Chem. Soc. 75:1515 (1953).

Ascorbic acid deficiency and cholesterol synthesis.
R. R. Becker, H. B. Burch, L. L. Salomon, T. Venkitasubramanian and C. G. King (Columbia University).
J. Am. Chem. Soc. 75:2020 (1953).

Kinetic analysis of enzyme reactions. II. The potassium activation and calcium inhibition of pyruvic phosphoferase.
J. F. Kachmar and P. D. Boyer (University of Minnesota).
J. Biol. Chem. 200:669 (1953).

The Vanderbilt Cooperative Study of Maternal and Infant Nutrition. IV. Dietary, Laboratory, and Physical Findings in 2129 Delivered Pregnancies.
W. J. Darby, et al.
J. Nutrition 51:565 (1953).

The Vanderbilt Cooperative Study of Maternal and Infant Nutrition. I. Background. II. Methods. III. Description of the Sample and Data.
W. J. Darby, et al.
J. Nutrition 51:539 (1953).

The Vanderbilt Cooperative Study of Maternal and Infant Nutrition. V. Description and Outcome of Obstetric Sample. VI. Relationship of Obstetric Performance to Nutrition.
W. J. McGanity, W. J. Darby, et al.
Am. J. Ob. and Gyn. 67:491-500, 501-527 (1954).

The Vanderbilt Cooperative Study of Maternal and Infant Nutrition. VII. Tocopherol in Relation to Pregnancy.
M. E. Ferguson, E. Bridgforth, M. L. Quaife, M. P. Martin, R. O. Cannon, W. J. McGanity, J. Newbill and W. J. Darby.
J. Nutrition 55:305 (1955).

The Vanderbilt Cooperative Study of Maternal and Infant Nutrition. VIII. Some Nutritional Implications.
W. J. McGanity, E. B. Bridgforth, M. P. Martin, J. A. Newbill and W. J. Darby.
J. Am. Diet. Assoc. 31:582 (1955).

The Vanderbilt Cooperative Study of Maternal and Infant Nutrition. IX. Some Obstetrical Implications.
W. J. Darby, E. Bridgforth, M. P. Martin and W. J. McGanity.
Obstetrics and Gynecology 5:528 (1955).

The Vanderbilt Cooperative Study on Maternal and Infant Nutrition. X. Ascorbic Acid.
M. P. Martin, E. Bridgforth, W. J. McGanity and W. J. Darby.
J. Nutrition 62:201 (1957).

The Development of Vitamin B_{12} Deficiency by Untreated Patients with Pernicious Anemia.
W. J. Darby, E. Jones, S. L. Clark, Jr., W. J. McGanity, J. Dutra de Oliveira, C. Perez, J. Kevany and J. le Brocquy.
Am. J. Clin. Nutrition 6:513 (1958).

Vitamin B_{12} Requirement of Adult Man.
W. J. Darby, E. B. Bridgforth, J. le Brocquy, S. L. Clark, Jr., J. Dutra de Oliveira, J. Kevany, W. J. McGanity and C. Perez.
Am. J. Med. XXV:726 (1958).

Vanderbilt Cooperative Study of Maternal and Infant Nutrition. XII. Effect of Reproductive Cycle on Nutritional Status and Requirements.
W. J. McGanity, E. B. Bridgforth and W. J. Darby.
J. Am. Med. Assn. 168:2138 (1958).

The effect on human serum-lipids of a dietary fat, highly unsaturated, but poor in essential fatty acids.
E. H. Ahrens, Jr., J. Hirsch, M. L. Peterson, W. Insull, Jr., W. Stoffel, J. W. Farquhar, T. Miller and H. T. Thomasson.
Lancet I:115 (1959).

The analysis of fatty acid mixtures by gas-liquid chromatography: construction and operation of an ionization chamber instrument.
J. W. Farquhar, W. Insull, Jr., P. Rosen, W. Stoffel and E. H. Ahrens, Jr.
Nutrition Reviews Supplement 17, pp. 1-30 (August 1959).

The oxidation state of the respiratory carriers and the partial reactions of oxidative phosphorylation.
C. L. Wadkins and A. L. Lehninger.
J. Biol. Chem. 234:681 (1959).

The use of high efficiency capillary columns for the separation of certain cis-trans isomers of long chain fatty acid esters by gas chromatography.
S. R. Lipsky, J. E. Lovelock and R. A. Landowne.
J. Am. Chem. Soc. 81:1010 (1959).

Serum magnesium, cholesterol, and lipoproteins in patients with atherosclerosis and alcoholism.
O. M. Jankelson, J. J. Vitale and D. M. Hegsted.
Am. J. Clin. Nutrition 7:23 (1959).

Interrelations between the kind and amount of dietary fat and dietary cholesterol in experimental hypercholesterolemia.
D. M. Hegsted, A. Gotsis, F. J. Stare and J. Worcester.

Appendix

Am. J. Clin. Nutrition 7:5 (1959).

Effect of mixed fat formula feeding on serum cholesterol level in man.
S. A. Hashim, R. E. Clancy, D. M. Hegsted and F. J. Stare.
Am. J. Clin. Nutrition 7:30 (1959).

Investigation of mechanisms by which unsaturated fats, nicotinic acid and neomycin lower serum lipid concentrations. Excretion of sterols and bile acids.
G. A. Goldsmith, J. G. Hamilton and O. N. Miller.
Transactions Association Am. Physicians LXXII:207 (1959).

The separation of some steroids by glass-paper chromatography.
J. G. Hamilton and J. W. Dieckert.
Archives Biochem. and Biophys. 82:212 (1959).

Cholesterol levels of maternal and fetal blood at parturition in upper and lower income groups in Guatemala City.
J. Mendez, B. S. Savits, M. Flores and N. S. Scrimshaw.
Am. J. Clin. Nutrition 7:595 (1959).

Prevention and control of chronic disease.
R. E. Olson.
Am. J. Pub. Health 49:1120 (1959).

Pathogenesis of atherosclerosis and myocardial infarction.
W. S. Hartroft, R. M. O'Neal and W. A. Thomas.
Fed. Proc. 18:36 (1959).

Modifications of diets responsible for induction of coronary thromboses and myocardial infarcts in rats.
W. A. Thomas, W. S. Hartroft and R. M. O'Neal.
J. Nutrition 69:325 (1959).

The function of cytidine diphosphate diglyceride in the enzymatic synthesis of inositol monophosphatide.
H. Paulus and E. P. Kennedy.
J. Am. Chem. Soc. 81:4436 (1959).

Pathological abnormalities of magnesium metabolism.
W. E. C. Wacker and B. L. Vallee.
Med. Clin. of N. Am. 44:1357 (1959).

Stimulating effect of thyroxine in contraction of rat liver mitochondria.
A. L. Lehninger.
Biochem. Biophys. Acta. 44:1357 (1960).

The phosphate-water oxygen exchange reaction of oxidative phosphorylation in submitochondrial preparations.
P. C. Chan, A. L. Lehninger and T. Enns.
J. Biol. Chem. 235:1790 (1960).

Swelling of liver mitochondria from rats fed diets deficient in essential fatty acids.
T. Hayashida and O. W. Portman.
Proc. Soc. Exp. Biol. & Med. 103:656 (1960).

Geographic differences in the severity of aortic and coronary atherosclerosis.
I. Gore, W. B. Robertson, A. E. Hirst, G. G. Hadley and Y. Koseki.
Am. J. Path. 36:559 (1960).

Spontaneous atheromatous embolization.
I. Gore and D. P. Collins.
Am. J. Clin. Path. 33:416 (1960).

The enzymatic synthesis of triglycerides.
S. B. Weiss, E. P. Kennedy and J. Y. Kiyasu.
J. Biol. Chem. 235:40 (1960).

The enzymatic synthesis of inositol monophosphatide.
H. Paulus and E. P. Kennedy.
J. Biol. Chem. 235:1303 (1960).

Composition of molecular distillates of corn oils: isolation and identification of sterol esters.
A. Kuksis and J. M. R. Beveridge.
J. Lipid Res. 1:311 (1960).

Serum lipids and protein-bound iodine levels of Guatemalan pregnant women from two different socioeconomic groups.
J. Mendez, N. S. Scrimshaw, M. D. Abrams and E. N. Forman.
Am. J. Obstet. and Gynocology 80:114 (1960).

Effect of saturated medium-chain triglyceride on serum-lipids in man.
S. A. Hashim, A. Arteaga and T. B. Van Itallie.
Lancet I:1105 (1960).

Diet and coronary artery disease.
R. E. Olson.
Circulation XXII:453 (1960).

The obese hyperglycemic syndrome in mice. Metabolism of isolated adipose tissue *in vitro*.
A. E. Renold, J. Christophe and B. Jeanrenaud.
Am. J. Clin. Nutrition 8:719 (1960).

Studies on the interrelationships between dietary magnesium, quality and quantity and quantity of fat, hypercholesterolemia and lipidosis.
E. E. Hellerstein, M. Nakamura, D. M. Hegsted and J. J. Vitale.
J. Nutrition 71:339 (1960).

The phosphate-water oxygen exchange reaction of

Appendix

oxidative phosphorylation in submitochondrial preparations.
P. C. Chan, A. L. Lehninger and T. Enns.
J. Biol. Chem. 235:1790 (1960).

Studies on the metabolic response to prolonged fasting.
F. C. Wood, Jr., L. Domenge, P. R. Bally, A. E. Renold and G. W. Thorn.
Med. Clinics of No. America 44:1371 (1960).

The nutritional status of children of pre-school age in the Guatemalan community of Amatitlan. 2. Comparisons of dietary, clinical and biochemical findings.
M. Behar, G. Arroyave, M. Flores and N. S. Scrimshaw.
Brit. J. Nutrition 14:217 (1960).

Sequence in which indispensable and dispensable amino acids become limiting for growth of rats fed diets low in fibrin.
U. S. Kumta and A. E. Harper.
J. Nutrition 71:310 (1960).

Riboflavin in red blood cells in relation to dietary intake of children.
V. A. Beal and J. J. Van Buskirk.
Am. J. Clin. Nutrition 8:841 (1960).

The unique role of ascorbic acid in peripheral vascular physiology as compared with rutin and hesperidin; a micromanipulative study.
R. E. Lee.
J. Nutrition 72:203 (1960).

The influence of sleep, work, diuresis, heat, acute starvation, thiamine intake and bed rest on human riboflavin excretion.
R. G. Tucker, O. Mickelson and A. Keys.
J. Nutrition 72:251 (1960).

Biochemical concomitants of hunger and satiety in man.
T. B. Van Itallie and S. A. Hashim.
Am. J. Clin. Nutrition 8:587 (1960).

Oral and dental lesions in vitamin B_6 deficient rhesus monkeys.
C. C. Berdjis, L. D. Greenberg, J. F. Rinehart and G. Fitzgerald.
Brit. J. Exper. Path. XLI:198 (1960).

Calcification, XXVI. Caries susceptibility in relation to composition of teeth and diet.
A. E. Sobel, J. H. Shaw, A. Hanock and S. Nobel.
J. Dental Research 39:462 (1960).

Diet and coronary artery disease.
R. E. Olson.
Circulation XXII:453 (1960).

Role of oleic acid in the metabolism of essential fatty acids.
G. A. Dhopeshwarkar and J. F. Mead.
J. Am. Oil Chem. Soc. XXXVIII:297 (1961).

Biosynthesis of complex lipids.
E. P. Kennedy.
Fed. Proc. 20:934 (1961).

Biosynthesis and metabolism of unsaturated fatty acids.
K. Bloch, P. Baronowsky, H. Goldfine, W. J. Lennarz, R. Light, A. T. Norris and G. Scheuerbrandt.
Fed. Proc. 20:921 (1961).

Alterations in the blood fatty acids in single and combined deficiencies of essential fatty acids and vitamin B_6 in monkeys.
L. D. Greenberg and H. D. Moon.
Arch. Biochem. Biophys. 94:405 (1961).

The blood ketone and plasma free fatty acid concentration in diabetic and normal subjects.
E. E. Werk, Jr., and H. C. Knowles, Jr.
Diabetes 10:22 (1961).

Diet and serum cholesterol levels among the "Black Caribs" of Guatemala.
N. S. Scrimshaw, J. Mendez, M. Flores, M. A. Guzman and R. de Leon.
Am. J. Clin. Nutrition 9:206 (1961).

The role of pyridoxine in the metabolism of polyunsaturated fatty acids in rats.
J. C. Kirschman and J. G. Coniglio.
J. Biol. Chem. 236:2200 (1961).

Influence of dietary fatty acids on serum lipids.
D. E. Pickering, D. A. Fisher, A. Perley, G. M. Basinger and H. D. Moon.
Am. J. Diseases of Children 102:42 (1961).

Pathology of lipid disorders: liver and cardiovascular system.
W. S. Hartroft.
Fed. Proc. (supplement 7) 20:135 (1961).

New approaches in the study of cardiovascular disease: aldosterone, renin, hypertension and juxtaglomerular cells.
W. S. Hartroft and P. M. Hartroft.
Fed. Proc. 20:845 (1961).

Nutrition in relation to arteriosclerosis.
F. J. Stare.
Postgrad. Med. 29:133 (1961).

Factors influencing serum cholesterol levels of Central American children. II. The effect of gross dietary changes.

Appendix

J. Mendez, N. S. Scrimshaw, M. Flores, R. de Leon and M. Behar.
Am. J. Clin. Nutrition 9:148 (1961).

Studies of patients with hyperglyceridemia.
L. W. Kinsell, G. D. Michaels, G. Walker, S. Splitter and R. E. Vistidine.
Am. J. Clin. Nutrition 9:1 (1961).

Glucose metabolism and mobilization of fatty acids by adipose tissue from obese mice.
B. Leboeuf, S. Lochaya, N. Leboeuf, F. C. Wood, Jr., J. Mayer and G. F. Cahill, Jr.
Am. J. of Physiol. 201:19 (1961).

Dietary intake of individuals followed through infancy and childhood.
V. A. Beal.
Am. J. Public Health 51:1107 (1961).

Serum and liver vitamin A and lipids in children with severe protein malnutrition.
G. Arroyave, D. Wilson, J. Mendez, M. Behar and N. S. Scrimshaw.
Am. J. Clin. Nutrition 9:180 (1961).

Amino acid balance and imbalance. VII. Effects of dietary additions of amino acids on food intake and blood urea concentration of rats fed low-protein diets containing fibrin.
U. S. Kumta and A. E. Harper.
J. Nutrition 74:139 (1961).

Efficiency of tryptophan as a niacin precursor in man.
G. A. Goldsmith, O. N. Miller and W. G. Unglaub.
J. Nutrition 73:172 (1961).

A genetic study of two new structural forms of tyrosine in neurospora.
N. H. Horowitz, M. Fling, H. Macleod and N. Sueoka.
Genetics 46:1015 (1961).

Effects of dietary methionine and vitamin B_{12} on the net synthesis of choline in rats.
K. K. G. Menon and C. C. Lucas.
Can. J. Biochem. Physiol. 39:683 (1961).

Enzymatic synthesis of the methyl group of methionine. II. Involvement of vitamin B_{12}.
S. Takeyama, F. T. Hatch and J. M. Buchanan.
J. Biol. Chem. 236:1102 (1961).

Serum ascorbic acid, riboflavin, carotene, vitamin A, vitamin E and alkaline phosphatase values in Central American school children.
M. A. Guzman, G. Arroyave and N. S. Scrimshaw.
Am. J. Clin. Nutrition 9:164 (1961).

Vitamin A transport in severe protein malnutrition.
G. Arroyave, D. Wilson, H. Castellanos and N. S. Scrimshaw.
Fed. Proc. 20:372 (1961).

Radiographic atlas of skeletal development of the foot and ankle. A standard of reference.
N. L. Hoerr, S. I. Pyle and C. C. Francis.
Charles C. Thomas, Publishers, Springfield, Illinois.

The interrelationships between dietary molybdenum, copper, sulfate, femur alkaline phosphatase activity and growth of the rat.
H. L. Johnson and R. F. Miller.
J. Nutrition 75:459 (1961).

Diet and heart disease—facts and unanswered questions.
T. B. Van Itallie and S. A. Hashim.
J. Am. Diet. Assn. 38:531 (1961).

Pathology of lipid disorders: liver and cardiovascular system.
W. S. Hartroft.
Fed. Proc. (Supplement 7) 20:135 (1961).

New approaches in the study of cardiovascular disease: aldosterone, renin, hypertension and juxtaglomerular cells.
W. S. Hartroft and P. M. Hartroft.
Fed. Proc. 20:845 (1961).

Nutrition in relation to arteriosclerosis.
F. J. Stare.
Postgrad. Med. 29:133 (1961).

The effects of chain length on the metabolism of saturated fatty acids by the rat.
S. L. Kirschner and R. S. Harris.
J. Nutrition 73:397 (1961).

Nutritional challenges for physicians.
Fredrick J. Stare.
J. Am. Med. Assn. 178:924 (1961).

Highlights on the cholesterol-fats, diets and atherosclerosis problem.
G. A. Goldsmith.
J. Am. Med. Assn. 176:783 (1961).

Contributions of technology to the nutritional value of food.
C. G. King.
Food Drug Cosmetic Law J. 16:8 (1961).

Science and food: today and tomorrow.
Food Protection Committee, Food and Nutrition Board, National Academy of Sciences—National Research Council, Pub. 877 (1961).

World food needs and food resources.
Fed. Proc. (Suppl. 7) 20:365 (1961).

Appendix

Diet and heart disease—facts and unanswered questions.
T. B. Van Itallie and S. A. Hashim.
J. Am. Diet. Assoc. 38:531 (1961).

Comparison of a natural and a purified diet with respect to reproductive ability and caries susceptibility.
J. H. Shaw and D. Griffiths.
J. Dental Research 42:1198 (1963).

Stoichiometric relationships between mitochondrial ion accumulation and oxidative phosphorylation.
C. S. Rossi and A. L. Lehninger.
Biochem. and Biophys. Research Commun. 11:411 (1963).

Primates in medical research with special reference to new world monkeys.
F. J. Stare, S. B. Andrus and O. W. Portman.
Proc. Conf. on Research with Primates (1963). Tektronix Foundation, Beaverton, Oregon.

Cali-Harvard Nutrition project. III. The erythroid atrophy of severe protein deficiency in monkeys.
J. Ghitis, E. Piazuelo and J. J. Vitale.
Am. J. Clin. Nutrition 12:452 (1963).

Dependence of respiration on phosphate and phosphate acceptor in submitochondrial systems. I. Digitonin fragments.
C. T. Gregg and A. L. Lehninger.
Biochem. Biophys. Acta 78:12 (1963).

Interrelations among magnesium, vitamin B_6, sulfur and phosphorus in the formation of kidney stones in the rat.
F. F. Faragalla and S. N. Gershoff.
J. Nutrition 81:60 (1963).

Intracellular distribution of some enzymes catalyzing reactions in the biosynthesis of complex lipids.
G. F. Wilgram and E. P. Kennedy.
J. Biol. Chem. 238:2615 (1963).

Carbohydrate and fat metabolism and response to insulin on vitamin B_6 deficient rats.
A. M. Huber, S. N. Gershoff and D. M. Hegsted.
J. Nutrition 82:371 (1964).

The zinc-binding groups of carboxy-peptidase A.
T. L. Coombs, Y. Omote and B. L. Vallee.
Biochemistry 3:653 (1964).

Sodium intake during pregnancy.
R. L. Pike.
J. Am. Diet. Assn. 44:176 (1964).

Changes in sulfhydryl groups of rat liver mitochondria during swelling and contraction.
M. V. Riley and A. L. Lehninger.
J. Biol. Chem. 239:2083 (1964).

Serum lipids in breast-fed infants and in infants fed evaporated milk.
C. W. Woodruff, M. C. Bailey, J. T. Davis, N. Rogers and J. G. Coniglio.
Am. J. Clin. Nutrition 14:83 (1964).

Treatment of chyluria and chylothorax with medium-chain triglyceride.
S. A. Hashim. H. B. Roholt, V. K. Babayan and T. B. Van Itallie.
New England J. of Med. 270:756 (1964).

The role of vitamin B_{12} in methyl transfer to homocysteine.
J. M. Buchanan, H. L. Elford, R. E. Loughlin, B. M. McDougall and S. Rosenthal.
Ann. N. Y. Acad. Sci. 112:756 (1964).

Effect of copper intake on concentration in body tissue and on growth, reproduction and production in dairy cattle.
R. W. Engel, W. A. Hardison, R. F. Miller, N. O. Price and H. T. Huber.
J. Animal Science 23:1160 (1964).

Effect of potassium on juxtaglomerular cells and the adrenal zona glomerulosa of rats.
P. M. Hartroft and Elizabeth Sowa.
J. Nutrition 82:439 (1964).

A new pteridine-requiring enzyme system for the oxidation of glyceryl ethers.
A. Tietz, M. Lindberg and E. P. Kennedy.
J. Biol. Chem. 239:4081 (1964).

A control mechanism for the activity of vitamin B_6-enzymes.
A. Novogrodsky, K. Soda and A. Meister.
Fed. Proc. 23:278 (1964).

Vitamin K induced prothrombin formation: antagonism by actinomycin D.
R. E. Olson.
Science 145:926 (1964).

Serum cholesterol levels in Central American population groups.
Jose Mendez, Lucila Sogandares and N. S. Scrimshaw.
Archivos Venezolanos de Nutricion 14:139 (1964).

Alterations in serum proteins during pregnancy and lactation in urban and rural populations in Guatemala.
G. H. Beaton, G. Arroyave and M. Flores.
Am. J. Clin. Nutrition 14:269 (1964).

Mode of action of selenium in relation to biological activity of tocopherols.
I. D. Desai and M. L. Scott.
Arch. Biochem. and Biophys. 110:309 (1965).

Appendix

Hepatic lesions in pyridoxine-deficient monkeys.
Joseph P. Wizgird, Louis G. Greenberg and Henry D. Moon.
Arch. Path. 79:317 (1965).

Certain organic substances and their effects upon the incidence of dental caries in the cotton rat.
D. T. Thompson, J. J. Vogel and P. M. Phillips.
J. of Dental Research 44:596 (1965).

Quantitative effects of dietary fat on serum cholesterol in man.
D. M. Hegsted, R. B. McGandy, M. L. Myers and F. J. Stare.
Am. J. Clin. Nutrition 17:281 (1965).

Nimiquipalg operation VIII. Comparative study of morality evolution between the City of New York and a rural Guatemalan village.
Helberto Luna-Jaspe, Joaquin Cravioto and Leopoldo Vega Franco.
Revista del Colegio Medico 16:45 (1965).

Further observations on the amino acid requirements of older men. II. Methionine and lysine.
Stewart G. Tuttle, Samuel H. Bassett, Wendel H. Griffith, Dorothy B. Mulcare and Marian E. Swendweid.
Am. J. Clin. Nutrition 16:229 (1965).

Metabolism of zinc and its deficiency in human subjects.
Ananda S. Prasad.
Zinc Metabolism, Charles C. Thomas, Springfield, Illinois, 1966

Dietary carbohydrate and serum cholesterol levels in man.
R. B. McGandy, D. M. Hegsted, M. L. Myers and F. J. Stare.
Am. J. Clin. Nutrition 18:237 (1966).

Catabolism and elimination of cholesterol in germfree rats.
Bernard S. Wostmann, Norbert L. Wiech and Elisabeth Kung.
J. Lipid Research 7:77 (1966).

Effect of amino acid imbalance on the fate of the limiting amino acid.
P. Yoshida, M.-B. Leung, G. R. Rogers and A. E. Harper.
J. Nutrition 89:80 (1966).

Metabolic patterns in preadolescent children: XIII. Zinc balance.
R. W. Engel, R. F. Miller and N. O. Price.
Zinc Metabolism, Chapter 18, Charles C. Thomas, Springfield (1966).

Prevalence of osteoporosis in high- and low-fluoride areas in North Dakota.
D. S. Bernstein, N. Sadowsky, D. M. Hegsted, C. D. Guri and F. J. Stare.
J. Am. Med. Assn. 198:499 (1966).

Comparative studies of spontaneous and experimental atherosclerosis in primates.
S. B. Andrus and O. W. Portman.
Some Recent Development in Comparative Medicine, Symposia of the Zoological Soc. of London 17:161 (1966). Academic Press.

Effect of amino acid imbalance on rats maintained in a cold environment.
A. E. Harper and Q. R. Rogers.
Am. J. Phys. 210:1234 (1966).

Protein-calorie malnutrition and psychobiological development in children.
Joaquin Cravioto.
Boletin de la Oficina Sanitaria Panamericana, English Edition, p. 34 (1966).
Boletin de la Oficina Sanitaria Panamericana, Spanish Ed. LXI, f4:285 (1966).

Obesity.
George Christakis and Robert K. Plumb.
The Nutrition Foundation, 15 pp. (1966).

Your diet: health is in the balance.
Marie M. Alexander and Fredrick J. Stare.
The Nutrition Foundation, 22 pp. (1966).

Copper, manganese, cobalt and molybdenum balance in preadolescent girls.
R. W. Engel, N. O. Price and R. F. Miller.
J. Nutrition 92:197 (1967).

Importance of zinc in human nutrition.
Ananda S. Prasad.
Am. J. Clin. Nutrition 20:648 (1967).

Dietary fats, carbohydrates and atherosclerotic vascular disease.
Robert B. McGandy, D. M. Hegsted and F. J. Stare.
New England J. Med. 277:417 and 469 (1967).

Factors affecting steroid excretion in the rat.
Thomas F. Kellogg and Bernard S. Wostmann.
Proceedings Indiana Acad. Sciences for 1966, 76:191 (1967).

Individual trends in the total serum cholesterol of children and adolescents over a ten-year period.
Virginia A. Lee.
Am. J. Clin. Nutrition 20:5 (1967).

Cellular response with increased feeding in neonatal rats.
Myron Winick and Adele Noble.
J. Nutrition 91:179 (1967).

Appendix

Cellular Growth in Human Placenta I. Normal Placental Growth.
Myron Winick, Anthony Coscia and Adele Noble.
Pediatrics 39:248 (1967).

II. Diabetes Mellitus.
Myron Winick and Adele Noble.
J. Pediatrics 71:216 (1967).

III. Intrauterine growth failure.
Myron Winick.
J. Pediatrics 71:390 (1967).

Better diet for brighter minds.
Medical World News, March 17, 1967.

Caloric and nutrient intakes of teen-agers.
Mary C. Hampton, Ruth L. Huenemann, Leona R. Shapiro and Barbara W. Mitchell.
J. Am. Diet. Assn. 50:385 (1967).

The chemical senses and nutrition.
Morley Kare and Owen Maller.
Based on a symposium sponsored by the Nutrition Foundation, June 1966.
Johns Hopkins Press, Baltimore (1967).

International cooperation by various disciplines to improve nutrition in developing countries.
Paul B. Pearson.
Proceedings of the Seventh International Congress of Nutrition, Vol. 3, Pergamon Press (1967).

Malnutrition, learning and behavior.
Nevin S. Scrimshaw.
Am. J. Clin. Nutrition 20:394 (1967).

Malnutrition, learning and behavior.
Nevin S. Scrimshaw and John E. Gordon.
Proceedings of a conference held in March, 1967, sponsored jointly by The Nutrition Foundation, the Ford Foundation and the Massachusetts Institute of Technology.
M.I.T. Press, 1968.

Putting nutrition to work.
Symposium organized by Horace L. Sipple, sponsored jointly by the Institute of Technologists and The Nutrition Foundation on May 15, 1967.
Food Technology 22:53 (1968).

Cellular recovery in rat tissues after a brief period of neonatal malnutrition.
Myron Winick, Irving Fish and Pedro Rosso.
J. Nutrition 95:4, 623 (1968).

A nutrition study of school children in a depressed urban district. II. Physical and biochemical findings.
Madge L. Meyers, Judith A. Mabel and Fredrick J. Stare.
J. Am. Diet. Assn. 53:3, 234 (1968).

Enzymes of glucose catabolism in hydra. II. Application of microfluorometric analyses to patterns of enzyme localization.
Charles L. Rutherford and Howard M. Lenhoff.
Arch. Biochem. Biophys. 133:1, 128 (1969).

Voluntary intragastric feeding: oral and gastric contributions to food intake and hunger in man.
Henry A. Jordon.
J. Comp. & Phys. Psych. 68:4, 498 (1969).

Pharmacological tests for the function of hypothalamic norepinephrine in eating behavior.
J. L. Slangen and N. E. Miller.
Physiology & Behavior 4:543 (1969).

Food intake: regulation by plasma amino acid pattern.
Phillip M.-B. Leung and Quinton R. Rogers.
Life Sciences 8, Part III: 1 (1969).

The ultrastructure of vertebrate taste buds.
P. P. C. Graziadei.
Olfaction & Taste, Rockefeller University Press IV:315 (1969).

Breast and formula feeding of infants.
Virginia A. Beal.
J. Am. Diet. Assn. 55:1, 31 (1969).

Stock diet for colony production of germ-free rats and mice.
Thomas F. Kellogg and Bernard S. Wostmann.
Am. Assn. for Laboratory Animal Science 19:6, 812 (1969).

Effect of maternal protein deficiency on cellular development in the fetal rat.
Frances J. Zeman and Ellen C. Stanbrough.
J. Nutrition 99:3, 274 (1969).

Experimental human magnesium depletion.
Maurice E. Shils.
Medicine 48:1, 61 (1969).

Relation of severity of atherosclerosis to chemical composition of human aorta.
Jose Mendez and Carlos Tejada.
Am. J. Clin. Pathology 51:1, 113 (1969).

Iron nutriture from infancy to adolescence.
Virginia A. Beal and Aldula J. Meyers.
Am. J. Public Health 60:4, 666 (1970).

Effect of protein deficiency during gestation on postnatal cellular development in the young rat.
Frances J. Zeman.
J. Nutrition 100:5, 530 (1970).

Zinc and wound healing: effects of zinc deficiency and zinc supplementation.
Harold H. Sandstead, Verne C. Lanier, Jr., Glenn

Appendix

H. Shephard and David D. Gillespie.
Am. J. Clin. Nutrition 23:5, 514 (1970).

Effect of Early Malnutrition on the Reaction of Adult Rats to Aversive Stimuli.
R. H. Barnes.
Nature 225:468 (1970).

Oral and Intragastric Feeding in Vagotomized Rats.
A. N. Epstein.
J. of Comp. & Phys. Psych. 71:59 (1970).

Taste Responses in Ruminants: 1) Reactions of Sheep to Sugars, Saccharin, Ethanol and Salts, 2) Reactions of Sheep to Acids, Quinine, Urea and Sodium Hydroxide, 3) Reaction of Pygmy Goats, Normal Goats, Sheep and Cattle to Sucrose and Sodium Chloride, 4) Reaction of Pygmy Goats, Normal Goats, Sheep and Cattle to Acetic Acid and Quinine Hydrachloride.
D. C. Church.
Technical Paper No. 2801, Oregon Agric. Exp. Sta. (1970).

Effect of Amino Acid Imbalance and Deficiency on Food Intake of Rats with Hypothalamic Lesions.
P. M.-B. Leung and Q. R. Rogers.
Nutr. Rep. Intern'l. 1: 1 (1970).

Infant Feeding and Weaning Practices in a Rural Pre-Industrial Setting—A Sociocultural Approach.
D. Sanjur, J. Cravioto, L. Rosales and A. van Veen.
Acta Paediatrica Scandinavia, Supplement 200 (1970) Stockholm, Sweden.

Puerto Rican Food Habits.
Diva Sanjur.
Cornell Univ. Notebook (1970).

Patterns of ^{35}S-Thiamine Hydrochloride Absorption in the Malnourished Alcoholic Patient.
Herman Baker, Carroll M. Leevy and A. D. Thompson.
J. Lab. Clin. Med. 76:34 (1970).

Enzymes and Metabolites of Intermediatry Metabolism in Urea-fed Sheep.
W. J. Visek, R. L. Prior, A. J. Clifford and D. E. Hogue.
J. Nutrition 100:938 (1970).

Tissue Amino Acid Concentrations in Rats During Acute Ammonia Intoxication.
R. L. Prior, A. J. Clifford and W. J. Visek.
Am. J. Physiol. 219:1680 (1970).

Effect of Glycine and Serine on Methionine Metabolism in Rats Fed Diets High in Methionine.
N. J. Benevenga and A. E. Harper.
J. Nutrition 100:1205 (1970).

Atropine induced prandial drinking.
H. W. Chapman and A. N. Epstein.
Physiol. Behav. 5:549 (1970).

The vital role of saliva as a mechanical sealant for suckling in the rat.
A. N. Epstein, E. M. Blass, M. L. Batshaw and A. D. Parks.
Physiol. Behav. 5:1395 (1970).

Drinking induced by injection of angiotensin into the brain of the rat.
A. N. Epstein, J. T. Fitzsimons and B. J. Simons.
J. Physiol. (London) 210:457 (1970).

Gastrointestinal sensory and motor control of food intake.
C. T. Snowdon.
J. Comp. Physiol. Psychol. 71:68 (1970).

Primary hyperdipsia in the rat following septal lesions.
E. M. Blass and D. Hanson.
J. Comp. Physiol. Psychol. 70:87 (1970).

Additivity of effect and interaction of a cellular and an extracellular stimulus of drinking.
E. M. Blass and J. T. Fitzsimons.
J. Comp. Physiol. Psychol. 70:200 (1970).

Effect of amino acid imbalance and deficiency on food intake of rats with hypothalmic lesions.
Philip M-B. Leung and Quinton R. Rogers.
Nutrition Reports Internat. 1:1 (1970).

Current concepts on trace minerals.
Harold H. Sandstead, Raymond F. Burk, Glenn H. Booth, Jr., and William J. Darby.
Medical Clinics of N. America 54:1509 (1970).

Effects of jejuno-ileal shunt on body composition in morbidly obese patients.
Harold H. Sandstead, A. Bertrand Brill, Edwin G. Stant, Jr., David H. Law IV and H. William Scott, Jr.
Surgical Forum Volume XXI (1970).

Lead Intoxication: Its effect on the renin-aldosterone response to sodium deprivation.
Harold H. Sandstead, Andrew M. Michelakis and T. Eugene Temple.
Arch. Environ. Health 20:356 (1970).

"Zinc and wound healing." Effects of zinc deficiency and zinc supplementation.
Harold H. Sandstead.
Am. J. Clin. Nutrition 23:514 (1970).

Liver phospholipids in choline-deficiency. I. Distribution of total lipid phosphorus.
Pirkko R. Turkki and Maria Teresita G. Silvestre.
Nutrition Report Internat'l. 1:378 (1970).

Appendix

Liver phospholipids in choline-deficiency II. Synthesis of phosphatidylethanolamine and its conversion to lecithin.
Pirkko R. Turkki and Maria Teresita G. Silvestre.
Nutrition Report Internat'l. 2:133 (1970).

Liver phospholipids in choline-deficiency III. Inhibition of the conversion of phosphatidylethanolamine into lecithin in vitro.
Pirkko R. Turkki and Maria Teresita G. Silvestre.
Nutrition Report Internat'l. 2:141 (1970).

Enzymes and metabolites of intermediary metabolism in urea-fed sheep.
R. L. Prior, A. J. Clifford, D. E. Hogue and W. J. Visek.
J. Nutrition 100:438 (1970).

Restoration of sodium balance in hypophysectomized rats after acute sodium deficiency.
Gerald Wolf.
Physiology & Behavior 5:1145 (1970).

Galactose toxicity in the chick: Oxidation of radioactive galactose.
Henry J. Wells, Maureen Gordon and Stanton Segal.
Biochim. Biophys. Acta 222:327 (1970).

Fetal Malnutrition.
Myron Winick.
Clinical Obstet. and Gynec. 13:526 (1970).

Differential cellular growth in the organs of hypothyroid rats.
Jo Anne Brasel and Myron Winick.
Growth 34:197 (1970).

Nutrition and mental development.
Myron Winick.
Medical Clinics of N. Amer. 54:1413 (1970).

Changes in brain weight, cholesterol, phospholipid, and DNA content in marasmic children.
Pedro Rosso, Julia Hormazabal and Myron Winick.
Am. J. Clin. Nutrition 23:1275 (1970).

Nutrition and nerve cell growth.
Myron Winick.
Fed. Proc. 29:1510 (1970).

Cellular growth of cerebrum, cerebellum, and brain stem in normal and marasmic children.
Myron Winick, Pedro Rosso and John Waterlow.
Experimental Neurology 26:393 (1970).

Hydrogen Sulfide from Heat Degradation of Thiamine.
Roy G. Arnold.
J. Agric. & Food Chem. 19:923 (1971).

Nutrition Studies During Pregnancy. I. Changes in Intakes of Calories, Fat, Protein, and Calcium. II. Dietary Intake, Maternal Weight Gain, and Size of Infant.
Virginia A. Beal.
J. Am. Diet. Assoc. 58:312 (1971).

Plasma Corticosterone levels and hepatic glycogen metabolism in young and old rats fed diets devoid of an essential amino acid.
A. J. Clark and M. C. Barron.
J. Nutrition 102:1407 (1971).

A lateralpreoptic osmosensitive zone for thirst in the rat.
E. M. Blass and A. N. Epstein.
J. Comp. Physiol. Psychol. 76:378 (1971).

Metabolism of tritiated angiotensin II in anaesthetized rats.
M. J. Osborne, N. Pooters, G. Angles d'Auriac, A. N. Epstein, M. Worcel and P. Meyer.
Pflüger's Arch. 326:101 (1971).

The complete dependence of beta-adrenergic drinking on the renal dipsogen.
K. A. Houpt and A. N. Epstein.
Physiol. Behav. 7:897 (1971).

The lateral hypothalamic syndrome: its implications for the physiological psychology of hunger and thirst.
E. Stellar and J. M. Sprague, eds.
Progress in Physiological Psychology, Academic Press 4:263 (1971).

An evaluation of the contribution of cholinergic mechanisms to thirst.
E. M. Blass and H. W. Chapman.
Physiol. Behav. 7:679 (1971).

The Cellular Approach to the Determination of Pyridoxine Requirements in Pregnant and Nonpregnant Rats.
Judy A. Driskell and Avanelle Kirksey.
J. Nutrition 101:661 (1971).

The role of homeostasis in adipose tissues upon the regulation of food intake of white leghorn cockerels.
S. Lepkovsky and F. Furuta.
Reprinted from Poultry Science: L:573 (1971).

Role of upper intestines in the regulation of food intake in parabiotic rats with their intestines "crossed" surgically.
S. Lepkovsky, Pamela Bortfeld, Mildred K. Dimick, S. E. Feldman, F. Furuta, I. M. Sharon and R. Park.
Reprinted from Israel Journal of Medical Sciences 7:639 (1971).

Appendix

Thirst and behavior in adipsic chickens with hypothalamic lesions before and after intravenous injection of hypertonic NaCl solution.
S. Lepkovsky, F. Furuta, I. M. Sharon and N. Snapir.
Physiol. and Behavior 6:477 (1971).

Density as a determinant of food and water intake.
Owen Maller and Harvey Wank.
Nutrition Report Internat. 4:49 (1971).

Evidence for hypothalamic a and b adrenergic receptors involved in the control of food intake of the pig.
H. M. Jackson and D. W. Robinson.
Br. Vet. J. 127:51 (1971).

Importance of prepyriform cortex in food-intake response of rats to amino acids.
P. M.-B. Leung and Quinton R. Rogers.
Am. J. Physiol. 221:929 (1971).

Effects of pituitary extract on food intake of intact and hypophysectomized rats fed imbalanced amino acid diets.
P. M.-B. Leung and Quinton R. Rogers.
Nutrition Report Internat. 4:207 (1971).

Experience with a new technic of intestinal bypass in the treatment of morbid obesity.
H. William Scott, Jr., Harold H. Sandstead, A. Bertrand Brill, Henry Burko, and Rachel K. Younger.
Annals of Surgery 174:560 (1971).

Nutritional deficiencies in disadvantaged preschool children.
Harold H. Sandstead, James P. Carter, Faye R. House, Freeman McConnell, Kathryn B. Horton, and Roger Vander Zwaag.
Am. J. Dis Child. 121:455 (1971).

Plasma renin activity in chronic plumbism.
Russell G. McAllister, Jr., Andrew M. Michelakis and Harold H. Sandstead.
Arch. Intern. Med. 127:919 (1971).

N-Nitrosamines not identified from heat induced D-glucose / L-alanine reactions.
Richard A. Scanlan and Leonard M. Libbey.
Agricul. and Food Chemistry 19:570 (1971).

Thiamine propyl disulfide: Absorption and utilization.
Oscar Frank, Herman Baker, Carroll M. Leevy and A. D. Thompson.
Annals of Internal Medicine, 74:529 (1971).

Intermediary metabolism and the response to insulin in ammonia intoxicated rats.
R. L. Prior, A. J. Clifford and W. J. Visek.
Am. J. Physiol. 220: (1971).

Reticulo-hypothalamic pathway in the rat.
Gerald Wolf.
The Anatomical Record, 169:547 (1971).

Lateral hypothalamic projections to the hypothalamic ventromedial nucleus in the albino rat: demonstration by means of a simplified ammoniacal silver degeneration method.
Gerald Wolf.
Brain Research 29:128 (1971).

Polyvinylpyrrolidone column chromatography of strawberry, rhubarb, and raspberry anthocyanins.
R. E. Wrolstad and Barbara J. Struthers.
J. Chromatog. 55:405 (1971).

Study of possible correlations between prenatal brain development and placental weight.
S. Zamenhof, L. Grauel and E. van Marthens.
Biol. Neonate 18:140 (1971).

DNA (Cell Number) and protein in neonatal rat brain: Alteration by timing of maternal dietary protein restriction.
S. Zamenhof, E. van Marthens and L. Grauel.
J. Nutrition 101:1265 (1971).

The effect of thymidine and 5-bromodeoxyuridine on developing chick embryo brain.
Stephen Zamenhof, Ludmila Grauel and Edith van Marthens.
Res. Comm. in Chem. Pathology and Pharmacology 2:261 (1971).

DNA (Cell Number) in neonnatal brain: Second generation (F^2) alteration by maternal (F) dietary protein restriction.
Stephen Zamenhof, Edith van Marthens and Ludmila Grauel.
Science 172:850 (1971).

Hormonal and nutritional aspects of prenatal brain development.
Stephen Zamenhof and Edith van Marthens.
Medical Sciences 14:329 (1971).

DNA (Cell Number) in neonatal brain: Alteration by maternal dietary caloric restriction.
Stephen Zamenhof, Edith van Marthens and Ludmila Grauel.
Nutrition Reports Internat'l. 4:269 (1971).

Prenatal cerebral development: Effect of restricted diet, reversal by growth hormone.
Stephen Zamenhof, Edith van Marthens and Ludmila Grauel.
Science 174:954 (1971).

Short-term retention of object discriminations in experienced and naive rhesus monkeys.

Appendix

Bela A. Balogh and Robert R. Zimmermann.
Perceptual and Motor Skills 33:543 (1971).

Performance of malnourished rats on the hebb-williams closed-field maze learning task.
Robert R. Zimmermann and Anne Marie Wells.
Perceptual and Motor Skills 33:1043 (1971).

Manipulatory responsiveness in protein-malnourished monkeys.
David A. Strobel and Robert R. Zimmermann.
Psychon. Sci. 24:19 (1971).

Cranial transillumination in early and severe malnutrition.
Jaime Rozovski N., Fernando Novoa S., Jorge Abarzua F. and Fernando Monckeberg B.
Br. Nutr. 25:107 (1971).

Enzymes of the sugar nucleotide pathway of galactose metabolism in chick liver.
Maureen Gordon, H. Wells and S. Segal.
Enzyme 12:513 (1971).

Galactose toxicity in the chick: Hyperosmolarity.
John I. Malone, Henry J. Wells and Stanton Segal.
Science 174:952 (1971).

Regulatory deficits in rats following unilateral lesions of the lateral hypothalamus.
Richard S. Wampler.
J. Comp. Phys. Psych. 75:190 (1971).

Cellular changes during placental and fetal growth.
Myron Winick.
Am. J. Obstet. Gynec. 109:167 (1971).

Efficiency of Utilization of Indispensable Amino Acids for Growth by the Rat.
Norlin J. Benevenga.
J. Nutrition 102:1199 (1972).

Effect of Cystein on Methionine Metabolism.
Norlin J. Benevenga.
Fed. Proc. 31:715 (1972).

Methylcysteine as a Methionine Analogue in Methionine Toxicity Studies.
Norlin J. Benevenga.
Fed. Proc. 31:715 (1972).

Chemistry of Thiamine Degradation: 4-methyl-5-(B-hydroxyethyl) thiazole from Thermally Degraded Thiamine.
B. K. Dwivedi, R. G. Arnold and L. M. Libbey.
J. Food Sci. 37:689 (1972).

Gas Chromatographic Estimation of Thiamine.
B. K. Dwivedi and R. G. Arnold.
J. Food Sci. 37:889 (1972).

Chemistry of thiamine degradation: Mechanisms of thiamine degradation in a model system.
B. K. Dwivedi and R. G. Arnold.
J. Food Sci. 37:886 (1972).

Effect of diet on RNA Polymerase activity in rats.
A. J. Clark and M. Jacob.
Life Sciences II:1147 (1972).

The partial purification and characterization of thiamine pyrophosphatase from rabbit brain.
J. R. Cooper and M. M. Kini.
J. Neurochemistry 19:1809 (1972).

Long-term follow-up of antibiotic-treated tropical sprue.
F. R. Rickles, F. A. Klipstein, J. T. Tomasini, J. J. Corcino and N. Maldonado.
Ann. Intern. Med. 76:203 (1972).

Nutritional status and intestinal function among rural populations of the West Indies. II. Barrio Neuvo, Puerto Rico.
F. A. Klipstein, I. Beauchamp, J. J. Corcino, M. Maldonado, J. T. Tomasini and E. A. Schenk.
Gastroenterology 63:758 (1972).

Lysine metabolism in rabbits.
J. A. Grove et al.
Arch. Biochem. & Biophys. 151:464 (1972).

Biosynthesis of acetolactate and its conversion to diacetyl and acetoin in cell-free extracts of Lactobacillus casei.
A. L. Branen and T. W. Keenan
Canadian Journal of Microbiology 18:4 (1972).

Aphagia and adipsia in pigs with induced hypothalamic lesions.
F. Khalaf and D. W. Robinson.
Res. Vet. Sci. 13:5 (1972).

Observations on the phagic response of the pig to infusions of dextrose and sodium pentobarbital into the ventromedial area of the brain.
F. Khalaf and D. W. Robinson.
Res. Vet. Sci. 13:1 (1972).

Isolation and properties of soluble elastin from copper-deficient chicks.
R. B. Rucker.
J. Nutrition 102:563 (1972).

The role of copper in the maturation of bone collagen and aortic elastin.
R. B. Rucker and R. S. Riggins.
Trace Substances in Environmental Health—VI (1972).

The relationship between alkaline and pyrophosphatase activity in quail bone.
M. Chan, R. B. Rucker, F. Zeman and R. S. Riggins.
Soc. Exp. Biol. Med. 141:822 (1971).

Appendix

Purification and properties of sheep plasma amine oxidase.
R. B. Rucker and W. Goettlich-Riemann.
Enzymologia 43:33 (1972).

Properties of rabbit aorta amine oxidase.
R. B. Rucker and W. Goettlich-Riemann.
Soc. Exp. Biol. Med. 39:286 (1972).

Zinc deficiency: effect on brain of the suckling rat.
Harold H. Sandstead, David D. Gillespie and Robert N. Brady.
Pediat. Res. 6:119 (1972).

Changes in body composition after jejunoileal bypass in morbidly obese patients.
A. Bertrand Brill, Harold H. Sandstead, Ron Price, R. Eugene Johnston, David H. Law, IV, and H. William Scott, Jr.
American Journal of Surgery 123:49 (1972).

Decreased RNA polymerase activity in mammalian zinc deficiency.
Harold H. Sandstead.
Science 177:68 (1972).

The availability of food folate in man.
E. L. R. Stokstad and T. Tamura.
British Journal of Haematology (1972).

Observations on the mechanism of thiamine hydrochloride absorption in man.
A. D. Thompson and C. M. Leevy.
Clinical Sciences 43:153 (1972).

The third western hemisphere nutrition congress.
Philip L. White and Nancy Selvey.
Am. J. of Clin. Nutrition 25:354 (1972).

Degradation of anthocyanins at limited water concentration.
J. A. Erlandson and R. E. Wrolstad.
J. Food Sci. 37:592 (1972).

Anthocyanin degradation in freeze-dried strawberries and strawberry puree.
J. A. Erlandson and R. E. Wrolstad.
M. S. Thesis (1972).

Quantitative determination of DNA in preserved brains and brain sections.
S. Zamenhof, Ludmila Grauel, Edith van Marthens and R. A. Stillinger.
J. Neurochemistry 19:61 (1972).

Studies on some factors influencing prenatal brain development.
Stephen Zamenhof, Edith van Marthens and Ludmila Grauel.
Reg. of Organ and Tissue Growth (1972).

Responsiveness of protein deficient monkeys to manipulative stimuli.
David A. Strobel and Robert R. Zimmermann.
Development'l. Psychobiology 5(4):291 (1972).

Abnormal social development of protein-malnourished rhesus monkeys.
Robert R. Zimmermann, Peter L. Steere, David A. Strobel and Harry L. Hom.
J. Abnormal Psych. 80:125 (1972).

Effect of protein-calorie malnutrition on food consumption, weight gain, serum proteins, and activity in the developing rhesus monkey (Macaca Mulatta).
Charles R. Geist, Robert R. Zimmermann and David A. Strobel.
Lab. Animal Sci. 22:369 (1972).

Protein preference in protein-malnourished monkeys.
P. L. Peregoy, R. R. Zimmermann and D. A. Strobel.
Perceptual and Motor Skills 35:495 (1972).

Responses of protein malnourished rats to novel objects.
Robert R. Zimmermann and Stephanie J. Zimmermann.
Perceptual and Motor Skills 35:319 (1972).

Adjusting retention scores: Reply to medin.
Robert R. Zimmermann and Bela Balogh.
Perceptual and Motor Skills 35:478 (1972).

Influence of environmental and nutritional factors on problem solving in the rat.
Annie Marie Wells, Charles R. Geist and Robert R. Zimmermann.
Perceptual and Motor Skills 35:235 (1972).

Abnormal social development of protein-malnourished rhesus monkeys.
Robert R. Zimmermann, Peter L. Steere, David A. Strobel and Harry L. Hom.
J. Abnormal Psych. 80:125 (1972).

Thiamin depletion induced by dietary folate deficiency in rats.
Allan D. Thomson, Oscar Frank, Barbara De Angelis and Herman Baker.
Nutr. Reports Internat'l. 6:107 (1972).

Cell migration and cortisone induction of sucrase activity in jejunum and ileum.
John J. Herbst and Otakar Koldovsky.
Biochem. J. 126:471 (1972).

Effects of proteins and polynucleotides on the activity of various hydrolases.
M. J. Palmieri and O. Koldovsky.
Biochem. J. 127:795 (1972).

Appendix

Nutritional and environmental interactions in the behavioral development of the rat: Long-term effects.
David A. Levitsky and Richard H. Barnes.
Science 176:68 (1972).

Malnutrition and mental development.
Fernando Monckeberg, Susana Tisler, Sonia Toro, Vivien Gattas and Lucy Vega.
Am. J. Clin. Nutrition 25:766 (1972).

Effects of dietary cholesterol and voluntary exercise on histopathology, plasma and hepatic lipids of the male rat.
Elaine R. Monsen, Marian T. Arlin and Ruth E. Rumery.
Int. Z. Angew. Physiol. 30:258 (1972).

Effects of graded dietary levels of cholesterol and cholic acid on plasma and hepatic lipids and histopathology of the young male rat.
Elaine Monsen, Carolyn T. Knutson and Ruth E. Rumery.
Int. Z. Angew. Physiol. 30:269 (1972).

Application of the erythroctye glutathione reductase assay in evaluating riboflavin nutrition status in a high school student population.
H. E. Sauberlich, J. H. Judd, Jr., G. E. Nichoalds, H. P. Broquist and W. J. Darby.
Am. J. Clin. Nutrition 25:756 (1972).

Nutrition teaching in preventive dentistry.
Abraham E. Nizel.
J. Am. College of Dent. 39:211 (1972).

Personalized nutrition counseling.
Abraham E. Nizel.
ASDC J. of Dentistry for Children 59:353 (1972).

Changes in brain and sciatic nerve composition with development of the rhesus monkey (Macaca Mulatta).
Oscar W. Portman, Manfred Alexander and D. Roger Illingworth.
Brain Research 43:197 (1972).

Decreased uptake of glucose by brain of the galactose toxic chick.
John I. Malone, Henry Wells and Stanton Segal.
Brain Research 43:700 (1972).

Weight regulation with palatable food and liquids in rats with lateral hypothalamic lesions.
Elliott J. Mufson and Richard S. Wampler.
J. Comp. Physiol. Psych. 80:382 (1972).

Failure to obtain sex differences in development of obesity following ventromedial hypothalamic lesions in rats.
David A. Rehovsky and Richard S. Wampler.
J. Comp. Physiol. Psych. 78:102 (1972).

Nutrition, environment, and behavioral development.
Myron Winick and John Coombs.
Annual Review of Medicine 23:149 (1972).

Chemistry of thiamine degradation. A review.
B. K. Dwivedi and R. G. Arnold.
J. Agric. & Food Chem. 21:54 (1973).

Lactose Malabsorption in Oklahoma Indians.
D. P. Bose and J. D. Welsh.
Am. J. Clin. Nutrition 26:1320 (1973).

A Skeletal Alteration Association with Silicon Deficiency.
E. M. Carlisle.
Fed. Proc. 32:930 (1973).

Nutrition Teaching at the Mount Sinai School of Medicine: a three-year experience.
G. Christakis, Reva Frankle, R. E. Brown, Ruth Jeffers, Joycelyn Walter and Kurt Deuschle.
Am. J. Clin. Nutrition 25:997 (1972).

Intestinal perfusion studies in tropical sprue. I. Transport of water, electrolytes and d-xylose.
J. J. Corcino, M. Maldonado and F. A. Klipstein.
Gastroenterology 65:192 (1973).

Cadmium toxicity in growing swine.
R. J. Cousins, A. K. Barber and J. R. Trout.
J. Nutrition 103:964 (1973).

Influence of cadmium on the metabolism of 25-hydroxycholecalciferol in chicks.
S. L. Feldman and R. J. Cousins.
Nutr. Reports Int'l. 8:251 (1973).

Effect of dietary cadmium on anemia, iron absorption, and cadmium binding protein in the chick.
J. H. Freeland and R. J. Cousins.
Nutr. Reports Int'l. 8:337 (1973).

Effect of cholecalciferol on cadmium uptake in the chick.
R. J. Cousins and S. L. Feldman.
Nutr. Reports Int'l. 8:363 (1973).

Nutrition and behavior and learning.
J. Cravioto and Elsa R. DeLicardie.
Food, Nutrition & Health. World Rev. of Nutr. & Diet. 16:80 (1973).

Additivity of dipsogens: angiotensin plus cell dehydration.
S. Hsiao and A. N. Epstein.
Fed. Proc. 32:384 (1973).

The thirsts of cellular dehydration and hypovolemia.

Appendix

A. N. Epstein, E. Stellar and J. Corbit (eds.)
NRP Bulletin on Motivation (1973).

Intestinal malabsorption in folate deficient alcoholics.
C. H. Halsted, E. A. Robles and E. Mezey.
Gastroenterology 64:526 (1973).

The distribution of ethanol in the human gastrointestinal tract.
C. H. Halsted and E. Mezey.
Am. J. Clin. Nutrition 26:831 (1973).

Newer concepts in the regulation of food intake.
S. Lepkovsky.
Am. J. Clin. Nutrition 26:271 (1973).

The plasma membranes of bovine taste papillae: Polyacrylamide gel electrophoresis of circumvallate membrane proteins.
Chai-Ho Lo and Tony Ma.
Biochim. Biophys. Acta 307:343 (1973).

Taste in acceptance of sugars by human infants.
J. A. Deosr, Owne Maller and Robert E. Turner.
J. Comp. Physiol. Psych. 84:496 (1973).

Hunger drive during starvation in rats enriched with odd-carbon fatty acids.
D. Quartermain, M. E. Judge and T. B. Van Itallie.
Proc. Soc. Exp. Biol. and Med. 143:929 (1973).

Properties of chick tropoelastin.
R. B. Rucker, W. Goettlich-Riemann and K. Tom
Biochim. Biophys. Acta 317:193 (1973).

Chick aorta pyrophosphatase.
M. Chen, J. McCarry, M. M. Chan, R. S. Riggins and R. B. Rucker.
Proc. Soc. Exp. Biol. and Med. 143:44 (1973).

Effect of fluoride on bone formation and strength in Japanese quail.
M. Chan, R. B. Rucker. F. Zeman and R. S. Riggins.
J. Nutrition 103:1431 (1973).

Identification of volatile compounds from heated L-cysteine-HCl/D-glucose.
Richard A. Scanlan, Stanley G. Kayser, Leonard M. Libbey and Max E. Morgan.
Agricul. and Food Chemistry 21:673 (1973).

Absorption and biotransformation of cholecalciferol in drug-induced osteomalacia.
R. Matheson, K. G. Tolman, J. J. Herbst, W. Jubiz and J. W. Freston.
Clin. Res. 21:244 (1973).

Calcium ATPase activity in drug-induced osteomalacia.
E. L. Watson and K. G. Tolman.
Res. Comm. Chem. Path. Pharm. 6:1079 (1973).

Effect of metal ions on the color of strawberry puree.
R. E. Wrolstad and J. A. Erlandson.
J. Food Sci. 38:460 (1973).

Gastrointestinal growth in the fetus and suckling rat pups: Effects of maternal dietary protein.
M. K. Younoszai and Jill Ranshaw.
J. Nutrition 103:454 (1973).

Reversal learning in the developing malnourished rhesus monkey.
Robert R. Zimmermann.
Behavioral Biol. 8:381 (1973).

Punishment of oral-genital self-stimulation in young rhesus monkeys.
Gerald R. Stoffer, Robert R. Zimmermann and David A. Strobel.
Perceptual and Motor Skills 36:199 (1973).

Shock thresholds of low-and high-protein-reared rhesus monkeys.
Larry A. Wise and Robert R. Zimmermann.
Perceptual and Motor Skills 36:674 (1973).

Effects of protein deprivation on dominance measured by shock avoidance competition and food competition.
Robert R. Zimmermann.
Behavioral Biol. 9:317 (1973).

Airblast avoidance learning sets in rhesus monkeys.
Robert R. Zimmermann.
Animal Learning & Behavior 1:211 (1973).

Airblast avoidance learning sets in protein-malnourished monkeys.
Robert R. Zimmermann.
Behavioral Biol. 9:695 (1973).

Nutrition and oral problems.
A. E. Nizel.
Food, Nutr. and Health. World Review of Nutr. and Dietetics 16:226 (1973).

Decrease in food intake following cortical spreading depression in static obese rats with ventromedial hypothalamic lesions.
Richard S. Wampler and David A. Rehovsky.
J. Comp. Physiol. Psych. 82:23 (1973).

Effects of lateral hypothalamic lesions on placentophagia in virgin, primiparous, and multiparous rats.
Mark B. Kristal.
J. Comp. Physiol. Psych. 84:53 (1973).

Food and water intake prior to parturition in the rat.
Mark B. Kristal and Richard S. Wampler.
Physiol. Psych. 1:297 (1973).

Effects of vascular insufficiency on placental ribonu-

Appendix

clease activity in the rat.
Elba G. Velasco, Jo Anne Brasel, Dirce M. Sigulem, Pedro Rosso and Myron Winick.
J. Nutrition 103:213 (1973).

Changes in alkaline ribonuclease activity during compensatory renal growth.
Pedro Rosso, James Diggs and Myron Winick.
Proc. Nat. Acad. Sci. 70:169 (1973).

Toxicities of Methionine and Other Amino Acids.
Norlin J. Benevenga.
Agricultural and Food Chemistry 22:2 (1974).

A Relationship Between Silicon, Glycosaminoglycans and Collagen Formation.
E. M. Carlisle.
Fed. Proc. 33:704 (1974).

Control of cadmium binding protein synthesis in rat liver.
K. S. Squibb and R. J. Cousins.
Environ. Physiol. Biochem. 4:24 (1974), Munksgaard, Copenhagen, Denmark.

Intestinal transport of tritiated folic acid (^{3}H-PGA) in the everted gut sac of different aged rats.
K. Bhanthumnavin, J. R. Wright and C. H. Halsted.
Johns Hopkins Med. J. 135:152 (1974).

Jejunal uptake of tritiated folic acid in the rat studied by in vivo perfusion.
C. Halsted, K. Bhanthumnavin and E. Mezey.
J. Nutrition 104:1674 (1974).

Intestinal transport of tritiated folic acid (^{3}H-PGA) in the everted gut sac of different aged rats.
K. Bhanthumnavin, J. Wright and C. H. Halsted.
Johns Hopkins Med. J. 135:152 (1974).

Hunger and Satiety in Humans During Parenteral Hyperalimentation.
Henry A. Jordan, Hamilton Moses, III, Bruce V. MacFayden, Jr. and Stanley J. Dudrick.
Psychosomatic Medicine 36:144 (1974).

An x-ray atlas of the sagittal plane of the chicken diencephalon and its use in the precise localization of brain sites.
S. Lepkovsky.
Phys. and Behavior 12:419 (1974).

Additional evidence for the binding of calcium ions t elastin at neutral sites.
R. B. Rucker, D. Ford, W. Goettlich-Riemann an K. Tom.
Calcified Tissue Research 14:317 (1974).

Calcium binding to elastin. In: Advances in Exper mental Biology and Medicine, Metal-protei Interactions.
R. B. Rucker.
M. Friedman, Ed., Plenum Publishing Co., (1974).

The influence of phenobarbital on metabolism of 25-hydroxycholecalciferol.
R. Burt, J. W. Freston and K. G. Tolman.
Clin. Res. 22:189A (1974).

High molecular weight complexes of folic acid in mammalian tissues.
Marilyn Zamierowski and Conrad Wagner.
Biochemical and Biophysical Research Comm. 60:81 (1974).

Regional distribution of homocarnosine and other ninhydrin positive substances in brains of malnourished monkeys.
C. O. Enwonwu and B. S. Worthington.
J. Neurochem. 22:1045 (1974).

Implementing behavioral objectives into your instruction.
B. S. Worthington.
Proc. National Nutrition Conference (1974).

Concentrations of histamine in brain of guinea pig and rat during dietary protein malnutrition.
C. O. Enwonwu and B. S. Worthington.
Biochem. J. 144:601 (1974).

Alterations of the aryl hydrocarbon hydroxylase system during riboflavin depletion and repletion.
Chung S. Yang.
Arch. Biochem. Biophys. 160:623 (1974).

Inhibition of hepatic mixed function oxidase by propyl gallate.
C. S. Yang and F. S. Strickhart.
Biochem. Pharmacol. 23:3129 (1974).

Inhibitions of the monoxygenase system by butylated hydroxyanisole and butylated hydroxytoluene.
C. S. Yang, F. S. Strickhart and G. K. Woo.
Life Sciences 15:1497 (1974).

Protective effect of ascorbic acid against cleft-palate formation in mice.
L. Y. Shih, C. Toliver and C. S. Yang.
Teratology 9:A-36 (1974).

Jejunal absorption of hexose in infants and adults.
M. K. Younoszai.
J. Ped. 85:446 (1974).

In vivo intestinal absorption of hexose in growth-retarded suckling rat pups.
M. K. Younoszai and Arlene Lynch.
J. Nutrition 104:671 (1974).

Gastrointestinal growth in normal male and female rats.
M. K. Younoszai and J. Ranshaw.

Appendix

Growth 38:225 (1974).

Deprivation of amino acids and prenatal brain development in rats.
S. Zamenhof.
J. Nutrition 104:1002 (1974).

Attention deficiencies in malnourished monkey.
Robert R. Zimmermann.
Sym. of the Swedish Nutr. Foundation XII (1974).

Piagetian object permanence in the infant rhesus monkeys.
Robert R. Zimmermann.
Development'l Psych., 10:429 (1974).

Cue-locus—A factor in the behavioral deficiency of the developing protein-malnourished monkey.
Robert R. Zimmermann.
Behavioral Biol. 10:473 (1974).

Absorption of intact protein by colonic epithelial cells of the rat.
B. S. Worthington and C. O. Enwonwu.
Am. J. Dig. Dis. 20:750 (1975).

Effects of high dietary cholesterol on the metabolism of tropoelastin and proteolytic enzymes in the chick aorta.
R. B. Rucker, W. Goettlich-Riemann, K. Tom, M. Chen, J. Poaster and S. Koerner.
J. Nutrition 105:46 (1975)

Influence of parenteral zinc and actinomycin D on tissue zinc uptake and the synthesis of a zinc-binding protein.
R. J. Cousins and M. P. Richards.
Bioinorganic Chem. 4:215 (1975).

Effect of low dietary calcium on chronic cadmium toxicity in rats.
R. J. Cousins and P. W. Washko.
Nutrition Reports Int'l. 11:113 (1975).

Perceptual and learning disabilities in children: Volume 2, research and theory.
W. M. Cruickshank and D. P. Hallahan, Editors.
Syracuse University Press (1975).

Feeding and drinking in suckling rats. Hunger: Basic mechanism and clinical implications.
A. N. Epstein.
BRI 1:15 (1975).

Nutritional significance of chromium in different chronological age groups and in populations differing in nutritional background.
C. T. Gurson.
Nutrition Reports Int'l. 12:9 (1975).

Jejunal perfusion of simple and conjugated folates in man.
C. H. Halsted, C. M. Baugh and C. E. Butterworth, Jr.
Gastroenterology 68:261 (1975).

Occurrence of celiac sprue in a patient with Fabry's disease.
C. H. Halsted and J. Rowe.
Ann. Intern. Med. 83:324 (1975).

Effects of amino acid imbalance and protein content of diets on food intake and preference of young, adult, and diabetic rats.
Y. Peng, L. L. Meliza, M. G. Vavich and A. R. Kemmerer.
Reprinted from the Journal of Nutrition 105:1395 (1975).

Characterization of an *in vitro* protein synthesis system from the cerebrum, cerebellum, and optic lobes of chick brain.
D. S. H. Liu, J. W. Yang and A. Richardson.
Transactions, Ill. State Acad. Sci. 68:2 (1975).

Amino acid imbalance in the liquid-fed lamb.
Quinton R. Rogers.
Aust. J. Biol. Science 28:168 (1975).

Maternal malnutrition and placental transfer of amino isobutric acid.
Pedro Rosso.
Science 187:648 (1975).

Changes in the transfer of nutrients across the placenta during normal gestation in the rat.
Pedro Rosso.
Am. J. Obstet. Gynec. 122:761 (1975).

Effect of maternal undernutrition or placental metabolism and function.
Pedro Rosso, M. Wasserman, J. Rozovski and E. Velasco.
Clin. Chem. (1975).

Interaction of infection and nutrition: some practical concerns.
I. H. Rosenberg., N. W. Solomons and D. Levin.
Ecology of Food and Nutrition, 4:203 (1975).

Genetic engineering.
S. E. Stumpf.
Vanderbilt Alumnus, Vol. 60 (1975).

Osteomalacia associated with anticonvulsant drug therapy in mentally retarded children.
K. G. Tolman, W. Jubiz, J. J. Sannella, J. A. Madsen, R. E. Belsey, R. S. Goldsmith and J. W. Freston.
Pediatrics 56:45 (1975).

Functional variations in the ultrastructure of the thyroid gland in malnourished infant monkeys.
B. S. Worthington and C. O. Enwonwu.
Am. J. Clin. Nutr. 28:66 (1975).

Appendix

Integration of nutrition in medical education.
  Eleanor Young and Elliot Wester.
  Journal of Nutrition Education 7:112 (1975).

In vivo D-Glucose absorption in the developing rat small intestine.
  M. K. Younoszai and A. Lynch.
  Pediat. Res. 9:130 (1975).

Appendix E

Future Leader Awardees
The Nutrition Foundation
1964-1975

November 1964
A. Kirksey
Purdue University

November 1964
L. W. Sullivan
N. J. College of Medicine & Dentistry

April 1965
T. F. Kellogg & B. S. Wostmann
University of Notre Dame

April 1965
Elaine R. Monsen
University of Washington, Seattle

November 1965
R. H. Feinberg
University of Tennessee

November 1965
Elveda Smith
Utah State University

April 1966
Myron Winick
Columbia University

November 1966
Aranella Kirksey
Purdue University

November 1966
J. L. Typpo
University of Missouri

April 1967
R. G. Brown
Drexel Institute of Technology

April 1967
G. E Bunce
Virginia Polytechnic Institute

April 1967
T. C. Campbell
Virginia Polytechnic Institute

April 1967
Quinton R. Rogers
University of California, Davis

April 1967
Barbara Underwood
Columbia University

April 1967
Frances Zeman
University of California, Davis

November 1967
R. A. Ahrens
University of Maryland

November 1967
W. G. Bergen
Michigan State University

November 1967
T. A. Borgese
*H. H. Lehman College of the
  City University of New York*

November 1967
T. W. Keenan
Purdue University

November 1967
Vernon R. Young
Massachusetts Institute of Technology

May 1968
Alfred J. Clark
University of California, Los Angeles

May 1968
Betty E. Haskell
University of California, Davis

Appendix

May 1968
Harold H. Sandstead
Vanderbilt University

November 1968
Dorice M. Czajka Narins
Michigan State University

November 1968
Susan M. Oace
University of California, Davis

November 1968
Oscar Pineda
Institute of Nutrition of Central America and Panama

November 1968
R. A. Scanlan
Oregon State University

November 1968
Pirkko R. Turkki
Syracuse University

May 1969
N. J. Benevenga
University of Wisconsin

May 1969
John A. Grove
South Dakota State University

November 1969
Roy G. Arnold
University of Nebraska

November 1969
Robert N. Brady
Vanderbilt University

November 1969
William S. Runyan
Iowa State University

November 1969
R. A. Wampler
Kansas State University

November 1969
R. E. Wrolstad
Oregon State University

May 1970
Robert G. Campbell
University of Rochester

May 1970
John W. Scott
Emory University

November 1970
Jose J. Corcino
University of Puerto Rico

November 1970
Johanna Dwyer
Harvard School of Public Health

May 1971
Helen L. Anderson
University of Missouri

May 1971
David A. Levitsky
Cornell University

May 1971
George E. Nicholads
Vanderbilt University School of Medicine

May 1971
M. K. Younoszai
University of Iowa

November 1971
Robert J. Cousins
Rutgers, The State University of New Jersey

November 1971
Robert B. Rucker
University of California, Davis

December 1972
James G. Bergan
University of Rhode Island

December 1972
Charles H. Halsted
The Johns Hopkins University

December 1972
Henry A. Jordan
University of Pennsylvania

December 1972
Roy J. Martin
Pennsylvania State University

December 1972
M. U. K. Mgbodile
Meharry Medical College

December 1972
Arlan Richardson
Illinois State University

December 1972
Chung-shu Yang
College of Medicine & Dentistry of New Jersey

May 1973
Joel A. Grinker
The Rockefeller University

May 1973
William C. MacLean, Jr.
The Johns Hopkins University

Appendix

May 1973
Pedro Rosso
Columbia University

November 1973
Michael C. Archer
Massachusetts Institute of Technology

November 1973
Gerald F. Russell
University of California, Davis

November 1973
Noel W. Solomons
University of Chicago and Pritzker School of Medicine

November 1973
Bonnie Sue Worthington
University of Washington, Seattle

May 1974
M. R. C. Greenwood
Columbia University

November 1974
Gordon Bailey
Chiang Mai Medical College, Thailand

Appendix F

Recipients of Awards Supported by The Nutrition Foundation

Recipients of The Babcock-Hart Award
(Formerly, 1948-1954, The Stephen M. Babcock Award)

Administered by the Institute of Food Technologists

1975
  Donald K. Tressler
  AVI Publishing Company

1974
  Bernard S. Schweigert
  The University of California, Davis

1973
  C. O. Chichester
  The University of Rhode Island

1972
  James W. Pence
  Western Marketing & Nutrition Research Division
  U.S. Department of Agriculture

1971
  Hisateru Mitsuda
  Kyoto University

1970
  Ricardo Bressani
  Institute of Nutrition of Central America and Panama

1969
  Samuel A. Goldblith
  Massachusetts Institute of Technology

1968
  A. I. Morgan, Jr.
  U.S. Department of Agriculture
    Western Regional Laboratory

1967
  W. B. Van Arsdel
  U.S. Department of Agriculture

1966
  Roderick K. Eskew
  U.S. Department of Agriculture
    Agricultural Research Service

1965
  Tetsuijiro Obara
  Tokyo University of Education

1964
  Robert R. Williams, President Research Corporation

1963
  M. A. Joslyn
  University of California, Berkeley

1962
  V. Subrahmanyan
  Central Food Technological Institute, Mysore, India

1961
  Emil M. Mrak
  University of California, Davis

1960
  Arnold Johnson
  National Dairy Products Corporation

1959
  Samuel Lepkovsky
  University of California, Berkeley

1958
  B. L. Oser
  Food and Drug Research Laboratories

1957
  E. M. Nelson
  Food and Drug Administration

Appendix

1956
Gail M. Dack
Food Research Institute, University of Chicago

1955
W. V. Cruess
University of California, Berkeley

1954
E. J. Cameron
National Canners Association

1953
C. N. Frey
Massachusetts Institute of Technology

1952
F. W. Tanner
University of Illinois

1951
S. C. Prescott
Massachusetts Institute of Technology

1950
Carl R. Fellers
University of Massachusetts

1949
Clarence Birdseye
Processes, Inc.

1948
F. C. Blanck
Mellon Institute, University of Pittsburgh

Recipients of The Joseph Goldberger Award
Administered by the Council on Foods and Nutrition of the American Medical Association

1975
Ananda S. Prasad
Wayne State University

1974
Robert Olson
Saint Louis University

1973
Clement A. Finch
University of Washington, Seattle

1972
George G. Graham
The Johns Hopkins University

1971
John E. Canham
The University of Iowa
Robert E. Hodges
U.S. Army Medical Research & Nutrition Laboratory

1970
Stanley J. Dudrick and Jonathan E. Rhoads
University of Pennsylvania

1969
Nevin S. Scrimshaw
Massachusetts Institute of Technology

1968
L. Emmett Holt, Jr.
New York University

1967
Cicely Williams
Institute of Social Medicine, Oxford

1966
William B. Castle
Thorndike Memorial Laboratory

1965
Grace A. Goldsmith
Tulane University

1964
William J. Darby
Vanderbilt University

1963
John B. Youmans
United Health Foundations, Inc.

1962
Edwards Albert Park
The Johns Hopkins Hospital

1961
Fredrick J. Stare
Harvard School of Public Health

1960
Richard W. Vilter
University of Cincinnati

1959
Carl V. Moore
Washington University

Appendix

1958
V. P. Sydenstricker
Medical College of Georgia

1957
Paul Gyorgy
Childrens Hospital of the University of Pennsylvania

1956
No recipient

1955
No recipient

1954
Russell M. Wilder
Mayo Clinic

1953
James S. McLester
McLester Clinic, Birmingham, Alabama

1952
William Henry Sebrell, Jr.
National Institutes of Health

1951
No recipient

1950
Fuller Albright
Harvard Medical School

1949
Randolph West
College of Physicians and Surgeons, Columbia University

Recipients of The Osborne & Mendel Award Administered by the American Institute of Nutrition

1975
B. Connor Johnson
College of Medicine, University of Oklahoma

1974
DeWitt S. Goodman
College of Physicians & Surgeons
Columbia University

1973
Hector F. DeLuca
University of Wisconsin

1972
Edwin T. Mertz
Purdue University

1971
Walter Mertz
U.S. Department of Agriculture

1970
Roslyn B. Alfin-Slater
University of California, Los Angeles

1969
Hamish N. Munro
Massachusetts Institute of Technology

1968
Charles H. Hill
North Carolina State University

1967
Samuel Lepkovsky
University of California, Berkeley

1966
Harold H. Mitchell
University of Illinois

1965
D. Mark Hegsted
Harvard School of Public Health

1964
L. Emmett Holt
N.Y.U. College of Medicine

1963
James B. Allison
Rutgers University

1962
William J. Darby
Vanderbilt University School of Medicine

1961
Max E. Horwitt
Elgin State Hospital

1960
Nevin S. Scrimshaw
Institute of Nutrition for Central America and Panama

1959
Grace A. Goldsmith
Tulane University

1958
Paul Gyorgy
Philadelphia General Hospital

Appendix

1957
George R. Cowgill
Yale University

1956
Albert G. Hogan
University of Missouri

1955
E. V. McCollum
The Johns Hopkins University

1954
Leonard M. Maynard
Cornell University

1953
Vincent du Vigneaud
Cornell University

1952
Icie Macy Hoobler
Children's Fund of Michigan

1951
Esmond E. Snell
University of Wisconsin

1950
Conrad A. Elvehjem
University of Wisconsin

1949
William C. Rose
University of Illinois

Recipients of The Mary Swartz Rose Award
Administered by the American Dietetic Association

1975
Judith L. Bonner

1974
Elizabeth Ann Schiller

1973
Charlotte May Thompson

1972
Leona R. Shapiro

1971
Betty Laura Beach

1970
Sister Mary Rosita Schiller

1969
Donna R. Watson

1968
Mary Bess Kohrs

1967
Lee Alyce Weller

1966
Marilyn Teschmacher Mower

1965
June Ann Krohn Clarke

1964
Rachel M. Ice Hubbard

1963
Annette T. Gormican

1962
Sara M. Hunt

1961
Gertrude Blaker

1960
Jerry M. Rivers

1959
Gladys Witt Strain

1958
Aimee L. Moore

1957
Elisabeth S. Yearick

1956
Aimee L. Moore

1955
Myrtle L. Brown

1954
Marjorie M. McKinley

1953
Margaret L. Ross

1952
Mary Kiefer Bloetjes

1951
Helen F. Barbour

1950
Pearl Jackson Aldrich

1949
Pearl Jackson

Appendix G

Reprint of The Food and Nutrition Board Twenty-Five Years in Retrospect 1940-1965

Introduction

A. G. Norman, *Chairman, Division of Biology and Agriculture*

There are certain milestones along the road traversed by men and by organizations. The Food and Nutrition Board reaches one of these milestones at this meeting. Twenty-five years have elapsed since its founding. It is therefore appropriate to mark the occasion by congratulations to the Board on its anniversary, by felicitations and expressions of deep respect and regard for its many distinguished accomplishments. This I do as Chairman of the Division of Biology and Agriculture of the National Academy of Sciences, within which administratively the Board rests. But I do it also, inadequately but sincerely, on behalf of President Seitz who deeply regretted his inability to be present, and charged me with the most pleasant task of expressing to you his appreciation of the multifarious services which the Board has performed to science and the nation through this 25-year period and his confidence that in the years ahead the Board will continue to occupy an important place in the Academy-Research Council structure.

When one pauses at one of these milestones, one may do several things—one can look back with some pride, perhaps not untouched by the powers of hindsight, at the road that has been traversed and the hills that have been scaled. One can stop to draw a breath and perhaps contemplate a little the contemporary scene and one's relevance to it. One can look ahead into a region of poor visibility and try to discern the features of the countryside to be surmounted. I hope that as individuals you will try each of these from your own vantage points; collectively as a Board, the agenda of your sessions makes provision for this.

It is notable that the Food and Nutrition Board has had a somewhat unusual sense of continuity and that some members have given of their service for many years. We should, I believe, pay special tribute to the small group of far-sighted scientists who were responsible for its creation and establishment a quarter of a century ago. Some of those are present today, as are others who were members in the early years when its efforts had to become recognized and gain acceptance. We do honor those of the Board who were its founding fathers and pioneering leaders. The circumstances under which it came into being will be referred to by Dr. Glen King and Dr. Maynard who speak with the authority of participants. It is not for me to do more than point out to you that the world of science in 1940 was indeed a very different place from the world of 1965—this far have we come in a single generation. At that time, the development and evolution of science depended in great measure on the separate efforts of individual scientists. There were no great federal programs, there was not as yet fully understood the great power of organized science and science-based technology. Federal expenditures for science were miniscule by present standards—and were expended primarily by the Department of Agriculture and for government installations such as the Bureau of Standards. Scientists were not mobile—they met together infrequently at professional society meetings and on similar occasions—west coast scientists rarely met with east coast scientists. It was therefore only quite serious business that would cause a geographically dispersed group to be brought together to address themselves to questions of mutual interest. The nation had emerged painfully from an extended economic depression, and was uneasily regarding the dark storm clouds of armed conflict in Europe that so soon were to spread to our shores. This, therefore, was the general context in which the Board was formed.

Appendix

Though I cannot speak with any assurance on this point, the Academy-Research Council under whose auspices it developed, had not yet found the place and role which has emerged for it since World War II, even though the unique advisory service which it provides to the government and other agencies was clearly recognized in its charter. More than a passive role was envisaged, more than willingness to respond if called upon. It is now the primary objective of the Academy and its Research Council to bring together the most competent scientists and engineers in the country in appropriate groups to deal with contemporary scientific problems of all sorts, and to exchange information in the furtherance of research and the strengthening of the national welfare. There is therefore a creative role for some of our Boards and Committees who exercise continuing surveillance over the scientific developments bearing on their field of interest, and as they deem to be appropriate, initiate studies, make recommendations or alert the proper groups or agencies to actions which might be taken.

The Food and Nutrition Board has traditionally operated in this way. It has not had the continuing program advisory relationship to a single agency that occupy some of our other Boards. It does include in its interests a broad range of problems stretching all the way from basic topics in nutritional science to applied problems of food technology.

Perhaps the one most important feature which has permitted the adoption of this desirably independent stance by the Board has been steady financial support at an adequate level. This, of course, has been supplemented many times for specific tasks which the Board has identified or have been brought to it, but unlike certain other of the Boards of the Academy, it has not been wholly dependent on acceptance of funds for a sequence of unrelated tasks, which of course presents difficulties in retaining a professional staff of quality.

It is appropriate, therefore, to acknowledge and pay tribute to those foundations and more recently those food industries, commercial laboratories and the like who have been willing and far-sighted enough to provide adequately for the continuing support of the Board and some of its major activities—those of the Food Protection Committee and the Codex, for example. Perhaps I am sufficiently old fashioned to think that we should not always have to turn to the Federal Government in such matters. We can, I think, feel gratified and comfortable about this aspect of the Board's support. To representatives of the sponsoring foundations and industrial groups that may be present, I would express thanks and commend them on their judgment.

One ought also not to allow this occasion to pass without reference to the fact that not only has there been an unusual degree of continuity on the Board, but also in the person of its executive staff, and particularly of course in that Roy Voris has for so many years served the Board loyally and devotedly. There is never any doubt as to where his primary interests lie—the Board and its programs come first every time. In asking me to open this program, he suggested that my remarks might be directed towards "the place of the Board in the National Academy of Sciences-National Researach Council and the Division of Biology and Agriculture." I was not sure just what he had in mind, being temporarily stunned by the ponderous quality of the title, and am definitely uneasy as to whether my remarks up to this point have conformed to his request.

Although the Academy traditionally and organizationally reflects the sharp disciplinary division of the basic sciences, its activities through the Research Council, its Divisions, and their Boards and Committees are overwhelmingly concerned with the application of science and its extension into technology. The problems studied and the advice rendered usually require diverse disciplinary inputs. Many of the recommendations or conclusions involve balanced judgments, the setting of standards, the weighing of risks, the prediction of probabilities. The welfare or interests of the public are frequently involved. Assignments of this sort seem to be competently and responsibly handled; in many ways we have something like a court of science with the impartiality and integrity that one demands of a court. When however one looks at those activities of the Division that relate more to the furtherance and development of science rather than to its application we seem to be less effective, at least in the Division of Biology. It is not at all clear to me why this is so; we are of course not a research organization, but the powerful combinations of minds that we bring together in our deliberations might well give a little more of their time and their talents to the identification of the scientific events involved in the applied problems and what should be done to elucidate them. In the Division at present the Executive Committee is addressing itself to a strengthening of this aspect of our role and I hope that this Board, as it stops to draw breath and contemplate a little the contemporary scene, will also do so. I await with great interest the remarks of the Chairman on this subject later this morning. I have an intuitive feeling that nutritional science is due for another burst of activity that might lead to giant strides forward. When I was a student in college the exciting things in biochemistry were those relating to nutrition, the discovery of the vitamins and their structure, the role of essential elements and the like. Some of you

Appendix

indeed played a great part in such work. Biochemistry has flowered almost unbelievably since then and the cellular and molecular biochemists look at metabolic events of great complexity with great understanding. It should be possible to analyze nutritional sequences with equal perception.

In closing let me again refer to the passage of milestones, which in the aggregate is history. This Board has a proud history and can look forward to performing for the next 25 year period with equal grace and distinction.

The History and Philosophy of the Food and Nutrition Board Including Its International Activities

C. G. King, *Vice Chairman, Food and Nutrition Board*

The Food and Nutrition Board now has a history of twenty-five years of steady growth in accomplishments. If experience is indicative of our future, the opportunities ahead should continue to challenge our best efforts for many years. Like each of our parent organizations, the National Academy of Sciences and the National Research Council, we were born in a period of war emergency. We may again be called upon to serve in international strife, but hopefully, the scene may change some day so that we can be as successful in preventing wars as we have been fortunate in serving to meet them during the past century.

As a result of the initiative shown by such leaders as Paul E. Howe, M. L. Wilson, Russell M. Wilder, and Thomas Parran in 1940, a Committee on Foods and Nutrition was established within the Division of Biology and Agriculture in the National Academy of Sciences-National Research Council, with Dr. Wilder serving as the first chairman. The driving force for its organization came directly from the Council on National Defense, and was guided largely by the personal interest and enthusiasm of M. L. Wilson, then Assistant Secretary of Agriculture. Dr. Wilder was brought into the picture on recommendation from the Division of Medical Sciences, but he quickly sensed the necessity of building a program wider in scope and with greater freedom of action within the Division of Biology and Agriculture.

Of the 21 members appointed in 1940, there were eight biochemists, seven physicians, two home economists, two agricultural economists, one food industry executive, and one food technologist:

John D. Black
Henry Borsook
Frank G. Boudreau
George R. Cowgill
Joseph S. Davis
Martha M. Elliot
Conrad A. Elvehjem
Icie Macy Hoobler
Phillip C. Jeans
Norman Jolliffe
Glen King
L. A. Maynard
James S. McLester
Helen Mitchell
S. C. Prescott
Lydia J. Roberts
William C. Rose
G. Cullen Thomas
Russell M. Wilder
Robert R. Williams
John B. Youmans

In 1941, nine additional members were appointed, including five biochemists, two physicians, one home economist, and one physiologist:

Franklin C. Bing
Paul E. Howe
E. V. McCollum
John R. Murlin
E. M. Nelson
W. H. Sebrell, Jr.
H. C. Sherman
Louise Stanley
Frederick F. Tisdall

From that time forward, there has been a slow but steady rotational change, averaging about two or three per year.

Although not regular members of the Committee, special acknowledgment for wholehearted administrative support is due Thomas Parran, then Surgeon General; Robert Griggs, chairman of the division, NAS-NRC; and Ross Harrison, chairman of the Executive Committee of the NRC. In addition, the Board has been continuously blessed with strong leadership in its chairmen, as shown by the successive terms of Dr. Boudreau, Dr. Maynard, Dr. Elvehjem, and Dr. Goldsmith. We have been equally fortunate in the succession of highly competent office staff as illustrated by the executive secretaries, Helen Mitchell, Frank Gunderson, and LeRoy Voris. All through the history of the Board, a key role has been exercised by the Executive Committee in relation to policies, committee appointments, finances, and long-range planning.

Dr. Wilder, then chairman of the Department of Medicine at the Mayo Clinic, had had extensive experience in clinical nutrition. He very adroitly maintained liaison with the Medical Sciences Division by continuing for a time as chairman of their subcommittee on nutrition. Thus he could report both ways and speak for both divisions until he was ready to release the subcommittee to Dr. James McLester.

Appendix

He was truly an inspiring leader, with endless enthusiasm and a saving sense of humor. His spontaneous warmth of spirit was sorely tried, however, on one occasion, when he discovered that a less dignified committeeman had brought to a dinner meeting of the Board a candid camera record of Dr. Wilder in the Academy foyer drinking lustily from a bottle of Coca Cola. Officially, he was a knight in armor, ever ready to attack the dangers hidden in the limited nutritive value of such foods as sugar, white flour, and corn meal, he loved to call vitamin B_1 "the morale vitamin."

The clouds of war were rolling up in ominous fashion, and the electrified spirit of the times was indicated by Dr. Wilder in his charge to the new Committee:

> It is no longer a question of a few experts in our colleges and research centers talking about vitamins and minerals. What we must do now is make people understand that nutrition is not an academic matter but a thoroughly practical consideration, concerning every person in the country—producers, processors, marketers, consumers, nutritional experts—everyone!

Under this broad directive, the Committee, which was soon given the status of a Board, established liaison representation with organizations inside and outside the Academy, including representation from Canada. Specific tasks were assigned to committees with a clear understanding that we were to exercise the combined sense of judgment and urgency of a nation girding for all-out war.

Immediately we were to take stock of the national situation with respect to the extent, nature, and causes of malnutrition, and to make recommendations for programs of correction. Questions of a direct military nature were given high priority in every respect.

Historically, in the United States, research and education in foods and nutrition had been chiefly in agricultural institutions instead of medical or public health schools. Hence, placement of the Board in the Division of Biology and Agriculture had general approval. Experience demonstrated that by having highly qualified medical and agricultural personnel on the Board, the problem of rapport between the various professional disciplines in nutrition was solved very satisfactorily.

Among other debated questions were:
(a) Should members of government agencies or from industry have Board membership or only liaison participation? Obviously there were risks of clashes on policy with a particular government agency, or
(b) a partisan interest for industrial advantage. In both instances, after serious debate, it was decided that the integrity and professional stature of the individual should be the deciding factor. Excellent illustrations of this point are seen in the early appointments of E. M. Nelson, from the Food and Drug Administration, W. H. Sebrell, Jr., from the Public Health Service, and Cullen Thomas, from the General Mills Company. Traditionally, however, the practice has been to select a chairman from an independent institution and to rotate in reasonable degree between the fields of medicine and biochemistry. The same policy has been followed with respect to committee chairmen.

Primarily to protect its independence, the Board also maintained a core budget from independent sources instead of being dependent on a single government agency or industry. Dr. Boudreau succeeded in obtaining such support from the Milbank Fund, the Williams-Waterman Fund, and the Nutrition Foundation. Funds for special projects, however, have been accepted much more freely. Large grants, for example, were used in support of the Committee on Food Composition, the Food Protection Committee, and the Committee on Protein Malnutrition.

Direct advisory services for the military forces included liaison representation from the respective Surgeons General and the Quartermaster General. In this area, Colonel Paul Howe gave outstanding leadership. He had in fact been one of the earliest persons to alert the Defense Commission to the urgency for a food and nutrition program. His private battles with representatives of the Quartermaster General added color and excitement to many meetings of the Board.

Two basic problems were of equal interest to civilians and military personnel:

(a) First was the need for a quantitative estimate of the human nutrient requirements for vigorous health, for all age groups, and under all normal or special circumstances; and

(b) second was the need for an estimate of the quantities of practical food materials that would furnish such requirements. Out of these studies came (a) the first Board report on Recommended Dietary Allowances, with Lydia Roberts serving as chairman of the Committee, and (b) a report on Food Composition, with Conrad Elvehjem serving as committee chairman.

Another major activity was the M-Day Committee, to handle urgent matters of procurement and personnel assignment, with Glen King as chairman. Problems of priorities for equipment, supplies, and scientific personnel called for constant attention, as illustrated by the crucial needs of the chemical and food

Appendix

industries, and the need to keep a balance between scientists needed in civilian service or in military establishments. The Merck Company, for example, had a real fight to get priorities for materials and personnel to construct as quickly as possible, a new plant to produce the vitamins essential to the flour and bread enrichment program. Incidental to this experience, Dr. James Crabtree and I were designated to draft a letter for General Parran to sign and forward to the President, setting the basis for War Order #1, which established the flour and bread enrichment program.

Dr. Boudreau guided a special committee on Industrial, In-Plant Feeding, and Dr. H. D. Kruse served as chairman of a special committee on techniques of identifying specific forms of clinical malnutrition. During this period, micro methods of blood analysis were advanced rapidly, especially by Dr. Otto Bessey and Dr. Oliver Lowry. Frequent reports were made of research progress of interest to the military forces, such as water sparing emergency rations, high protein diets during convalescence from burns and other forms of injury, and low fat-high carbohydrate rations for maximum altitude tolerance.

Even in dealing with such serious matters, there were lighter moments. On one occasion Dr. McLester chided our research-minded committeemen and intoned that what the military personnel needed was immediate answers from experts instead of a slow reply based on research. Then he submitted two lists of food for the Air Force—one giving foods they should eat, and another, foods they should not eat—but he yielded, when we pointed out that he had placed some of the foods in both lists. Again, after repeated and heated debates on whether rum should be included in our lifeboat rations, a strong plea was made that even though there was no physiological basis to support the practice, we should follow the British in furnishing rum because they had had so much experience at sea. A few days later word came from London that the British had discontinued the practice.

One of the shocking observations from medical examinations of enlisted men was the high incidence of rejections because of tooth decay. This stimulated the Board to prepare, with the assistance of Gerald Cox, a much needed monograph on "A Survey of the Literature on Dental Caries," and a brochure on "Control of Tooth Decay."

The Food Protection Committee proved to be one of the most significant of the Board's activities. The successive chairmen, Dr. H. E. Longenecker and Dr. W. J. Darby, and the secretarial staff guided by Dr. Voris and Dr. Johnson, have served remarkably well. Long before Congressman Delaney created the unfortunate political myth of zero tolerance, or the public was denied cranberries for Thanksgiving and Christmas, on the assumption that some people might eat more than one ton per day for a long time, or the publication of *Silent Spring*, Dr. Elmer M. Nelson in the Food and Drug Administration had reported promptly and accurately to the Board on the need for new measures to safeguard the public food supply. His reports on finding minute quantities of penicillin and DDT in milk supplies spearheaded the appointment of the Food Protection Committee.

International cooperation has always been a strong feature of the Board's program, particularly in working with Canadian, Latin American, and British groups. We shall always be indebted to Dr. Boudreau for his experience and guidance in international affairs, and his bringing to the Board such guests as Lord Boyd Orr and others from all over the world. During the war years, the need for working closely with our allies was clear and urgent, both in military matters and in relation to civilian health. From 1946 onward this aspect of the Board's service continued to have strong emphasis in keeping with a similar trend throughout the Academy. For example, publications on Recommended Dietary Allowances, policies on food enrichment, industrial feeding management, Tables of Food Composition, Heat Injury to Proteins, Maternal Nutrition and Child Health, Literature of Dental Caries, Control of Tooth Decay, Therapeutic Nutrition, Analytical Methods for Pesticides, Safety of Intentional Chemical Additives to Food, Safety of Artificial Sweeteners, Safety of Mono- and Diglycerides, The Role of Dietary Fat in Human Health, Evaluation of Protein Nutrition, The Role of Nutrition in International Programs, Meeting Protein Needs of Infants and Children, Radionuclides in Foods, Evaluation of Protein Quality, and Recommendations on Administrative Policies for International Food and Nutrition Programs, all have had a broad interest internationally.

One of the most important functions of the Board, internationally, has been the research and educational work of the Committee on Protein Malnutrition. The Committee was organized under the chairmanship of Dr. Sebrell to request and administer two grants totaling $550,000, from the Rockefeller Foundation, with which to support the work of outstanding nutrition scientists in a coordinated, international program to combat protein malnutrition, particularly in mothers and pre-school children. The work was planned and conducted primarily in cooperation with independent nutrition scientists, but also with the advice and cooperation of the Protein Advisory Group and staff members of FAO, WHO, and UNICEF.

Appendix

Just preceding the Sixth International Congress in Edinburgh, the Rockefeller Foundation was host to a special conference at the Villa Serbelloni, Lake Como, Italy, organized by Paul Gyorgy, to accelerate action programs on "Prevention of Malnutrition in the Pre-School Child." A brief summary of the conference was presented by Maurice Pate, Executive Director of UNICEF, at the Edinburgh meeting, and wide distribution of this report was made possible by UNICEF.

Toward the end of the study, in December, 1964, an international conference was held in Washington, under the chairmanship of Dr. Sebrell, to review progress and to establish a basis for worldwide action programs to prevent protein-calorie malnutrition. The Proceedings will appear soon in a special monograph. Meanwhile, for educational purposes, a layman's summary of the monograph was published and given wide distribution, during the summer of 1965.

Members of the Board have represented both the National Academy of Sciences and the American Institute of Nutrition in each of the six successive International Congresses of Nutrition. Dr. F. B. Morrison and I were privileged to serve as delegates to the first organizing Congress held in London in 1946, under the chairmanship of Sir Joseph Barcroft.

Plans for the Seventh International Congress of Nutrition in Hamburg, Germany, August 3-10, 1966, are developing well under the presidency of Professor Dr. J. Kuhnau, as indicated by preliminary announcements from the General Secretary, Professor Dr. U. Ritter, Martinistrasse 52, Hamburg 2, West Germany. The Board is represented in planning for the Congress by myself as a vice-president and by Dr. O. L. Kline as chairman of the U.S. National Committee for the IUNS.

The U.S. National Committee, as the adhering body from the National Academy of Sciences and the American Institute of Nutrition, has forwarded draft copies of suggested by-law revisions for the IUNS. If approved by the IUNS, the new by-laws will accompany a petition of the IUNS for membership in the International Council of Scientific Unions, to be presented by Sir David Cuthbertson, president of the IUNS, at their next meeting in Bombay, India. Dr. Harrison Brown and Mr. E. C. Rowan in the Academy office have been very helpful in preparing the draft copy.

Participation of the Board in the forthcoming International Biological Program is represented formally by the former chairman of the Biology and Agriculture Division of the National Research Council, Dr. T. C. Byerly, and by Dr. George K. Davis, chairman of the Subcommittee on Use and Management of Biological Resources. Dr. Davis has a major responsibility for developing a nutrition program as an integral part of the IBP. Thus far only preliminary plans for the program have been released.

The Board is grateful for the strong support we have had from the presidents of the Academy, and the chairmen of the National Research Council, in forwarding our communications on national and international programs to high ranking government officials. We have been assured, for example, that the recently improved policies on foods and nutrition within the Agency for International Development and the Food For Peace program resulted substantially from recommendations prepared and submitted by the Board. These changes urged by the Board and put into action are almost certain to mean fewer deaths, less blindness, less sickness, less stunting of physical and mental development, and higher standards of living for many millions of people in areas where malnutrition is now a major challenge to human health and survival.

The worldwide improvements in nutrition that the Board is working toward should have their greatest direct effect on the health of pre-school children. This alone would be rewarding enough, but we are justified also in the belief and hope that the prospect of peace among the nations has been at least favored by the enlightened policies and programs that we have recommended.

Contributions of the Food and Nutrition Board to National Nutrition Programs

L. A. Maynard

From the outset the Board was concerned with national nutrition programs. At its first meeting, November 26-27, 1940, Dr. M. L. Wilson, recently appointed to head a National Program of Nutrition, raised specific questions both as to nutritional policies and procedures for carrying them out, stating that the Government would rely on the Board for guidance.

As an immediate need Dr. Wilson mentioned food standards for government planning. Accordingly, Dr.

Appendix

Wilder appointed a committee headed by Dr. Lydia Roberts to make recommendations the next morning on "desirable levels of known food factors with suggestions for ways of reaching these levels"—some assignment! The next day she reported dietary requirements for calories and nine nutrients, for consideration by the Board. Following much further study, with the assistance of many nutritionists throughout the country, a table of Recommended Daily Allowances was approved at the Board meetings in March and May, 1941, distributed to government agencies and others, and published in early 1943. Naturally, particularly in view of the limited knowledge at the time, decisions involved much debate. One Board member said the thiamine allowance should be 10 mg.!

Upon release, these allowances found immediate use in food production and nutrition education programs, and as guides for rationing as shortages occurred. As you know, there have been repeated revisions of the RDA, as new information has developed, the last, issued in 1964. Each revision has represented the work of several subcommittees. The Allowances have made outstanding contributions in nutrition education programs, in helping to assess nutritional status and, most of all perhaps, in stimulating further research. They have also formed the basis for standards set up by several foreign countries.

At the first meeting of the Board, the question of the enrichment of white flour and bread came under discussion and a proposal of the Council on Foods of the AMA, previously given at a Food and Drug Hearing, was endorsed. The Board presented a statement on flour and bread enrichment at the National Nutrition Conference for Defense held in May, 1941, a Conference which the Board had helped organize and conduct. The Conference endorsed the proposals of the Board, and an active national program to carry them out was initiated. So began a program in which the Board continued active for many years under the guidance of the Committee on Cereals appointed early in 1941. There was compulsory enrichment of flour and bread during the war years, followed by voluntary enrichment by the large millers and bakers and, later, by the enactment of compulsory legislation in most states. The Board actively supported these developments and also turned its attention to other cereals, notably corn and rice, with constructive results.

At the same time it actively opposed proposed food fortifications which it did not consider nutritionally needed or desirable. In late 1941, in response to a request from the Food and Drug Administration, it issued a "Statement of Policy in the Matter of Addition of Specific Nutrients to Foods." This statement approved the addition of certain nutrients to specific foods and opposed others. Guidelines for future decisions were laid down. This policy statement was reissued with minor revisions in 1948, 1953, 1958, and 1961. It has had a very salutary influence on food manufacturing and marketing practices, and on public education as well.

Evidence of the nutritional and health benefits from the enrichment program has become clear from clinical and dietary surveys. The program has reached almost every member of the population—a unique overall contribution to national nutrition. The effective leader in achieving this contribution was the Chairman of the Cereal Committee, Dr. R. R. Williams.

At the first meeting of the Board, Dr. Wilson stated that there might be problems in industrial feeding needing attention, and shortly thereafter a Committee on Nutrition of Industrial Workers was organized, with Dr. Boudreau as Chairman. Initially the committee made investigations by questionnaires and plant visits, and found that little attention was being given to the nutrition of industrial workers. It recommended a federal program of nutrition education, and also controlled studies to get evidence that would forestall opposition from both labor and management to action programs. It prepared a pamphlet entitled, "The Food and Nutrition of Industrial Workers in Wartime," published in April 1942 and widely distributed.

As a result of a request from Dr. Wilson's office for a detailed program for attacking the problems of nutrition in industry, it submitted a statement including 12 points and recommendations. These recommendations were utilized by an Industrial Nutrition Unit which had been created in Dr. Wilson's office. In October 1943 an Interdepartmental Committee for Food for Workers was established to coordinate and intensify programs. To assist in these programs the Committee prepared a "Manual on Industrial Feeding."

By these activities, the Committee was responsible in large measure for developing an awareness of the importance of the better nutrition of industrial workers, and for spelling out procedures which proved effective in accomplishing the objective.

Upon our entry into World War II the problem of producing and distributing a food supply adequate for the armed forces and the civilian population and for sharing with our allies became of crucial importance. Thus in 1942 the Board was called upon by various government agencies for recommendations on the following questions:

Appendix

1. Guides for the rationing of milk, with particular reference to the vulnerable groups; the utilization of skim milk.
2. The role of sugar in the diet and directions for its rationing both to civilians and the food industries.
3. The nutritive value of fats, and the oleo-butter problem.
4. Nutritional implications of meat rationing, minimum desirable daily allowances, and the usefulness of various vegetable sources of protein.
5. Civilian needs for synthetic vitamins and vitamin concentrates, to guide allocations of raw materials to industry for their increased production.

There were many other questions of lesser general significance.

These questions could not be answered off the cuff, but strenuous activity by the Board's committees already functioning and new ones appointed quickly resulted in recommendations which made large contributions to the war effort. The work of these committees later resulted in the publication of extensive reports which had long-time value as guides to research in food and nutrition.

By government request as an aid to production planning, in 1942 the Board classified some 120 foods and food groups into three categories for wartime emergency conditions as follows: 1. Essential for continuance in the wartime emergency; 2. Intermediate in essentiality; 3. Dispensable or non-essential, at least during the emergency.

By a request from the Army in 1942, the Board submitted a documented report: "Minimum Allowances of Dietary Essentials for the Armed Services." It also answered several specific questions concerned with the nutritive value of army rations, and set up a Committee on Food Composition to obtain further information, under the chairmanship of Dr. C. A. Elvehjem. This committee of 16 members was concerned with: the tabulation of data on food composition, the analysis of army rations and studies of dehydrated foods. The composition data, except those for army rations, were included in a joint publication of the committee and the Bureau of Human Nutrition and Home Economics.

From January 1942 to June 1945 the Board held 23 full two-day meetings interspersed by meetings of the Executive Committee and committees serving specific fields.

For some time after the war the Board continued to be concerned with questions of food allocation, particularly in view of the continuing needs of our allies and efforts to alleviate semi-starvation in several European countries. With rationing still in effect it supplied the Government, by request, a detailed report: "ND Allowances for Temporary Food Shortages Necessitating Rationing."

The Board also began studies of new problems, in part highlighted by the war emergency and its aftermath. A bulletin prepared by the Committee on Diagnosis and Pathology of Nutritional Deficiencies, and published in late 1943, had reported evidence of widespread deficiencies as revealed both by dietary surveys and clinical data. As rationing was put into practice the need became urgent for current data on nutritional status, a need emphasized by questions from the War Production Board in 1944. A Committee on Nutrition Surveys, with Dr. King as Chairman, was appointed to consider methods of measuring nutritional status and to promote action programs. In 1949, a report was published: "Nutrition Surveys: Their Techniques and Value." There were later activities of the committee through 1954 under the chairmanship of Dr. R. E Shank. The reports had a large influence in emphasizing the importance of continuing dietary and clinical surveys and in stimulating their undertaking by individuals and later by government agencies.

The Committee on Milk continued active after the war, centering its attention on the greater use of skim milk, the production of which was being little utilized as human food. In 1946 it published a report: "Need for a Program to Effect Wider Use of Skim Milk Solids in Food," which had a wide influence on making the public aware of their nutritive values and in promoting their use accordingly. Among later activities in this field, a very important contribution was made in supervising a two-year, nationwide survey of milk regulations and the quality of milk as marketed. A comprehensive report, published in 1953, had a substantial influence for the improvement of market practices.

Recognizing that the special nutritional needs in pregnancy and lactation were not receiving adequate attention, in 1946 the Board appointed a Committee on Maternal and Child Feeding under the chairmanship of Dr. Icie M. Hoobler. In 1950 a bulletin was published entitled: "Maternal Nutrition and Child Health," which proved of great value to public health agencies and others concerned with the broad problem. In the same year, with a revision in 1953, a comprehensive bulletin on the composition of milks—human, cow, and goat, with data for calories, proteins, fats, 19 fatty acids, 31 mineral elements, 18 amino acids and 17 vitamins, was issued. These comparative data proved of great value for the devis-

Appendix

ing of milk formulas for infants and for studies of their usefulness. Special consideration of the problem of infant nutrition was renewed with the appointment of a new committee in 1959, under the chairmanship of Dr. R. L. Jackson. It reviewed methods and results of studies of infant nutrition and, as a result, contributed importantly to the solution of the controversial problem of protein requirements.

During the war period and its aftermath the Committee on Protein Foods under the chairmanship of Dr. W. C. Rose, was very active in dealing with problems of the supply and nutritional quality of protein foods. Around 1950 the Board's activities in the field of protein nutrition concentrated on the amino acids, and a committee with Dr. J. B. Allison as chairman made many studies which resulted in two comprehensive publications: "The Evaluation of Protein Nutrition with Emphasis on Amino Acid Proportionalities," in 1957, and "The Evaluation of Protein Nutrition," in 1962. These publications provided fine summaries of current knowledge and highlighted questions needing further research.

The Board's wartime Committee on Fat dealt with problems of supply, body needs and the controversial margarine-butter problem. In 1955 questions in debate as to the possible role of fat and specific fatty acids in promoting circulatory troubles caused the Board to give special attention to these questions, since both important foods and health were involved. In 1958 the Board published a judicial and well documented bulletin, "The Role of Fat in Human Nutrition," which set forth present knowledge on the questions at issue, did much to quell undue concern and, most important, stimulated further and better controlled research. As the general problem grew in importance and in complication, the Board appointed a new committee under the chairmanship of Dr. C. S. Davidson, to revise the previous report as needed, particularly in the light of new medical findings. In 1962 it was reprinted in revised form. Since then the Committee has been working on a new publication, "Dietary Fat in Human Health," covering the manifold aspects of the overall problem. When issued it should make a very important contribution in this perplexing field.

Such is the story, condensed into the time alloted me, of important contributions of the Board to national nutrition, except those discussed by others in this program.

Basic Science Contributions of the Board

Grace A. Goldsmith, *Chairman, Food and Nutrition Board*

The science of nutrition is both a basic and an applied science. We have difficulty defining it as it cuts across many areas. The Food and Nutrition Board has made contributions to many of these areas, and perhaps I can point out a few of these.

In the course of the Board's activities and deliberations, current knowledge of the basic aspects of the science of nutrition has been summarized, unsolved problems delineated, and new research stimulated. Acting on its own initiative or in response to questions directed to it by various agencies, the Board has examined many areas of nutrition science through its appointed committees of experts in diverse fields. It has carried out extensive search for data, has evaluated and interpreted findings, and has provided an accurate picture of existing information. Numerous monographs have been prepared, and you have heard about a number of them from the previous speakers. These monographs have served, and continue to serve, as references or texts in specific areas of the science of nutrition.

Questions often arose in the course of deliberations of the Board's committees which could not be answered. In such instances, research was stimulated by the Board or its committees or by the publications of the Board. This research has often resulted in the needed answers. I believe that many of these investigations might not have been undertaken without an advisory group of this kind.

One of the first challenges to the Board—perhaps it was even one of the reasons for its appointment—was the development of recommendations for nutrient intakes that would provide good nutrition, health, and working capacity for the population of the United States during the exigencies of war. This initial activity resulted in publication of Recommended Dietary Allowances in 1943. Development of this dietary standard or nutritional goal was not easy. It necessitated evaluation of all of the basic nutrition research which could contribute information relative to nutritive requirements of man. This review indicated serious gaps in knowledge. One of the activities of the Board, a most interesting one, which was started in 1942, has assisted greatly in filling some of these gaps.

Appendix

This was a collaborative effort of the Food and Nutrition Board and the Elgin State Hospital. The studies that have been conducted at Elgin have significantly extended knowledge of human nutritional requirements. The laboratory there has been, and still is, under the direction of Dr. Max Horwitt. Dr. Wilder was Chairman of the first committee dealing with the activities at Elgin State Hospital, and he appreciated that this particular setting provided an unusual opportunity for carrying out long-term studies of human nutritional needs under controlled conditions. This project resulted in the establishment of the L. B. Mendel Research Laboratory, which has been a model for human metabolic experiments ever since, and was the forerunner of developments elsewhere of similar nature.

The investigations carried out at Elgin have made numerous important contributions to knowledge of the human requirements for thiamine, riboflavin, and niacin. The early investigations, entitled Human Requirements of the B Complex Vitamins, were published as Bulletin No. 116 of the National Research Council. Subsequent studies from this laboratory have appeared in many professional journals. In recent years, studies of requirements for vitamin E were carried out, including relationships of this vitamin to polyunsaturated fatty acids. In association with the human studies, there were many animal experiments and many basic biochemical investigations, all of which shed light on the metabolism of the vitamins being studied.

Recently, the Food and Nutrition Board's Committee on Studies at Elgin State Hospital has been discontinued. The L. B. Mendel Laboratory has so thoroughly established its role in research that sponsorship by the Board is no longer needed. We are most grateful for the many activities of the Elgin State Hospital.

Another consequence of the development of Recommended Dietary Allowances in 1943 was the necessity for provision of tables of food composition, so that allowances might be met by diets of ordinary food. This was accomplished by a Committee on Food Composition. In 1950 a bulletin on the Composition of Milks (No. 119) was compiled and published by the Board.

Recommended Dietary Allowances have been revised every five years since 1943, so that new information might be incorporated as it became available. On several occasions the Board has had to stimulate research to add to knowledge of nutrient requirements. When the importance of vitamin B_6 in human nutrition became apparent, a conference was called to summarize existing information and to point out areas for future research. On another occasion, it appeared that the protein requirements of infants has not been adequately studied and further work was fostered in this area. This work has resulted in more precise data for this age group. Calcium requirements were also the subject of investigation of a special committee and currently iron requirements are receiving attention.

Another aspect of the Board's activities in the area of human needs was the development of recommendations of nutrient intake for survival during periods of emergency.

The Board has made numerous contributions to the medical aspects of the science of nutrition and some of these are basic as well as applied. In 1943, the Committee on Diagnosis and Pathology of Nutritional Deficiencies published a bulletin on the prevalence and significance of nutritional deficiencies in the United States. In 1944, a request was received for information concerning methods by which the nutritional wellbeing of the public could be tested periodically. This resulted in the appointment of a Committee on Nutrition Surveys, and in 1949 a bulletin was published entitled "Nutrition Surveys: Their Techniques and Value." This publication summarized objectives, methods, findings, and their interpretation, and usefulness of dietary, clinical, and biochemical aspects of nutrition surveys. Since then, many other groups have contributed to this important subject of the evaluation of nutritional status.

In 1950 a comprehensive textbook, Clinical Nutrition, edited by Drs. Norman Jolliffe, Frederick Tisdale, and Paul Cannon, was published under the sponsorship of the Food and Nutrition Board. Subsequently, the application of nutritional therapy in the recovery from disease, surgery, and injury was reviewed by a Committee on Therapeutic Nutrition, with emphasis on military applications. The Board also reviewed the subject of nutrition and dental caries, and the role of fluoride in the prevention of caries, as has been mentioned by previous speakers. A brochure on maternal and child nutrition sponsored by the Board has also been mentioned this morning. Another publication dealing with medical nutrition was one on sodium-restricted diets.

In the 1950's, the importance of protein and specific amino acids in nutrition became the subject of extensive research. The Board, accordingly, appointed a Committee on Amino Acids and a bulletin was published in 1959 entitled "The Evaluation of Protein Nutrition." This dealt with basic concepts of amino acid and protein requirements, the effect of deficiency of amino acids and protein, amino acid imbalance, the protein and amino acid content of diets, and problems of improving protein nutrition by amino acid supplementation and other methods. This compila-

Appendix

tion of information pointed out the needs for future research and has been an important stimulus to further study. Currently, the Committee on Amino Acids is undertaking a revision of this document. Last year this committee sponsored and assisted in planning a conference at Rutgers on the significance of changes in plasma amino acid patterns for the evaluation of protein nutrition.

The importance of protein-calorie malnutrition throughout the world, particularly in infants and children in developing countries, led to the establishment of the Committee on Protein Malnutrition in 1956. This committee initiated and carried out a worldwide research program in cooperation with UNICEF, FAO, and WHO with the support of a very generous grant from the Rockefeller Foundation. In 1960 this committee sponsored an international conference with the assistance of the Nutrition Study Section of NIH to discuss the problems of meeting the protein needs of infants and children. This conference provided an opportunity for exchange of information and ideas among research workers in various parts of the world, and indicated the areas of greatest promise for new research activities. The proceedings of the conference summarize the progress that has been made in this research program and was published as NAS-NRC Pub. No. 843.

In 1963, another conference was convened to consider methods for evaluation of protein quality because it had become evident that research was being hindered by inconsistencies in methodology and terminology. The deliberations of this body were published as NAS-NRC Publication 1100, "Evaluation of Protein Quality." In this bulletin, current methods were discussed, recommendations were made, and the problems which needed more research were delineated.

In 1964, in the terminal phase of the research program of the Committee on Protein Malnutrition, it appeared that the most prominent deterrent to progress in developing countries was the failure of healthful development in pre-school children resulting from malnutrition and disease. In cooperation with the Board's Committee on Child Nutrition, another international conference was organized on the Prevention of Malnutrition in the Pre-School Child. This meeting provided evidence of the magnitude of the problem of malnutrition in pre-school children and described the physical and behavioral consequences of such malnutrition. It surveyed the experiences with malnutrition in pre-school children in various geographic areas in terms of deficiency diseases, agricultural resources, and trained personnel, and considered practical alleviative measures, with emphasis on educational, social, and economic implications. A brief summary of this conference, "Pre-School Child Malnutrition, Primary Deterrent to Human Progress," has been published and the complete proceedings, which will bear the same title, are in the process of publication.

The impact of these worldwide studies has been gratifying. In the United States, many government agencies, such as Food For Peace and the Agency for International Development, have been alerted to the importance of nutrition in their overall practical programs. This adventure of the Food and Nutrition Board in specific sponsorship of basic scientific research should have immeasurable practical consequences.

In the 1950's, the importance of fat in human nutrition and possible relationships of dietary fat to the pathogenesis of artherosclerosis were being widely investigated. The Board felt that this was an area to which it should direct its attention. A committee was appointed to critically review the role of dietary fat in human health. In a monograph on this subject, the following were considered: the chemistry and metabolism of fats, their nutritional role, and their possible implication in cardiovascular disease. Specific needs for expanded research were indicated. Currently, another review of this subject has been completed by the Committee on Fats.

A current activity of the Board is that of advising the Bureau of Commercial Fisheries on research and processing procedures necessary for the production of fish protein concentrates and other fish products from whole fish for human consumption. This is an important program in the development of practical measures for relief of protein malnutrition throughout the world. The program thus far has dealt essentially with research: research on product development, quality, and safety. The nutritional value of the products must be tested in animals and man. Some animal studies have already been carried out. Acceptability and practability for human use will be the subject of future investigation.

Another committee of the Board at the present time is one on geographic nutrition. This was established to develop a report pointing out differences in existing nutritional disease patterns in various areas of the world, and reasons for these differences. This report should stimulate further research in the etiology, epidemiology, and clinical aspects of many unsolved nutritional problems of medical and public health importance.

The Food Protection Committee has made numerous contributions to basic nutrition knowledge. Information has been collected and critically evaluated in many areas of food technology and food protection that have important relationships to public

Appendix

health. Research has been stimulated where insufficient data were available. Among the problems considered have been the use and safety of chemical additives and pesticides in foods, including procedures for evaluation of safety, information on radionuclides and carcinogens in foods, and evaluation of public health hazards from microbiological contamination and from naturally occurring toxicants in foods. This committee has developed guidelines for the use of human subjects in the safety evaluation of pesticides and food chemicals. It has sponsored the development of a Food Chemicals Codex, which is a scientific endeavor of great merit and usefulness that probably would not have been undertaken by any other group.

The Committee on Child Nutrition is currently concerned with stimulating research to obtain longitudinal data in children that will provide more information about nutritional requirements, better criteria for evaluating infant and child development, and a more accurate picture of the influence of nutrition on health in various age groups.

Recently, the Food and Nutrition Board appointed an ad hoc Committee on Nutrition Research and Training. This committee was given the responsibility of reviewing the whole field of nutrition research and training in the United States, and was asked to report to the Board on the current situation, the needs for development and expansion, and general recommendations for meeting these needs.

From this brief review, it is obvious that the Food and Nutrition Board has made many contributions to the science of nutrition, particularly in the aspects of this science that are related to human health. The Board has been concerned also with nutrition education at all levels: the general public, elementary and high school students and training of nutrition scientists in all areas—agriculture, biochemistry, animal experimentation, dietetics, medicine, and public health.

It is anticipated that the Board will continue to give stimulation, guidance, and advice in basic nutrition, as well as in the application of nutrition knowledge to the solution of current problems. One important activity in the next few years will undoubtedly be cooperation in the International Biological Program to the fullest possible extent for the advancement of the science of nutrition.

Committee Histories

THE COMMITTEE ON FOOD COMPOSITION
1942-1945

In November 1942, the Committee on Food Composition was established in response to a request of the Quartermaster Corps for assistance in problems concerning food composition. Although the Quartermaster Corps was already availing itself of the services of regular civilian agencies and its own technical consultants, it expressed a need for further immediate aid in the assembling, coordination, critical appraisal, evaluation, and distribution of information on food composition.

C. A. Elvehjem, Ph.D., Department of Biochemistry, University of Wisconsin at Madison, Wisconsin, was asked by the officers of the Food and Nutrition Board to act as chairman of the committee. Paul L. Pavcek, Ph.D., was named secretary. The standing committee was maintained at approximately ten members, and the following individuals served at some time during the Committee's existence:

C. A. Elvehjem, Chairman of Committee, Dept. of Biochemistry, University of Wisconsin, Madison, Wisconsin;

Paul L. Pavcek, Secretary of Committee, November 1942-April 1945, National Research Council, Washington, D.C.;

L. J. Teply, Secretary of Committee, April-August 1945, National Research Council, Washington, D.C;

Lura Mae Odland, Nutritionist, January-August 1945; Acting Secretary of Committee, August 1945, National Research Council, Washington, D.C.;

Georgian Adams, Office of Experiment Stations, U.S. Dept. of Agriculture, Washington, D.C.;

Charlotte Chatfield, War Food Administration, U.S. Dept. of Agriculture, Washington, D.C.;

C. N. Frey, Fleischmann Laboratories, Standard Brands, Inc., New York, New York;

Ancel Keys, Laboratory of Physiological Hygiene, Minneapolis, Minnesota;

L. A. Maynard, U.S. Plant, Soil and Nutrition Laboratory, Cornell University, Ithaca, New York;

E. M. Nelson, Vitamin Division, Food and Drug Administration, Washington, D.C.;

Appendix

L. B. Pett, Division of Nutrition, Department of National Health and Welfare, Ottawa, Canada;

H. K. Stiebeling, Bureau of Human Nutrition and Home Economics, U.S. Dept. of Agriculture, Washington, D.C.;

E. L. Phipard, Bureau of Human Nutrition and Home Economics, U.S. Dept. of Agriculture, Washington, D.C.;

Sybil Smith, Office of Experiment Stations, U.S. Dept. of Agriculture, Washington, D.C.;

Charles Woodbury, Agricultural Research Administration, U.S. Dept. of Agriculture, Washington, D.C;

John B. Youmans, Vanderbilt University, Nashville, Tennessee, and Surgeon General's Office, War Dept., Washington, D.C.

Ex officio members included:

Robert F. Griggs, Chairman, Division of Biology and Agriculture, National Research Council, Washington, D.C.; and

Frank G. Boudreau, H. C. Sherman, Russell M. Wilder, and Frank L. Gunderson, Chairman, Vice-Chairman, Vice-Chairman and Executive Secretary, respectively, Food and Nutrition Board, National Research Council.

Close contact was maintained with all branches of the military services, with several allied nations, and with interested government agencies. Liaison representatives of these organizations attended the sixteen meetings of the committee and received copies of mimeographed reports.

One of the first tasks undertaken by the committee was the compilation of tables of food composition listing proximate, mineral and vitamin data for some 250 foods designated by the army. In response to an appeal from the committee, information was generously furnished by academic institutions, federal departments, industrial laboratories, and allied nations. Nutritionists were employed by the committee and through the cooperation of the Bureau of Human Nutrition and Home Economics, U.S. Dept. of Agriculture, were assigned to gather data from the extensive files of that agency. To fill in the gaps in food composition data, it was necessary to solicit samples and submit them for analysis to a number of laboratories throughout the country which offered their services. Most of the vitamin determinations were made at the laboratories of the Food and Drug Administration, Washington, D.C., and the Department of Biochemistry, University of Wisconsin, Madison, Wisconsin. Proximate and mineral analyses were obtained through the cooperation of the University of Maryland and the National Canners Association.

Many of the original data were distributed as "advance releases" which obviated any delay in the distribution of needed information and yet expressed the reservation that the committee had not had time to carefully appraise the figures.

The first Tables of Food Composition on a Per-Pound Basis were issued in March 1943, and after that there were three revisions. The dates of issue were as follows:

1st	Issuance,	March 1, 1943
1st	Revision,	Nov. 1, 1943
2nd	Revision,	Sept. 1, 1944
3rd	Revision,	May 1, 1945

A supplement to the army tables which included many new items was issued on August 1, 1945.

On March 1, 1944, the Committee on Food Composition mimeographed tables giving data on a per-100 gram basis and these were made available to professional workers throughout the country. Printed "Tables of Food Composition in Terms of 11 Nutrients," embodying data on both the per-pound and per-100 grams' were published jointly by the committee and the Bureau of Human Nutrition and Home Economics. Distribution was made through the Superintendent of Documents, U.S. Dept. of Agriculture, and the tables were listed as Miscellaneous Publication 572.

From time to time it was necessary to investigate and improve certain methods for measuring vitamins to establish their reliability. Collaborative studies were made comparing the fermentation, thiochrome and fungus grown methods for determining thiamine. Joseph H. Roe, Ph.D., George Washington University, Washington, D.C., compared his phenylhydrazine method with the indophenol titration method in the determination of vitamin C in foods. There was close agreement in the values obtained by the two methods. A number of collaborative studies were made on carotene and vitamin A. Instruments were compared through the use of a standard dichromate solution and identical samples of dehydrated eggs and canned egg products were tested for vitamin A potency by both chemical and biological methods in a number of laboratories. During 1945 the committee was engaged in supervising

Appendix

the collaborative assay of three canned vegetable products by more than thirty laboratories in the United States, Canada and England.

New ration items were routinely analyzed as they were developed. As a result of the committee's report on components of the C and K rations, some of the items, notably the biscuits, were changed. Some one hundred canned items in the army's B-ration were analyzed both in the original and cooked form by the laboratories of the U.S. Public Health Service and the Food and Drug Administration.

Studies at the Universities of Chicago, Minnesota and Wisconsin indicated that there was serious loss of thiamine during storage of canned and dehydrated meat products. Components of the B-ration were analyzed after storage at 115°F. for eight months. Ten-in-one ration items were analyzed after storage for various periods ranging up to a year at 77° and 100°F. The results showed nicotinic acid and riboflavin to be very stable. There was serious loss of thiamine in the canned meat products but much greater stability was observed in cereal products. Vitamin C was assayed only in the B-ration items and there was definite loss on storage. Vitamin A was stable in canned dairy products but not in canned egg products. The data furnished by these studies aided the armed forces in their planning of food purchasing, shipping and storage.

If the composition of food as actually consumed is to be known, the fate of certain nutrients during both storage and cooking must be studied. Much information on losses during cooking was obtained from several projects sponsored by the Office of Scientific Research and Development (under the technical supervision of the Committee on Food Composition) and the National Cooperative Projects of the U.S. Dept. of Agriculture Experiment Stations. Other data were collected through the cooperation of the Bureau of Human Nutrition and Home Economics. On May 12, 1943, a mimeographed bulletin was issued which summarized available information and a revision was issued on June 1, 1944. On June 7, 1945, a revised and simplified table was released. To facilitate the collection and appraisal of cooking loss data and their condensation into a form which can be useful to the military services, a Working Group on Cooking Losses was established and the first meeting was held on August 3, 1945.

During World War II, the variety and production of dehydrated foods increased tremendously. The committee was interested in the effect of various types of blanching, drying and packaging on the retention of certain nutrients. Proximate, mineral and vitamin analyses were made in 89 different samples of 16 dehydrated food products. The vitamins found to be most affected were thiamine and vitamin C.

The Committee on Food Composition had under its technical supervision the following projects financed by the Office of Scientific Research and Development:

"Vitamin Losses in the Preparation of Dehydrated Vegetables;" Faith Fenton, Ph.D., Responsible Investigator, Cornell University;

"Vitamin Losses in Raw, Cooked and Dehydrated Vegetables and in Dehydrated Meats, Fish and Pork Scrapple;" Agnes Fay Morgan, Ph.D., Responsible Investigator, University of California;

"Nutrients in Dehydrated Vegetables;" Jet C. Winters, Ph.D., Responsible Investigator, University of Texas;

"A Study on Cooking Losses;" Esther L. Batchelder, Ph.D., Responsible Investigator, Bureau of Human Nutrition and Home Economics;

"A Study on Cooking Losses at the Pentagon Post Restaurant;" Major Fred G. Koch, Responsible Investigator.

These projects provided special information at a time when it was most vitally needed.

For some time it was hoped that a single set of figures for each food could be arrived at for use by all countries but it seemed that the variation in foods from one country to another made it impracticable to compile such tables. It appeared rather to be desirable to have individual tables for each country, all compiled in the same manner so that comparison might be facilitated. The Committee on Food Composition stood ready to cooperate in the evolution of such tables. With the interest in the Far East increasing by 1945, there was need for much study of foods indigenous to that region and the committee became engaged in that work.

The committee continued to aid the Office of the Quartermaster General and other branches of the military forces in solving any special food problems relating to composition, nutrient stability under varied packaging and storage conditions, and analytical methods for nutrient appraisal during the remainder of its existence.

COMMITTEE ON NUTRITION STUDIES AT ELGIN STATE HOSPITAL

This report will attempt to summarize for the record the unique collaboration between the Food and Nutri-

Appendix

tion Board and the Elgin State Hospital during the past 23 years.

On April 17, 1942, Dr. M.K. Horwitt, in charge of the Biochemical Research Laboratory at Elgin State Hospital, wrote to Dr. Frank L. Gunderson, Executive Secretary of the Food and Nutrition Board, suggesting the possibility of conducting studies in human nutrition at Elgin. This initiated an exchange of correspondence and credentials which stimulated a visit to Elgin on June 20, 1942, by Dr. Gunderson and Dr. Frank G. Boudreau, Chairman of the Food and Nutrition Board.

At that time, the Biochemical Research Laboratory, which occupied four rooms in an old building called Wing Cottage, was only four years old. Although this laboratory had achieved some minor recognition in the graduate educational scheme of the University of Chicago and the University of Illinois as a place to study human metabolism and brain chemistry, the furnishings and equipment of the laboratory were quite primitive, having been improvised with the help of the hospital carpenters and mechanics from bits and pieces found around the institution. That such a laboratory was permitted to develop at all in a State Hospital in those days was due to the superior academic attitudes of the late and remarkable Dr. Charles F. Read, who, as superintendent of the hospital, had created at Elgin a teaching institution for young clinicians which produced many eminent psychiatrists. By coincidence, Dr. Horwitt, who had been brought to Elgin in 1937 to study any physiological changes which may exist in patients with mental diseases, had obtained his doctorate in the nutritional sciences. Except for a survey on the ascorbic acid levels and requirements of the hospital patients, using the medical staff as controls, and some early studies on microbiological assay of the vitamins, most of his work at Elgin had not been directly related to nutrition. The primary aim of the laboratory was, and still is, to study the metabolism of schizophrenic patients. To date, no differences have been confirmed in such patients which are not a part of their environment or of the stress of the disease.

Dr. Boudreau and Dr. Gunderson were apparently satisfied, after their project site visit, that the Elgin State Hospital had a favorable environment for conducting long-term human nutritional experiments and a new committee of the Food and Nutrition Board was organized, which had its first meeting at Elgin on August 29, 1942. The membership of the Committee on Nutritional Aspects of Aging, which changed only slightly during the next four years, included E. S. G. Barron, C. A. Elvehjem, A. Baird Hastings, M. K. Horwitt, E. Liebert, W. D. B. MacNider, C. F. Read, Lydia J. Roberts, T. D. Spies, R. D. Williams with R. M. Wilder as chairman. It was a great credit to Dr. Wilder's leadership that the *ex officio* members, R. F. Griggs, F. G. Boudreau, F. L. Gunderson, P. Pavcek, and F. Fremont-Smith, were also faithful in attending meetings and providing important assistance.

The first Elgin Project produced auspicious clues of that which was to follow in future projects. No important differences were found in comparing the nutritional needs of the healthy young and the healthy older individual. Although the older men did utilize their nutritional components at a slower rate, there was no evidence that their daily requirements per unit of active tissue was different from that for the younger men. Of possibly greater significance was the development of methods which made it feasible to fix more accurately the human requirements for thiamine and to provide information about the amino acid and riboflavin requirements, which were to be studied more thoroughly later. In addition, information obtained about the more exaggerated psychotic behavior of the thiamine-deficient patient was to prove important.

By 1945, the laboratory had grown sufficiently to necessitate a move out of Wing Cottage, and with Dr. Read's assistance it was possible to rejuvenate an old one story building into what was then considered to be a well-equipped laboratory.

The second Elgin Project, which was designed specifically to evaluate the riboflavin requirements of adult men, was initiated in March, 1947 under the auspices of a new Committee on Vitamin Deficiency Studies at Elgin State Hospital. Dr. Russell M. Wilder was again designated as chairman, and the members included E. S. G. Barron, E. A. Elvehjem, M. K. Horwitt, A. C. Ivy, E. Liebert, D. L. Steinberg, D. Vail and R. D. Williams.

Of all the Elgin Projects, this one went most nearly according to plan. The excellent correlations obtained between dietary intake, urinary excretion of riboflavin, and clinical signs of ariboflavinosis gave considerable weight to conclusions reported about the riboflavin requirements of adult men. No confirmation was obtained that corneal vascularization was part of the syndrome of ariboflavinosis, but signs of angular stomatitis and seborrheic dermatitis were quite positively confirmed. The only surprise was the specificity and high frequence of a form of scrotal dermatitis which responded dramatically to riboflavin supplementation. This scrotal dermatitis was apparently identical to that which had been observed by others on pellagra-producing diets, but in this present instance the diet was adequate both in protein and in niacin. In general, the study confirmed the impression that some traumatic experience to the skin must precede the development of clinical signs of

Appendix

ariboflavinosis and that healing was inhibited and the wound aggravated when the supply of flavoproteins was inadequate. In addition, whereas early thiamine deficiency studied previously had produced severe disturbances of function as reflected by metabolic, neurological, and psychic inadequacies, early riboflavin deficiency had relatively minor effects on the comfort of the patient and there were fewer subjective complaints.

In May 1950, the Elgin Committee agreed to attempt a more complete evaluation of the relative roles played by riboflavin, niacin and tryptophan in the pellagra syndrome. Dr. Wilder continued as chairman and new members included O. A. Bessey, P. Bailey, R. M. Kark, and R. S. Goodhart.

The plans of the various Elgin Projects differed from similar studies which have been attempted elsewhere in one important respect, i.e., in addition to having a supplemented control group which consumed the same basal diet as the experimental group, another group of subjects approximately equal in number, ate the regular hospital diet *ad libitum*. Time and again, errors of interpretation and procedure became apparent to the investigators only because this Hospital Diet (HD) group was available for simultaneous biochemical and clinical study. This proved especially true during one phase of Elgin Project No. 3 when liver dysfunctions and enlarged livers were noted in both the depleted and the supplemented subjects but not in the HD group. This inadequacy of hepatic function proved to be a consequence of the poor amino acid balance of the basic ration. It is noteworthy that replacement and/or supplementation of the protein in the diet with methionine, choline, and lactalbumin for two to six months had no apparent effect in ameliorating this liver dysfunction; but when the subjects were given a ration that included liberal amounts of meat and milk, a marked decrease in liver size was noted within four months. Protein in the initial basal diet was largely supplied by flour, zein, and gelatin in an effort to decrease the tryptophan. The effects of this diet on liver function could not be repaired by adding 30 grams of lactalbumin to the diet, although a balanced ration providing the same amount of protein apparently cured those parts of the liver dysfunction syndrome which could be studied.

Of some significance was the observation that higher than normal basal blood levels of lactic and pyruvic acid were noted in the experimental subjects, despite adequate thiamine supplementation, after two months on the basal niacin-tryptophan low diet, although clinical signs of pellagra did not become apparent. These elevated levels of lactic and pyruvic acids persisted throughout the depletion period but were rapidly repaired after supplementation with animal protein foods.

Possibly, the most important contribution of Elgin Project No. 3 was the accumulation of data which made possible a tentative arithmetical relationship between tryptophan and niacin in man so that we are now able to speak of niacin equivalents instead of niacin *per se*. Fortunately, Dr. Grace Goldsmith's studies on pellagra, which were being conducted at the same time in New Orleans, provided very important clinical and biochemical data which dovetailed perfectly with those from the Elgin Projects so that some of the doubts that might have normally been raised about the Elgin niacin-tryptophan ratios were at least partially resolved.

Elgin Project No. 4 did not materialize until after a rather detailed evaluation of the literature convinced the Board that it was time to make a thorough study of the tocopherol requirements of man. For this purpose, a new Committee on Nutritional Studies at Elgin State Hospital was organized in 1952. The members included: W. J. Darby, Chairman; M. K. Horwitt, Executive Secretary; P. Bailey, J. Campbell, G. A. Goldsmith, R. S. Goodhart, R. M. Kark, K. E. Mason, and D. Haffron. Dr. Haffron was later succeeded by Dr. E. S. Klein. In 1956, Dr. Grace Goldsmith assumed the chairmanship. When, in 1958, she became Chairman of the Food and Nutrition Board, Dr. R. W. Vilter became Chairman of this Elgin Committee; he served until he retired from the Board in 1963. In 1964, Dr. J. F. Mueller was appointed chairman, and new members appointed in 1964 were A. E. Harper, Philip Harris, R. T. Holman, and W. H. Sebrell, Jr.

At the start of the new dietary phase in the fall of 1953, it was thoroughly understood that working with a fat-soluble vitamin in adults would require a long depletion period. The absence of information about human requirements made it necessary to proceed cautiously. Accordingly, a complete deficiency with maximum stress was out of the question in a preliminary evaluation of human requirements for vitamin E. Nevertheless, despite the fact that the diet was not particularly low in tocopherol content and the subjects had quite considerable stores of this fat-soluble vitamin in their tissues, hematological signs of tocopherol depletion appeared within five years. The decrease in tocopherol levels in the plasma and the related increase in susceptibility of erythrocytes to peroxide hemolysis became quite evident after only one year, but a statistically significant decrease in erythrocyte survival times did not become apparent until after five years, at which time it was considered necessary to terminate the depletion period. A reticulocyte response was detected after supplementa-

Appendix

tion with tocopherol. Since there was no apparent anemia, the response was relatively small. This small reticulocyte response, which had been noted earlier in the study in previous instances of supplementation, would not have been considered significant except for the unusual special precautions taken to eliminate possible errors of procedure and interpretation with the last four subjects tested; in addition, no such responses were obtained when subjects who had not been depleted were given the tocopherol supplement.

The slow decrease in tocopherol stores of adult men stimulated a simultaneous study of rates of change in the fatty acid composition of the depot fats on different diets. This investigation began in September 1960 and is still continuing. In general, the slow changes in stored tocopherol are similar to the slow changes noted in the adipose tissue fatty acids when attempts are made to alter the ratio of the fatty acids by dietary means.

As there is no reason to believe that human requirements for a-tocopherol are significantly different from animal requirements (differences in the incidence of deficiency being a function of differences in the type of food consumed), work on growing animals proceeded simultaneously with the study of humans. Such animal studies have provided unusually specific correlations between the a-tocopherol requirement and the potential level of peroxidizability of the fatty acids in the tissues; the latter will, of course, vary with the diet and the tissue studied. The amount of selenium in the diet has a major effect on the tocopherol requirement in animals and may also be important in human nutrition.

Over the years considerable time and effort have been directed toward improvement of methods for analyzing the various tocopherols in biological materials. It is pertinent to note, that although pure tocopherol samples can be quantitated with precision, when plasma extracts are chromatographed on paper or on thin-layers, unless extraordinary precautions are taken, there are large oxidative losses of tocopherol. This seems to be particularly true if the levels of tocopherol in the plasma are low. Consequently, more consistent results are obtained by using the older reducing techniques (like Quaifé and Harris) and subtracting a figure for the reducing material which is not tocopherol. This is important because publications have recently appeared which erroneously cast doubt on the older procedures and leave the impression that many individuals are lower in tocopherol than they really are. When properly conducted, the chromatographic techniques show that about 0.1 mg % of the "apparent total tocopherol" in the plasma is not tocopherol. For example, plasma tocopherol levels of 1.0, 0.5, and 0.2 mg % should be corrected to read 0.9, 0.4, and 0.1 mg %, respectively, in previous Elgin papers. This does not alter any of the conclusions reached.

A directive that the Elgin tocopherol studies be recorded in a National Research Council bulletin has not been acted upon, mainly because too many controversial areas of the problem remain to justify giving official approval to current conclusions. Moreover, there seems to be good reason to believe that in the future a-tocopherol requirements will be considered less in terms of preventing deficiency diseases and more in terms of the maintenance of optimum tissue metabolism as a function of its activities as an antioxidant.

No report of the Elgin Projects would be complete without mentioning our debt to the many scientists, technicians, and consultants who participated actively in the research procedures. During the 23-year tenure of the Elgin Committees, many of these individuals have graduated to mature positions of responsibility in other institutions, so it is probably proper to say that the educational aspects of the Elgin Projects were also an important contribution. The assistance of Dr. LeRoy Voris has been particularly important.

The laboratory itself was moved into a new building in 1959 and its name was changed to the L. B. Mendel Research Laboratory at that time. This building, which combines the assets of a large metabolic ward and a well-equipped laboratory under one roof, houses over 50 well trained workers of whom nine are considered senior investigators and four have faculty rank at the University of Illinois College of Medicine.

The need for a sponsoring national Research Council committee is no longer a critical requirement and the research work of the Elgin Projects continues.

Bibliography of Elgin Projects

The following list of references is a selection of publications of the L. B. Mendel Research Laboratory (previously the Biochemical Research Laboratory) at the Elgin State Hospital which pertain to the work of the Elgin Committees of the Food and Nutrition Board. Additional papers are now being prepared for publication.

1. M. K. Horwitt, E. Liebert, O. Kreisler, and P. Wittman: Studies of vitamin deficiency. Science *104*: 407-408, 1946.
2. G. E. F. Brewer, W. S. Brown, C. C. Harvey, and M. K. Horwitt: Variations of the individual blood plasma amino acid nitrogen level. J. Biol. Chem. *168*: 145-150, 1947.

Appendix

3. O. Kreisler, E. Liebert, and M. K. Horwitt: Psychiatric observations on induced vitamin B complex deficiency in psychotic patients. Am. J. Psychiat. *105*: 107-110, 1948.

4. M. K. Horwitt, E. Liebert, O. Kreisler, and P. Wittman: Investigations of human requirements for B-complex vitamins. National Research Council Bulletin, No. 116: pp. 1-106, Washington, 1948.

5. M. K. Horwitt, O. W. Hills, and O. Kreisler: Lactic and pyruvic acids in the blood after glucose and exercise in diabetes mellitus. Am. J. Physiol. *156*: 92-99, 1949.

6. C. C. Harvey and M. K. Horwitt: Excretion of essential amino acids by men on a controlled protein intake. J. Biol. Chem. *178*: 953-962, 1949.

7. M. K. Horwitt and O. Kreisler: The determination of early thiamine-deficient states by estimation of blood lactic and pyruvic acids after glucose administration and exercise. J. Nutrition *37*: 411-427, 1949.

8. M. K. Horwitt, Gordon Sampson, O. W. Hills, and D. L. Steinberg: Dietary management in a study of riboflavin requirements. J. Am. Dietet. Assoc. *25*: 591-594, 1949.

9. M. K. Horwitt, O. W. Hills, C. C. Harvey, E. Liebert, and D. L. Steinberg: Effects of dietary depletion of riboflavin. J. Nutrition *39*: 357-373, 1949.

10. M. K. Horwitt, C. C. Harvey, O. W. Hills and E. Liebert: Correlation of urinary excretion of riboflavin with dietary intake and symptoms of ariboflavinosis. J. Nutrition *41*: 247-264, 1950.

11. M. K. Horwitt: Studies of thiamine and riboflavin requirements in man. Currents in Nutrition, Nutr. Symp. Series, Nat. Vit. Found. *2*: 1-17, 1950.

12. O. W. Hills, E. Liebert, D. L. Steinberg, and M. K. Horwitt: Clinical aspects of dietary depletion of riboflavin. Arch. Int. Med. *87*: 682-693, 1951.

13. M. K. Horwitt: Dietary requirements of the aged. J. Am. Dietet. Assoc. *29*: 443-448, 1953.

14. M. K. Horwitt: Report on Elgin Project No. 3 with emphasis on liver dysfunction. Nut. Symp. Series, Nat. Vit. Found. *7*: 67-83, 1953.

15. R. M. Kark, M. K. Horwitt, and W. S. Rothwell: Production and repair of experimental liver dysfunction in man by modifications of dietary protein. J. Lab. and Clin. Med. *42*: 823, 1953.

16. M. K. Horwitt: Niacin-tryptophan relationships in the development of pellagra. Am. J. Clin. Nutrition *3*: 244-245, 1955.

17. M. K. Horwitt: Implications of observations made during experimental deficiencies in man. Ann. N.Y. Acad. Sci. *63*: 165-173, 1955.

18. O. A. Bessey, Ruth H. Love, and M. K. Horwitt: Dietary deprivation of riboflavin and blood riboflavin levels in man. J. Nutrition *58*: 367-383, 1956.

19. M. K. Horwitt, C. C. Harvey, W. S. Rothwell, J. L. Cutler, and D. Haffron: Tryptophan-niacin relationships in man: Studies with diets deficient in riboflavin and niacin, together with observations on the excretion of nitrogen and niacin metabolites. J. Nutrition *60*: Supplement 1, 1-43, 1956.

20. M. K. Horwitt, C. C. Harvey, G. D. Duncan, and W. C. Wilson: Effects of limited tocopherol intake in man with relationships to erythrocyte hemolysis and lipid oxidations. Am. J. Clin. Nutrition *4*: 408-419, 1956.

21. M. K. Horwitt: Nutritional problems in the aged. Geriatrics *12*: 683-686, 1957.

22. M. K. Horwitt: Niacin-tryptophan requirements of man: Designation in terms of niacin-equivalents. J. Am. Dietet. Assoc. *34*: 914-919, 1958.

23. B. Century, M. K. Horwitt, and P. Bailey: Lipid factors in the production of encephalomalacia in the chick. A.M.A. Arch. Gen. Psychiat. *1*: 420-424, 1959.

24. M. K. Horwitt and P. Bailey: Cerebellar pathology in an infant resembling chick nutritional encephalomalacia. A.M.A. Arch. Neurol. *1*: 312-314, 1959.

25. M. K. Horwitt, C. C. Harvey, and B. Century: Effect of dietary fats on fatty acid composition of human erythrocytes and chick cerebella. Science *130*: 917-918, 1959.

26. B. Century and M. K. Horwitt: Effect of fatty acids on chick encephalomalacia. Proc. Soc. Exp. Biol. and Med. *102*: 375-377, 1959.

27. B. J. Meyer, B. Century, A. C. Meyer, and M. K. Horwitt: Effects of triiodothyronine in schizophrenic patients: Correlations of changes in basal metabolism with urinary creatine and cholesterol and tocopherol levels in the blood. A.M.A. Arch. Gen. Psychiat. *2*: 528-533, 1960.

28. M. K. Horwitt: Vitamin E and lipid metabolism in man. Am. J. Clin. Nutrition *8*: 451-461, 1960.

29. B. Century and M. K. Horwitt: Role of diet lipids in the appearance of dystrophy and creatinuria in the vitamin E-deficient rat. J. Nutrition *72*: 357-367, 1960.

30. M. K. Horwitt: Vitamin E in Human Nutrition—An Interpretative Review. Borden's Review of Nutrition Research *22*: 1-17, 1961.

Appendix

31. M. K. Horwitt, C. C. Harvey, B. Century, and L. A. Witting: Polyunsaturated lipids and tocopherol requirements. J. Am. Dietet. Assoc. *38*: 231-235, 1961.
32. L. A. Witting, C. C. Harvey, B. Century, and M. K. Horwitt: Dietary alterations of fatty acids of erythrocytes and mitochondria of brain and liver. J. Lipid Res. *2*: 412-417, 1961.
33. B. Century, L. A. Witting, C. C. Harvey, and M. K. Horwitt: Compositions of skeletal muscle lipids of rats fed diets containing various oils. J. Nutrition *75*: 341-346, 1961.
34. Coy D. Fitch, J. S. Dinning, L. A. Witting, and M. K. Horwitt: Influence of dietary fat on the fatty acid composition of monkey erythrocytes. J. Nutrition *75*: 409-413, 1961.
35. M. K. Horwitt and C. C. Harvey: Rate of fatty acid change in plasma, erythrocyte and depot fat in humans ingesting different fats. Am. J. Clin. Nutrition *10*: 351-352, 1962.
36. M. K. Horwitt: Interrelations between vitamin E and polyunsaturated fatty acids in adult human beings. "Vitamins and Hormones," Vol. 20. Academic Press, N.Y., 1962, pp. 541-558.
37. M. K. Horwitt, B. Century, and A. A. Zeman: Erythrocyte survival time and reticulocyte levels after tocopherol depletion in man. Am. J. Clin. Nutrition *12*: 99-106, 1963.
38. M. K. Horwitt: Nutrition and Metabolism in Mental Disease. Am. J. Clin. Nutrition *12*: 259-260, 1963.
39. B. Century and M. K. Horwitt: Effect of dietary lipids upon mitochondrial composition and swelling. J. Nutrition *80*: 145-150, 1963.
40. B. Century, L. A. Witting, C. C. Harvey, and M. K. Horwitt: Interrelationships of dietary lipids upon fatty acid composition of brain mitochondria, erythrocytes and heart tissue in chicks. Am. J. Clin. Nutrition *13*: 362-368, 1963.
41. L. A. Witting and M. K. Horwitt: Effect of degree of fatty acid unsaturation in tocopherol-deficiency induced creatinuria. J. Nutrition *82*: 19-33, 1964.
42. R. Sivarama Krishnan, L. A. Witting, and M. K. Horwitt: Analysis of fatty derivatives by gas-liquid chromatography. J. Chromatog. *13*: 22-25, 1964.
43. B. Century and M. K. Horwitt: Role of arachidonic acid in nutritional encephalomalacia: interrelationship of essential and nonessential polyunsaturated fatty acids. Arch. Biochem. and Biophys. *104*: 416-422, 1964.
44. M. K. Horwitt: Effect of diet on lipid composition of brain in "Progress in Brain Research," Vol. 9, eds. W. A. Himwich and H. E. Himwich, Elsevier Publishing Co., Amsterdam, 1964, pp. 217-219.
45. L. A. Witting and M. K. Horwitt: The biopotency of 1-a-tocopheryl acetate for the rat. Proc. Soc. Exp. Biol. Med. *116*: 655-658, 1964.
46. B. Century and M. K. Horwitt: The effect of dietary selenium on the incidence of nutritional encephalomalacia in chicks. Proc. Soc. Exp. Biol. Med. *117*: 320-322, 1964.
47. L. A. Witting and M. K. Horwitt: Effects of dietary selenium, methionine, fat level and tocopherol on rat growth. J. Nutrition *84*: 351-360, 1964.
48. M. K. Horwitt: Symposium paper: Role of vitamin E, selenium and polyunsaturated fatty acids in clinical and experimental muscle disease. Fed. Proc. *24*: 68-72, 1965.
49. B. Century and M. K. Horwitt: Symposium paper: Biological availability of various forms of vitamin E with respect to different indices of deficiency. Fed. Proc. *24*: 906-911, 1965.
50. L. A. Witting: Symposium paper: Biological availability of tocopherol and other anti-oxidants at the cellular level. Fed. Proc. *24*: 912-916, 1965.
51. L. A. Witting: Lipid Peroxidation *In Vivo*. J. Am. Oil Chem. Soc. (In press).
52. M. K. Horwitt: Nutrition in Mental Health. Nutrition Reviews *23*: 289-291, 1965.
53. E. M. Harmon, L. A. Witting, and M. K. Horwitt: Relative rates of depletion of a-tocopherol and linoleic acid after feeding polyunsaturated fats. Am. J. Clin. Nutrition (In press).

THE FOOD PROTECTION COMMITTEE: 1950-1965

Background

At the end of World War II there was a sudden upsurge in the number of chemicals that found useful application in food production, processing, and storage. The attention of many groups began to be directed to the public health implications of the increasing use of these chemicals. The fact that the Food and Drug Administration hearings concerning standards of identity for bread and bakery products were resumed after having been interrupted by the War, and the discovery that flour bleached with Agene (NCl$_3$) caused running fits in dogs that consumed enough of it served to focus this attention. At any rate, in May, 1948, the National Health Assembly met in Washington. One of the resolutions from that meeting was

Appendix

referred to the Food and Nutrition Board. In it the Assembly recommended that:

1. Studies be continued to determine to what extent pesticides or other toxic substances now occur in food products;
2. That a plan be developed by which the non-toxic nature of these chemical substances be established beyond reasonable doubt before food substances in which they are present are offered for human consumption.

The Board responded to the resolution by asking an ad hoc Committee to advise it on actions it should take with regard to the matter of possible public health hazards associated with chemicals in foods. The ad hoc Committee consisted of H. E. Longenecker, Chairman; F. C. Bing, F. C. Blanck, P. R. Cannon, E.M. Nelson, and J.R. Wilson. It recommended in May 1949 that the Board establish a permanent Committee, possibly jointly with the Agricultural Board of the National Research Council, to survey all aspects of the problem. It viewed as important aspects: 1) the necessity of protecting food crops and stored foods from pests, and of protecting the consumer from hazardous residues of pest-control chemicals; 2) the effects on nutritive quality of foods resulting from chemical treatments or from other treatments during handling, processing, and storage.

By the spring of 1949 there existed some thirty different groups interested in the same general problems. They were organized both on official bases and as volunteer groups. This fact influenced the Board to question whether anything useful would be accomplished by appointing the recommended committee. Instead it suggested that a national conference encompassing the views of government, public health, agriculture, manufacturing chemists, food manufacturers, and academic and private research organizations be called to formulate a course of action. The conference was held in December 1949. It resulted in the formation of an organizing committee, made up primarily of representatives of industrial concerns, to assist in establishing a permanent committee and to raise funds for its support. The membership of the organizing committee was:

Ernest W. Reid, Vice President, Corn Products Refining Company, Chairman

Thomas Carswell, Vice President, Commercial Solvents Corporation

Leland Cox, Beechnut-Packing Company

Charles N. Frey, Standard Brands

Per K. Frolich, Vice President, Merck and Company

H. T. Grady, California Spray Chemicals Corporation

C. G. King, Scientific Director, The Nutrition Foundation

H. E. Longenecker, University of Pittsburgh

Roy C. Newton, Swift and Company

Thomas Rector, General Foods

Norman A. Shepard, American Cyanamid

Cullen Thomas, General Mills

LeRoy Voris, Food and Nutrition Board

This group (Mr. Thomas could not attend, and Mr. Rector died before the committee met) recommended to the Board:

> "That a food protection advisory committee, with a fulltime secretary, be set up within the framework of the National Research Council. That the membership of the committee be composed of individuals with the scientific competence to advise on the various phases of food protection and include in its membership representation from the Public Health Service, the Food and Drug Administration, and the U.S. Department of Agriculture. That the function of the committee be: (1) to consider and evaluate available scientific data on chemicals proposed for addition to food, or for use that will affect food products; (2) to organize such data for use, and to point out missing data; (3) to recommend models of further experimental study, kind of evidence, or data required; (4) to organize panels of scientists and experts competent in the various phases of the problem to advise the committee as requested."

The Board acted upon the recommendation in May 1950 by establishing the Food Protection Committee.

Early Activities of FPC

The Food Protection Committee was organized just at the time of intense public involvement in the question of chemicals in foods. In August 1950 the Food and Drug Administration set forth the findings of facts derived from the long hearings concerning standards of identity for bread and bakery products. During the hearings there was conflicting testimony dealing with inclusion of some of the newer chemical substances in the standards, for example that concerning competing emulsifiers.

At about the same time, FDA was holding hearings dealing with tolerances for spray residues on food. And a Select Committee of the House of Representatives, the "Delaney" Committee, began its investiga-

Appendix

tion of the safety of foods. These hearings elicited conflicting statements about the number and identity of chemicals used in food and led to concern about the safety of such use.

The Food Protection Committee immediately became involved in questions associated with these various hearings. To deal with them it established four subcommittees: 1) on pesticides; 2) on toxicology; 3) on chemistry; and 4) on food technology. In addition, its Liaison Panel consisting of representatives of contributing industries, trade associations, scientific and technical organizations, and government agencies was organized as a means to facilitate exchange of information.

The first published reports of the committee stemmed directly from interests in the public hearings mentioned. Statements of usefulness of intentional chemical additives and pesticides and basic principles for assessing their safety appeared in 1951 (NAS-NRC Pub. 1951) and 1952 (NAS-NRC Pub. 1952). The hearings on standards of identity for bread included testimony on the usefulness and safety of some of the newer functional chemicals. FPC expressed its judgment concerning certain of the emulsifiers used or proposed for use when it published evaluations of the safety of mono- and diglycerides (Pub. 251) and of polyoxyethylene stearates (Pub. 280). The Subcommittees on Pesticides, Toxicology, and Food Technology were active in preparing these statements. At the same time, the Subcommittee on Chemistry was compiling an annotated bibliography of analytical methods for pesticides (Pub. 241).

By 1954, the committee had prepared a definitive statement of principles and procedures for evaluating the safety of chemicals for use in foods (NAS-NRC Pub. 1954), and had adopted the principle that it would devote little of its time to reviewing data related to safety of individual food chemicals, but rather would try to deal with broad principles. It had underway, however, a study of the safety of non-nutritive sweeteners and published its findings on this subject in 1955 (Pub. 386). It also was considering the general characteristic of surface activity of chemicals as it might relate to their safety as food additives (Pub. 463).

Later Activities of FPC

As indicated, about 1954 the committee decided to devote most of its efforts to general rather than specific problems. It undertook in sequence two long-range projects to compile information about chemicals used in food processing and about food packaging materials. The compilation on food chemicals was completed in 1956 (Pub. 398), and almost immediately plans were made to revise it. The revision has just been completed (Pub. 1274). The second compilation, "Food Packaging Materials: Their Composition and Uses," was published in 1958 (Pub. 645).

During this period the committee revised and brought up to date its statements on safe use of pesticides (Pub. 470), and principles and procedures for evaluating safety of food chemicals (Pub. 750). It also undertook to discuss specifically the problem of the carcinogenic hazard from use of food additives. To this end, it asked a small ad hoc group to advise it on this matter, and then in accordance with recommendations of the ad hoc subcommittee formed a permanent Subcommittee on Carcinogenesis. This group produced in 1959 the important and widely used "Problems in the Evaluation of Carcinogenic Hazard from Use of Food Additives" (Pub. 749).

A problem that interested the committee and its liaison panel rather early was the matter of how to deal administratively with levels of chemicals in foods that are insignificant toxicologically although demonstrable chemically. An ad hoc subcommittee discussed this matter in 1958.[1] This was one of the early attempts to explore the difficulties of using "zero" tolerances as an administrative device.

The committee during this period arranged or participated in public symposia dealing with the general subjects of toxicology and use of chemicals in foods,[2] (Pub. 877) and also published a general review of the technologic reasons for use of chemicals in food production, processing, storage, and distribution and the responsibilities of industry and government in assuring that these uses are safe (Pub. 887).

Recent Activities of FPC

The committee up to 1960 had been concerned almost entirely with public health implications of the use of chemicals in food production, processing, storage, and packaging. This interest continued, of course, but broader implications of food safety and protection gradually were brought to its attention. These included the matter of the contamination of foods with radionuclides and the hazards of microbiologic contamination. First ad hoc subcommittees, then permanent subcommittees were organized to serve as advisory groups in these fields, and important publications have resulted from their deliberations (Pubs. 988, 1195). Further, the committee is cur-

---

1. Insignificant Levels of Chemical Additives in Food. Food-Drug-Cosmetic Law Journal 15: 477-479, 1958.
2. Problems in Toxicology. Proceedings of a Symposium. Fed. Proc., Vol. 19, No. 3, part II, Supplement No. 4, 1960.

Appendix

rently involved in producing a monograph on *naturally* occurring toxicants in foods.

The most ambitious project undertaken by FPC is that of preparing a Food Chemicals Codex. The project was begun in 1961 after a lengthy period of study by FPC and advisory groups representing government, industry, and public interests. The purpose of the project is to compile specifications of identity and purity for the important chemicals used intentionally for functional purposes in foods. The monographs are published and distributed in a loose-leaf edition (Pub. 1143) as they are prepared. The first phase of the project will end in 1966 with the publication of the monographs then available (about 500 of them) as the first bound edition of the Codex. Plans for periodic revision of FCC are being developed.

The committee continues to be concerned with the adequacy of safety evaluation and plans revision of its existing statements of principles and procedures. The use of human subjects in safety evaluation has not had critical evaluation, but FPC has tried to bring perspective to this facet of the problem by asking an ad hoc subcommittee to "define needs, principles, and justified procedures for use of human subjects in safety evaluation of food chemicals and pesticide residues." The subcommittee's report has recently been published (Pub. 1270).

Finally, among its activities the committee continues to sponsor public and limited attendance conferences and symposia on important aspects of food protection. Proceedings of one such symposium were published by NAS-NRC (Pub. 1082). Another, "Research Needs and Approaches to the Use of Agricultural Chemicals from a Public Health Viewpoint," was sponsored cooperatively with the Environmental Sciences and Engineering and the Toxicology Study Sections of NIH in 1964. Proceedings are in preparation. Also in 1964, FPC, the Food Law Institute, and the Graduate School of Public Law of The George Washington University sponsored a symposium on "The Legal Basis and Regulatory Use of Food Standards."[3]

National and International Influence of FPC

It is difficult to assess the influence of a single organization in a field when many governmental, industrial, and institutional groups are active in the field. However, the influence of FPC can be discerned nationally in a number of areas.

The early deliberations of FPC and its Pesticide Subcommittee are clearly reflected in some of the provisions of the 1954 Miller Pesticide Amendment to the Federal Food, Drug, and Cosmetic Law. The recognition that safe levels of even the most toxic chemicals can be defined and that, if pesticide residues are at or below such levels in foods, they can be permitted, formed the basis of the amendment and of some of the early FPC statements.

The committee's statements of general principles and procedures for evaluating safety are recognized as guides by FDA and are so specified in FDA regulations.

The background for recognizing that "zero" tolerances are illogical was in part developed by the committee, and this conclusion is stressed in the report recently made by a NAS-NRC advisory committee to the Departments of Agriculture and Health, Education and Welfare.[4]

The apparent influence of the perspective given to the matter of microbiological hazards in foods is already noticed in official activities. It is perhaps too early to see an influence from the statement on use of human subjects, but one reviewer has stated that "the Report will long be regarded as a landmark in the progress of toxicology."[5]

The national influence of the Food Chemicals Codex is likely to be far-reaching in that it may well become to manufacturers and users of food chemicals what the USP and National Formulary are to pharmaceutical manufacturers and formulators.

Finally, the influence of the committee may be most important in its existence as a deliberative body. From time to time it has been called upon by Congressional committees and executive and regulatory groups in government to provide advice and information either directly or by organizing panels of scientists. Indeed, when the committee was first asked by a Congressional committee to organize an advisory panel of scientists to meet with the committee, it was only the second time such a panel had been requested. (The first was on polio vaccine.)

Internationally the committee's influence has been perhaps more direct than it has nationally. Two of the four American delegates to the first FAO/WHO Conference on Food Additives in 1955 were representatives of FPC and its Liaison Panel. The FAO/WHO Joint Expert Committee on Food Additives, which resulted from that Conference, has subsequently included representatives of the committee in each of its

---

3. Food, Drug, Cosmetic Law Journal, Vol. 20, No. 3, March, 1965, pp. 149-176, and Vol. 20, No. 4, April, 1965, pp. 180-196.

4. Report of the Pesticides Residues Committee. NAS/NRC. June, 1965.
5. The Proper Study—When is it a Proper Study? Editorial, Information Bulletin, British Industrial Biological Research Association, Vol. 4, No. 3, April, 1965, pp. 128-130.

Appendix

meetings and has at times depended heavily on the committee's reports as basic documents for its own deliberations. In another related area, FPC cooperated closely with the Foreign Agricultural Service in 1963 in planning and staffing the first Food Science Mission.

THE COMMITTEE ON FOOD HABITS

Simultaneously with the establishment of the Committee on Food and Nutrition within the Division of Biology and Agriculture, there was established a Committee on Food Habits within the Division of Anthropology and Psychology. Dr. Margaret Mead has summarized the history of the Committee on Food Habits in NAS-NRC Pub. No. 1225, 1964, entitled "Food Habits Research: Problems of the 1960's."

Beginning of the Recommended Dietary Allowances [1]

LYDIA J. ROBERTS, Ph.D.
Visiting Professor, University of Puerto Rico, Rio Piedras

The Recommended Dietary Allowances are now familiar to everyone in the field of nutrition and so widely used that newcomers to the field are inclined to accept them as if they had always been, and to use them as absolute standards of what is essential for good nutrition (1). It might be profitable for us to look back to the beginning of the Recommended Dietary Allowances and learn something of when, why, and how they came to be. Since I was present at their birth and helped in the labor that produced them, I was chosen as the one to review briefly their history.

We must first remember that the dietary allowances are only a little over sixteen years old. They officially came into being in May 1941, at the National Nutrition Conference which met in Washington at the call of President Franklin D. Roosevelt. Of course, the allowances did not spring into being all at once at that time. They were rather the result of more than a year's hard labor on the part of a group of devoted nutrition workers. It is of these early beginnings—the prenatal period it might be called—that I shall speak.

Most of you will remember the National Nutrition Program that was initiated during the years of World War II to insure that the nutrition of the people would be safeguarded. You may have been members of state or local nutrition committees which were organized during that period and which in many places are still continuing. As one part of this national program, a Food and Nutrition Board[2] was set up within the framework of the National Research Council. Its membership consisted of representatives from the various fields of nutrition with Dr. Russell Wilder as its chairman. The function of the Board was to advise government agencies on all problems relating to food and the nutrition of the people. The Board early realized that one of its functions would be to recommend the amounts of the various nutrients that should be provided for the armed forces and also for the general population. For this, it needed to adopt standards. How little the size of this problem was realized is shown by the fact that at the close of one day's meeting, Dr. Wilder appointed a committee of three—Dr. Helen Mitchell, Dr. Hazel Stiebeling, and myself—to prepare such a set of standards during the evening and be ready to present them to the group the next morning! We three spent the evening threshing over the problem (while the men, we felt sure, were out seeing the town). The result was, of course, that the only report we could bring in the next morning was that it couldn't be done, that the evidence was too scanty and too conflicting.

The First Committee

A special Committee was, therefore, appointed to work on the problem. As chairman of that Committee, I can testify that the members worked hard and long for more than a year and enlisted the efforts of scores of other nutrition specialists before they arrived at the allowances that were finally accepted by the Board and later adopted by the Nutrition Conference.

To be sure, some standards had previously been proposed for some nutrients by different workers. Sherman (2) had set his classic standards for protein, calcium, phosphorus, and iron for adults; and Lucy Gillett (3) had worked out calorie standards for children. The Nutrition Committee of the League of Na-

---

[1]Presented at the History of Nutrition Luncheon, 40th Annual Meeting of The American Dietetic Association in Miami, on October 25, 1958. Reprinted from the *Journal of the American Dietetic Association*, Vo. 34, No. 9, September, 1958.

[2]At first it was called the "Nutrition Committee," but the name was later changed to Food and Nutrition Board.

Appendix

tions (4) had proposed standards for some of the dietary factors. Individual workers doing research with vitamins had also suggested requirements for the particular vitamins they had studied, usually only for the adult or the infant. These values varied greatly. For example, requirements suggested for ascorbic acid ranged from 10 to 100 mg. a day and even higher, and estimates for vitamin A need ranged from 1,000 to 10,000 international units a day. Thus the existing standards were not only few, but conflicting, and there were none that covered all nutrients for all ages and conditions. This was what was desired by the Board.

How then was the first table of dietary allowances derived?

First, the Committee surveyed all research reports in the literature that threw light on the requirements for any of the nutrients. This in itself was a sizable task. From this evidence, they formulated a tentative set of values for the various nutrients for different ages and conditions. These were to be used as a "trial balloon."

The Democratic Approach

As a second step, the Committee then sent copies of these tentative allowances to a large group of nutrition workers throughout the country as well as to all members of the Board, with the request for their criticism and suggestions. They did this because they believed that any accepted allowances should represent not just the thought of a small group of workers, however competent they might be, but that all persons who had done research on any factor or had other bases for judgment should have a part in their formulation. Thus the tentative allowances were sent to more than fifty persons in various fields, with the request for their judgment on any items on which they felt qualified to give an opinion. The response was excellent. Most of these busy workers took time to reply and to express in detail their judgments about the requirement for one or more of the nutrients, with the evidence on which they based it.

The Committee studied these submissions, tabulated them, and tried as best they could to evaluate and reconcile them. They then prepared a revised set of allowances which were again sent to all contributors, together with the summary of all suggestions that had been submitted. Comments were again requested and received, and some further revisions made to harmonize as fully as possible with the judgments of specialists. This revised set was considered by the Board and with some modifications was adopted.

As a final test, the allowances were presented to the members of the American Institute of Nutrition at their annual meeting that year. The wide interest in the problem was evidenced by the fact that the room was packed. It was with some trepidation that I, as chairman of the Committee, faced that group of distinguished research workers to present the allowances. We fully expected criticism and disagreement, if not attack, on their validity. I remember that as I sat in front of the room waiting for the audience to assemble, Dr. Tom Spies, who was a member of the Board and sensed my feeling, stepped quietly up and whispered, "Remember you are among friends!"

There were questions and some comments, but to our surprise, no serious disagreements or attack. Why? For one reason, many of those present had already had their say in the matter. Others who might have held different opinions had no evidence to support them and being scientists would not speak until they had.

Whatever the reason, the group as a whole seemed willing to accept the allowances for the time being at least. These allowances, so derived, were the ones presented at the National Nutrition Conference in May 1941 and formally accepted as goals at which to aim until further research should justify changes.

I emphasize this procedure because I want you to realize that the first allowances were developed democratically, that all persons who had a basis for judgment concerning them had an opportunity to express it, and also that the accepted allowances represented as fully as possible the consensus of scientific judgment at the time of their adoption. I am sure that the main reason they have stood the test of time as well as they have is that they were developed by this democratic procedure.

I should like now to give you some idea of the varied types of evidence from which the first allowances were pieced together. This is shown in Table 1. I shall comment only briefly on the various factors. Further data are given elsewhere (5).

Calories

The calorie allowances for adults were the ones then in common use for the 70-kg. man and 56-kg. woman. When they were being discussed by the Board, Dr. Norman Jolliffe suddenly asked, "Where did you get that 70-kg. man?" Looking around the room, he added, "I don't believe there is a 70-kg. man in this room!" Dr. J. R. Murlin came to the rescue and explained that the 70 and 56 kg. for men and women were derived from averages by Voit (6) and Rubner (7) in the early days of their dietary studies. The question then arose as to whether they were now applicable to people in the United States. Dr. Wilder volunteered to investigate the matter. At the following meeting, he reported that statistics from measurements taken by

Appendix

TABLE 1
THE FIRST RECOMMENDED ALLOWANCES
First (1941) Recommended Dietary Allowances and bases for their derivation

	CALORIES Allowance	Ref. source	PROTEIN Allowance	Ref. source	CALCIUM Allowance	Ref. source	IRON Allowance	Ref. source	VITAMIN A Allowance	Ref. source	THIAMINE Allowance	Ref. source	RIBOFLAVIN Allowance	Ref. source	NIACIN Allowance	Ref. source	ASCORBIC ACID Allowance	Ref. source
			gm.		gm.		mg.		I.U.		mg.		mg.		mg.		mg.	
Adults																		
Man (70 kg.)			70		0.8		12		5000									
Sedentary	2500										1.5		2.2		15		75	
Moderately active	3000										1.8		2.7		18			
Very active	4500										2.2		3.3		23			
Woman (56 kg.)		6,7,8	60	2	0.8	2,15,16	12	2	5000	28,29 30,31		32		33,34			70	36,37 38,39
Sedentary	2100										1.2		1.2		12			
Moderately active	2500										1.5		1.5		15			
Very active	3000										1.8		1.8		18			
Pregnancy (last half)	2500	9	85	13	1.5	13	15		6000		1.8		2.5		18		100	
Lactation	3000	10	100	14	2.0	14	15		8000		2.3		3.0		23		150	
Children																		
Under 1 year	100/kg.*		3-4/kg.*				6		1500		0.4		0.6		4	35	30	
1-3 years	1200		40		1.0		7	21,22	2000		0.6		0.9		6		35	
4-6 years	1600		50		1.0	17,18	8	23,24,	2500		0.8		1.2		8		50	40,41
7-9 years	2000		60		1.0	19	10	25,26,	3500		1.0		1.5		10		60	
10-12 years	2500		70		1.2		12	27	4500		1.2		1.8		12		75	
Girls		11,12		11						31								
13-15 years	2800		80		1.3		15		5000		1.4		2.0		14		80	
16-20 years	2400		75		1.0		15		5000		1.2		1.8		12		80	
Boys																		
13-15 years	3200		85		1.4		15		5000		1.6		2.4		16		90	
16-20 years	3800		100		1.4		15		6000		2.0		3.0		20		100	

*Calories and protein for infants based on values in common pediatric use for artificial feeding of infants. No standards needed for breast-fed babies.

the Selective Service Board showed the average weight of American men to be 69.8 kg., of women, 55.9 kg. Thus the 70 and 56 kg. averages were validated.

Calorie allowances for pregnancy and lactation were based largely on the studies from the laboratories of Shukers et al. (9) and Coons (10). Those for children were derived from unpublished studies of intakes of large numbers of healthy children from ages two to twenty by Roberts, Blair, and Wait (11) and from others found in the literature (12).

Protein

The protein allowances for adults were based on the 1 gm. per kilogram advocated by Sherman (2) which was in common use; those for pregnancy and lactation on the work of Macy et al. (13) and of Coons (14). The allowances for children came from a compilation by Roberts, Blair, and Wait (11) of the intake of children in all balance studies found in the literature which resulted in positive balance.

Minerals

For *calcium*, there was the then widely used 0.67 gm. per day as found by Sherman (2) for the adult. Leitch (15), however, had shown from a statistical evaluation of the literature that a somewhat higher value of 0.85 gm. seemed indicated. Moreover, workers in Mitchell's laboratory at the University of Illinois found (16) that ten out of thirteen subjects were in balance on 10 mg. per kilogram or less and concluded that this was a reasonable standard. This 10 mg. per kilogram would amount to 0.70 gm. for the 70-kg. man. Since, however, a few subjects had required more, some margin above this seemed desirable, and the allowance was set at 0.80 gm., which was close to the level advocated by Leitch.

For children, the most specific evidence on calcium was that of Outhouse et al. (17) for pre-school children, plus some work of Daniels et al. (18) for this same age group. Studies of Wang and co-workers (19) provided some indication of the needs for the early school age. For upper ages, allowances were largely esti-

Appendix

mates based on the assumption of increased need during this period of rapid growth.

For *iron*, the allowance for adults was set at the 12 mg. advocated by Sherman (2), which was in common use. Recent work of McCance and Widdowson (20) had shown that the actual requirement is much lower—for adult males, practically zero—but since this work was new and not yet accepted by all and since the 12 mg. could easily be obtained in an otherwise good diet, there seemed no need for lowering this figure at that time. Women, although smaller on the average, were given the same allowance because of their need to replace losses in menstruation. The value for pregnancy was based on Sherman's estimate that an increase of 3 mg. was needed during this period. Since milk contains little iron, no increase was made for lactation.

For iron needs of children, there were chiefly the studies from the laboratory of Stearns (21) on infants, and of several groups of workers for preschool and early school age children (Rose *et al.* [22]; Leichsenring and Flor [23]; Ascham [24]; Daniels and Wright [25]; Porter [26]; Johnston and Roberts [27]). For older ages, the values were set empirically on the assumption that the needs would increase with age and be even higher at adolescence than for adults.

Vitamins

For *vitamin A*, the evidence was scanty. There was as yet no generally accepted method of determining the requirement, and few studies were available. The 5,000 I.U. set for adults was a compromise value derived from studies of Booher *et al.* (28); Blanchard and Harper (29); and Guilbert *et al.* (30) on various species of animals and the critical evaluation of the literature made by With (31). These studies indicated the requirement to be from 25 to 55 I.U. per kilogram or 2,000 to 4,000 I.U. daily, or twice this if the source was carotene. The 5,000 I.U. allowed for the adult assumed that about two-thirds of the vitamin A value of the American diet came from carotene, one-third from true vitamin A. Arbitrary increases above this were made for pregnancy and lactation. Allowances for children were calculated on the kilogram basis, but modified somewhat by estimates of workers in the field. The values were admittedly doubtless above actual needs, but since they could be easily attained in a good general diet, there seemed no need to lower them.

The main evidence for the *thiamine* requirement at that time was the comprehensive work of Williams, Mason, Smith, and Wilder (32) of the Mayo Clinic. These workers induced thiamine deficiency in human subjects and then made step-wise additions of thiamine until all objective and subjective evidences of deficiency disappeared. They concluded that about 0.6 mg. per 1,000 calories was the amount of thiamine desirable. Although there was some scattered evidence that the need was lower, the first allowance was set at this 0.6-mg. level, making the daily allowance for the 3,000-calorie level, 1.8 mg., and for the sedentary person, 1.5 mg. Values for children were derived purely by calculation on the basis of 0.5 mg. per 1,000 calories.

For *riboflavin*, there were only two lines of evidence. Sebrell and Butler (33) had induced riboflavin deficiency in a group of women and returned them to normal by step-wise additions of riboflavin. They estimated the need to be in the neighborhood of 3 mg. per day. Strong *et al.* (34), at Wisconsin, on the basis of human experiments had arrived at the same estimate. There was a general belief that this was too high, especially because it would be difficult to attain from natural foods. However, believing it better to set values too high than too low until further evidence was obtained, the allowance was reduced only to 2.7 mg. for the moderately active man and 2.2 for the average woman. Higher allowances were set for upper calorie levels. Values for children were reached by calculation per 1,000 calories.

For *niacin*, there were no human studies of requirement. The allowances were obtained from Elvehjem's (35) experience with animals. He had found that with rats, the niacin requirement was ten times that of thiamine. Since there was then no other basis for an estimate, the allowances were derived by multiplying the thiamine values by ten. It is surprising how closely later research has substantiated these values.

There was more evidence on which to base allowances for ascorbic acid than for any other vitamin. Methods of study had been better developed, and studies had been made by a number of workers, both on adults and children. Moreover, it was possible to get together the chief workers in this field at the time of the meeting of the American Institute of Nutrition. This group included Hazel M. Hauck (36), E. Neige Todhunter(37), M. L. Fincke (38), C. G. King and O. A. Bessey (39), M. Hathaway (40), V. Roberts (41), and a few others. After a give-and-take discussion, the allowances in the table were accepted as compromises by this group. I believe these values have not been changed to any significant degree in later revisions.

It can be seen from this review how much assumption and judgment of workers of necessity entered into the formulation of this first set of dietary allowances.

Some workers thought it a mistake to assign values for all ages for the various factors in view of the incomplete evidence. Others argued that someone would have to make estimates in practical usage, and

Appendix

it seemed that values derived by consensus of scientific judgment would be better than for each worker to set his own standard. In presenting the table, however, it was emphasized:

(a) That they were recommended allowances, not standards. They were goals, not necessarily absolute requirements.

(b) That they were based on the best knowledge available at the time they were formulated.

(c) That they would be subject to change as soon as more evidence became available.

Revisions in the B-Vitamin Allowances

The allowances have indeed gone through several editions, and a number of changes have been made in the sixteen years since they were first adopted. The first major revisions were made in 1944. These pertained to the B vitamins. It was the general belief that the values for these nutrients were too high, and some work had been done in the meantime to justify this belief. A meeting was therefore called to consider the revision, and all workers who had done research on any of them were invited.

About twenty-five persons attended. These included the members of the Committee (Drs. G. Cowgill, C. A. Elvehjem, P. C. Jeans, C. G. King, R. Wilder, F. Bing, and L. J. Roberts) and others distinguished for research on either thiamine or riboflavin or both (Drs. A. Keys, N. Jolliffe, E. Holt, W. H. Sebrell, H. Parsons, H. D. Kruse, H. Oldham, A. Ivy, T. Friedemann, K. O. Elsom, C. A. Morrell, M. Horwitt, D. Melnick, H. C. Sherman, R. Griggs, and R. R. Williams). Some of these workers held widely divergent views on the requirements. For example, Williams and Wilder believed the thiamine requirement to be about 0.6 mg. per 1,000 calories; Keys had shown that 0.23 mg. per 1,000 appeared adequate for adult men, and that even on 0.18 mg. they did not develop deficiency signs. Moreover, Holt had shown experimentally on human beings that thiamine could be synthesized in the intestinal tract and had suggested that perhaps one did not need any in the diet. Similar differences existed in respect to the riboflavin needs.

It was the task of this meeting to reconcile these divergent views and to reach a common ground for agreement. During the day each person had the opportunity to present his evidence and point of view, to listen to others while they presented theirs, and to participate in the general discussion. As a result, the group was able to arrive at compromise values that all were willing to accept as reasonable. For thiamine, 0.5 mg. per 1,000 calories was agreed on as a value for adults at moderate caloric intakes, with the provision that the day's total thiamine intake should never be less than 1.0 mg. For caloric intakes above 3,000, a lower value for the additional calories was accepted, i.e., 0.23 mg. per 1,000 calories. Lower compromise allowances were also decided upon for riboflavin.

To me, this conference stands out as a striking testimony to the fact that many differences can be worked out and agreements reached if the persons concerned can sit down together and thresh out the problem in a spirit of give and take and a willingness to compromise.

The revisions decided on at this meeting were the most drastic of any that have been made. Later revisions have, however, made some changes, and a few others have been made in the 1958 edition. That is as it should be. As fast as more knowledge is available on requirements for any nutrient, it should be reflected in the allowances.

Accomplishments of the Allowances

There can be no question, I believe, that the allowances have served a useful purpose. In the first place, they have been used as official guides in practically all nutritional enterprises in this country. They have served as the accepted yardstick for feeding the armed forces. The Quartermaster Corps has made a great effort to see that the foods provided for men in service measure up to the allowances.

They have unified nutrition allowances. For the first time in history, all groups working for nutritional betterment have used a common allowance instead of the varied and conflicting ones which previously obtained.

One of the greatest services they have rendered has been to stimulate research to determine requirements for the various nutrients. The review of evidence by the Committee had revealed great gaps in our knowledge, and workers were challenged to fill in those gaps. Some workers, moreover, who were convinced that the allowances were too high went into their laboratories and carried out research to produce evidence for their beliefs. As I have indicated, some of them have found it. Others have confirmed the values originally set. The surprising thing is that the early allowances have stood the test of time as well as they have and that so few important changes have been made in them.

Why have the recommended allowances been so widely accepted and used? For one reason, because they were put out by the National Research Council, a body whose reputation for scientific caution and dependability is outstanding. Even more important, I believe, is the democratic procedure by which they were derived, which gave all persons who had a basis

Appendix

for judgment as to requirements an opportunity to contribute to their development. All have realized that the consensus of judgment of nutrition authorities should prevail and have therefore been willing to accept allowances so derived until further evidence should justify changes.

Some persons are inclined to object to changes in the allowances. They ask, "Why can't they make up their minds?" Others resent the lowering of the allowance for any factor. They look on such action as a lowering of standards. They should remember that evidence for some factors was very scanty—for example, for riboflavin—and the allowances were admittedly probably too high. The lowering of values merely means that more evidence for the amount needed has become available and a more realistic value can be set. There is still too little evidence for some factors, and further changes in allowances for them may be expected as research reveals more closely the need for them. In the meantime, the allowances can continue to be used, as they were meant to be, as *goals at which to aim* in providing for the nutritional needs of groups of people.

REFERENCES

1. FOOD AND NUTRITION BD.: Recommended Dietary Allowances, Revised 1953. Natl. Acad. Sci.—Natl. Research Council Pub. No. 302, 1953.
2. SHERMAN, H. C.: Chemistry of Food and Nutrition. 3rd ed. N. Y.: Macmillan Co., 1926.
3. GILLETT, L. H.: A Survey of Evidence Regarding Food Allowances for Healthy Children. N. Y. Assn. for Improving the Condition of the Poor, Pub. No. 115, 1917.
4. TECH. COMMISSION OF THE HEALTH COMMITTEE, LEAGUE OF NATIONS: The Problem of Nutrition. Report on the Physiological Bases of Nutrition. Vol. II. N. Y.: Columbia Univ. Press, 1936.
5. ROBERTS, L. J.: Scientific basis for the Recommended Dietary Allowances. New York J. Med. 44: 59, 1944.
6. VOIT, E.: Collected papers.
7. RUBNER, M.: Collected papers.
8. ATWATER, W. O., AND BENEDICT, F. G.: Experiments on the Metabolism of Matter and Energy in the Human Body. U.S.D.A. Bull. No. 69, 1899.
9. SHUKERS, C. F., MACY, I.G., DONELSON, E., NIMS, B., AND HUNSCHER, H. A.: Food intake in pregnancy, lactation, and reproductive rest in the human mother. J. Nutrition 4: 399, 1931.
10. COONS, C. M.: Studies in Metabolism in Pregnancy. Okla. Agric. Exper. Sta. Bull. No. 223, 1935.
11. ROBERTS, L. J., BLAIR, R., AND WAIT, B.: Unpublished data.
12. White House Conference on Child Health and Protection. N. Y.: Century Co., 1932.
13. MACY, I. G., HUNSCHER, H. A., McCOSH, S. S., AND NIMS, B.: Metabolism of women during the reproductive cycle. 3. Calcium, phosphorus, and nitrogen utilization in lactation before and after supplementing the usual home diets with cod liver oil and yeast. J. Biol. Chem. 86: 59, 1930.
14. COONS, C. M., AND BLUNT, K.: The retention of nitrogen, calcium, phosphorus, and magnesium by pregnant women. J. Biol. Chem. 86: 1, 1930.
18. LEITCH, I.: The determination of the calcium requirements of man. Nutr. Abstr. & Rev. 6: 553, 1937.
16. MITCHELL, H. H.: Personal Communication.
17. OUTHOUSE, J., KINSMAN, G., SHELDON, D., TWOMEY, I., SMITH, J., AND MITCHELL, H. H.: The calcium requirements of five pre-school girls. J. Nutrition 17: 199, 1939.
18. DANIELS, A. L., HUTTON, M. K., KNOTT, E., EVERSON, G., AND WRIGHT, O.: Relation of ingestion of milk to calcium metabolism in children. Am. J. Dis. Child. 47: 499, 1934.
19. WANG, C. C., KERN, R., AND KAUCHER, M.: Minimum requirement of calcium and phosphorus in children. Am. J. Dis. Child. 39: 768, 1930.
20. McCANCE, R. A., AND WIDDOWSON, E. M.: The absorption and excretion of iron following oral and intravenous administration. J. Physiology 94: 148, 1938.
21. STEARNS, G., AND STINGER, D.: Iron retention in infancy. J. Nutrition 13: 127, 1937.
22. ROSE, M. S., VAHLTEICH, E. McC., ROBB, E., AND BLOOMFIELD, E. M.: Iron requirement in early childhood. J. Nutrition 3: 229, 1930.
23. LEICHSENRING, J. M., AND FLOR, I. H.: The iron requirement of the preschool child. J. Nutrition 5: 141, 1932.
24. ASCHAM, L.: A study of iron metabolism in preschool children. J. Nutrition 10:337, 1935.
25. DANIELS, A. L., AND WRIGHT, O. E.: Iron and copper retentions in young children. J. Nutrition 8: 125, 1934.
26. PORTER, T.: Iron balances on four normal preschool children. J. Nutrition 21: 101, 1941.
27. JOHNSTON, F. A., AND ROBERTS, L. J.: The iron requirement of children of the early school age. J. Nutrition 23:181, 1942.
28. BOOHER, L. E., CALLISON, E. C., AND HEWSTON, E. M.: An experimental determination of the minimum vitamin A requirements of normal adults. J. Nutrition 17: 317, 1939.

Appendix

29. BLANCHARD, E. L., AND HARPER, H. A.: Measurement of vitamin A status of young adults by the dark adaptation technique. Arch. Int. Med. 66: 661, 1940.
30. GUILBERT, H. R. HOWELL, C. E., AND HART, G. H.: Minimum vitamin A and carotene requirements of mammalian species. J. Nutrition 19: 91, 1940.
31. WITH, T. K.: Vitamin A requirement of man and warm blooded animals; the absorption, metabolism, and storage of vitamin A and carotenoids in warm blooded animals. 2. Requirements of the foetus and during pregnancy and lactation. Hospitalstidende 81: 1153 (Dec. 6), 1938.
32. WILLIAMS, R. D., MASON, H. L., SMITH, B. F., AND WILDER, R. M.: Induced thiamine (vitamin B_1) deficiency and the thiamine requirement of man: further observations. Arch. Int. Med. 69: 721, 1942.
33. SEBRELL, W. H., AND BUTLER, R. E.: Riboflavin deficiency in man. A preliminary note. Public Health Rep. 53: 2282, 1938.
34. STRONG, F. M., FEENEY, R. E., MOORE, B., AND PARSONS, H. T.: The riboflavin content of blood and urine. J. Biol. Chem. 137: 363, 1941.
35. ELVEHJEM, C. A.: The vitamin B complex in normal nutrition. J. Am. Dietet. A. 16: 646, 1940.
36. BELSER, W. B., HAUCK, H. M., AND STORVICK, C. A.: A study of the ascorbic acid intake required to maintain tissue saturation in normal adults. J. Nutrition 17: 513, 1939.
37. TODHUNTER, E. N., AND ROBBINS, R. C.: Observations on the amount of ascorbic acid required to maintain tissue saturation in normal adults. J. Nutrition 19: 263, 1940.
38. FINCKE, M. L., AND LANDQUIST, V. L.: The daily intake of ascorbic acid required to maintain adequate and optimal levels of this vitamin in the blood plasma. J. Nutrition 23: 483, 1942.
39. BESSEY, O. A., AND KING, C. G.: The distribution of vitamin C in plant and animal tissues and its determination. J. Biol. Chem. 103: 687, 1933.
40. HATHAWAY, M. L., AND MEYER, F. L.: Studies of the vitamin C metabolism of four preschool children. J. Nutrition 21: 503, 1941.
41. ROBERTS, V. M., AND ROBERTS, L. J.: A study of the ascorbic acid requirements of children of early school age. J. Nutrition 24: 25, 1942.

MEMBERS OF THE FOOD AND NUTRITION BOARD 1940-1965

Name	Appointment	Termination	Name	Appointment	Termination
ALLISON, J. B.	1956	1964*	ELVEHJEM, C. A.	1940	1961[a]
BENNETT, M. K.	1954	1957	EMERSON, Gladys	1959	1964
BING, Franklin C.	1941	1945	ENGEL, R. W.	1960	
BLACK, John D.	1940	1953	FINCKE, Margaret L.	1948	1951
BORSOOK, Henry	1940	1945	FREY, Charles N.	1944	1945
BOUDREAU, Frank G.	1940	1954	GOLDSMITH, Grace A.	1948	
CANNAN, R. Keith	1952	1954	GOODHART, Robert S.	1946	1950
CANNON, Paul R.	1947	1951	GORDON, Harry H.	1955	1959
CASSELLS, John M.	1943	1945	GRIFFITH, W. H.	1950	1962
CHELDELIN, Vernon	1964		GRIGGS, Robert F.	1947	1950
CLARK, B. S.	1953	1957	GUERRANT, N. B.	1949	1952
COWGILL, George R.	1940	1946	GUNDERSON, Frank	1945	1946
DARBY, William J.	1949		GYORGY, Paul	1956	1964
DAVIDSON, C. S.	1953		HAND, David B.	1949	
DAVIS, George K.	1961		HARPER, Alfred E.	1961	
DAVIS, John H.	1957	1959	HARRISON, Harold	1964	
DAVIS, Joseph S.	1940	1945	HASTINGS, A. Baird	1942	1946
DAY, Paul	1953	1959	HEGSTED, D. M.	1962	
DOFT, Floyd S.	1963		HEINEMAN, H. E. O.	1950	
ELIOT, Martha M.	1940	1945	HOOBLER, Icie Macy	1940	1950

Appendix

Name	Appointment	Termination	Name	Appointment	Termination
HOWE, Paul E.	1941	1945	SEBRELL, W. H., Jr.	1941	1949
JACKSON, Robert L.	1960			1956	
JEANS, Philip C.	1940	1952*	SEVERINGHAUS, E. L.	1947	1950
JOLLIFFE, Norman	1940	1947	SHANK, R. E.	1950	
	1952	1956	SHERMAN, H. G.	1941	1945
KEYS, Ancel	1949	1955		1947	1949
KING, C. Glen	1940		STANLEY, Louise	1941	1945
KRAUSS, William E.	1943	1949	STARE, Fredrick J.	1947	1954
KRUSE, H. D.	1942	1947		1955	1962
LONGENECKER, H. E.	1943	1956[b]	STIEBELING, Hazel K.	1942	1951
MAYNARD, L. A.	1940	1949	SYDENSTRICKER, V. P.	1943	1945
	1950	1955	THOMAS, G. Cullen	1940	1950
McCOLLUM, E. V.	1941	1946	TISDALL, F. F.	1941	1949*
McLESTER, James S.	1940	1946	TODHUNTER, E. Neige	1957	
MITCHELL, Helen	1940	1945	VILTER, R. W.	1956	1964
MUELLER, John F.	1964		WILDER, Russell M.	1940	1947
MURLIN, John R.	1941	1945		1948	1959*
NELSON, E. M.	1941	1950	WILLIAMS, Robert R.	1940	1960
NEWTON, R. C.	1946	1953	WILLIAMS, Roger J.	1949	1953
OHLSON, Margaret	1951	1957	YOUMANS, John B.	1940	1945
PETERS, F. N.	1957	1964			
PETT, L. B.	1942	1946			
POLLOCK, Herbert	1950	1955	**CHAIRMEN OF THE BOARD:**		
PRESCOTT, S. C.	1940	1945			
ROBERTS, Lydia J.	1940	1948	WILDER, Russell M.	1940	1941
ROBINSON, Herbert	1964		BOUDREAU, Frank G.	1941	1951
ROSE, W. C.	1940	1947	MAYNARD, L. A.	1951	1955
RUSSELL, Walter C.	1952	1954*	ELVEHJEM, C. A.	1955	1958
SCHULTZ, T. W.	1962	1965	GOLDSMITH, Grace A.	1958	

*Appointment terminated by death.
[a]Did not serve on the Board during 1949.
[b]Did not serve on the Board from 1949 until 1950.
(NOTE: No date in "Terminated" column indicates that appointment still continues.)

PUBLICATIONS OF THE FOOD AND NUTRITION BOARD 1940-1965

Title	Year of Publication	Identification
The Food and Nutrition of industrial Workers in Wartime	1942	NRC-RC Series No. 110
The NATION'S Protein Supply	1942	NRC-RC Series No. 114
Food Charts—Foods as Sources of the Dietary Essentials	1942	Brochure AMA/FNB
Recommended Dietary Allowances	1943	NRC-RC Series No. 115
A Report on Margarine	1943	NRC-RC Series No. 118
Inadequate Diets and Nutritional Deficiencies in the United States—Their Prevalence and Significance	1943	NRC Bulletin No. 109

Appendix

Title	Year	Reference
Food Charts—Foods as Sources of the Dietary Essentials	1944	Brochure AMA/FNB Revised edition
Principles Underlying Studies of Nutrition Pertaining to the Influence of Supplements on Growth, Physical Fitness and Health	1944	FNB/AMA
The Facts About Enrichment of Flour and Bread	1944	Brochure
Enrichment of Flour and Bread—A History of the Movement	1944	NRC-RC Series No. 110
Rehabilitation: The Man and The Job	1945	NRC-RC Series No. 121
The Nutritional Improvement of White Rice	1945	NRC Bulletin No. 112
Recommended Dietary Allowances, Revised 1945	1945	NRC-RC Series No. 122
The Nutrition of Industrial Workers, Second Report	1945	NRC-RC Series No. 123
Industrial Feeding Management	1945	USDA WFA NFC-14
Manual on Institutional Feeding in Industry	1945	WFA
Supplement to The Facts About Enrichment of Flour and Bread	1946	Brochure
Bread and Flour Enrichment 1946-47	1947	Brochure
Outlook for Bread and Flour Enrichment—Review of Events During 1947-48	1948	Brochure
Tables of Food Composition	1948	USDA Misc. Pub. No. 572
Investigations of Human Requirements for B-Complex Vitamins	1948	NRC Bulletin No. 116
Recommended Dietary Allowances, Revised 1948	1948	NRC-RC Series No. 129
Survey of Food and Nutrition Research in The United States 1947	1948	FNB/NRC
Nutrition Surveys: Their Techniques and Value	1949	NRC Bulletin No. 117
The Composition of Milks	1950	NRC Bulletin No. 119
Survey of Food and Nutrition Research in The United States, 1948-1949	1950	FNB/NRC
The Problem of Heat Injury to Dietary Protein	1950	NRC-RC Series No. 131
Sanitary Milk and Ice Cream Legislation in the United States	1950	NRC Bulletin No. 121
Flour and Bread Enrichment, 1949-50	1950	Brochure
Maternal Nutrition and Child Health	1950	NRC Bulletin No. 123
Therapeutic Nutrition—With Special Reference to Military Situations, A Report to the Medical Research and Development Board, D.O.D.	1951	
A Survey of the Literature of Dental Caries	1952	Pub. No. 225
The Safety of Mono- and Diglycerides for Use as Food Additives (FPC)	1952	Pub. No. 251
Safe Use of Chemical Additives in Foods	1952	Food Protection Committee
Annotated Bibliography of Analytical Methods for Pesticides—Section I, Aldrin and Dieldrin, Benzene Hexachloride, Chlordane and Heptachlor, DDT (FPC)	1952	Pub. No. 241
Therapeutic Nutrition	1952	Pub. No. 234
Sanitary Milk Control and its Relation to the Sanitary, Nutritive and Other Qualities of Milk	1953	Pub. No. 250
Control of Tooth Decay	1953	Brochure
The Safety of Polyoxyethylene Stearates for Use as Intentional Additives in Foods (FPC)	1953	Pub. No. 280
The Problem of Providing Optimum Fluoride Intake for Prevention of Dental Caries	1953	Pub. No. 294
Recommended Dietary Allowances, Revised 1953	1953	Pub. No. 302
Statement of General Policy in Regard to The Addition of Specific Nutrients to Foods	1953	Brochure
Survey of Food and Nutrition Research in the United States of America 1952-1953	1954	FNB/USDA
Annotated Bibliography of Analytical Methods for Pesticides—Section II, Insecticides, Herbicides, Fungicides, Rodenticides (FPC)	1954	Pub. No. 241

Appendix

Sodium-Restricted Diets—The Rationale, Complications and Practical Aspects of Their Use	1954	Pub. No. 325
Principles and Procedures For Evaluating the Safety of Intentional Chemical Additives in Foods	1954	Food Protection Committee
The Safety of Artificial Sweeteners For Use in Foods (FPC)	1954	Pub. No. 386
Policy Statement on Artificial Sweeteners	1955	Brochure
Safety of Artificial Sweeteners (FPC)	1955	Pub. No. 386
Grouping of Raw Agricultural Commodities for Residue Comparisons and the Simplification of Applications for Tolerances	1955	Food Protection Committee
The Relation of Surface Activity to the Safety of Surfactants in Foods (FPC)	1956	Pub. No. 463
Safe Use of Pesticides in Food Production (FPC)	1956	Pub. No. 470
Supplementation of Dietary Proteins With Amino Acids	1957	Reprint Public Health Reports
Cereal Enrichment in Perspective, 1958	1958	Brochure
Recommended Dietary Allowances, Revised 1958	1958	Pub. No. 589
The Role of Dietary Fat in Human Health	1958	Pub. No. 575
Food Packaging Materials—Their Composition and Uses (FPC)	1958	Pub. No. 645
The Safety of Polyoxyethylene (8) Stearate for Use in Foods	1958	Pub. No. 646
Evaluation of Protein Nutrition	1959	Pub. No. 711
Problems in the Evaluation of Carcinogenic Hazard from Use of Food Additives (FPC)	1959	Pub. No. 749
Principles and Procedures for Evaluating the Safety of Food Additives (FPC)	1959	Pub. No. 750
The Safety of Mono- and Diglycerides for Use as Intentional Additives in Foods (FPC)	1960	Pub. No. 251
Statement of General Policy in Regard to Addition of Specific Nutrients to Foods	1961	Brochure
The Role of Nutrition in International Programs, dealing with: agriculture/public health/education/economic development/food for peace/foreign aid	1961	Brochure
Meeting Protein Needs of Infants and Children	1961	Pub. No. 843
Science and Food: Today and Tomorrow (FPC)	1961	Pub. No. 877
The Use of Chemicals in Food Production, Processing, Storage and Distribution (FPC)	1961	Pub. No. 887
The Nutritional Significance and Safety of Milk and Milk Products in the National Diet	1962	Brochure
Radionuclides in Food (FPC)	1962	Pub. No. 988
Recommendations on Administrative Policies for International Food and Nutrition Programs	1963	Brochure
New Developments and Problems in the Use of Pesticides (FPC)	1963	Pub. No. 1082
Evaluation of Protein Quality	1963	Pub. No. 1100
Recommended Dietary Allowances, Revised 1963	1963	Pub. No. 1146
Food Chemicals Codex (FPC)	1963 (*et seq.*)	Pub. No. 1143
An Evaluation of Public Health Hazards from Microbiological	1964	Pub. No. 1195
Summary: Pre-School Child Malnutrition, Primary Deterrent to Human Progress	1965	Brochure
Pre-School Child Malnutrition, Primary Deterrent to Human Progress (in press)	1965	Pub. No. 1282
Some Considerations in the Use of Human Subjects in Safety Evaluation of Pesticides and Food Chemicals (FPC)	1965	Pub. No. 1270